Praise for Sara Gottfried, MD, and *The Hormone Cure*

"Gottfried takes a comprehensive look at the most common physical and emotional ailments affecting women and explains why a hormone imbalance may be at their root. Her premise is simple: when a woman's hormones are in sync, she's a powerhouse, but when they're out of whack, they wreak havoc on her body and mind. The book is both fun and an informative read, [and] Gottfried's take on the female body is eye-opening and empowering."

—*Spirituality and Health*

"Gottfried, a beautiful Harvard Medical School graduate, board-certified gynecologist, and yoga teacher, looks like an advertisement for healthy living and convincingly pushes women to make lifestyle changes rather than immediately asking for conventional prescription drugs to treat problems such as depression. Most of her tips are solid and helpful. . . . A valuable title."

—*Booklist*

"[A] scientifically advanced yet deeply humane guide to hormonal heath. Readers . . . will be cheered by [Sara Gottfried's] appealir and disarming candor. And likely, many of them will Gottfried's sympathetic understanding to stay the cours

—*Publishers Weekly*

"You don't have to accept the hormonal hell of being weight, and never in the mood for sex as you grow new book, the brilliant Dr. Gottfried gives you an ef plan to balance your hormones and become lean, er again. Stop settling and reclaim your sexy!"

—JJ Virgin, nutritionist and fitness expert,
author of *The Virgin Diet*

"Gottfried is a rare breed of physician who can discuss progesterone replacement and the power of chanting in the same paragraph—and with equal authority. Her engaging and well-researched book, *The Hormone Cure,* offers women an excellent resource for the sometimes wild ride from peri to menopause."

—Dr. Daphne Miller, MD, author of *The Jungle Effect: A Doctor Discovers the Healthiest Diets from Around the World—Why They Work and How to Bring Them Home*

"Dr. Sara is a rare combo of Harvard Medical School graduate, yoga teacher, and integrative physician. She's smart, she's hip, she writes in a user-friendly way! Learn all about your hormones—what they do, how they can ruin your life, how you can make them hum. Run, don't walk, to your computer or bookstore to buy this book—and throw more in the cart for your girl-friends, mother, sisters, and daughters. The life you save may be your own."

—Hyla Cass, MD, author of *8 Weeks to Vibrant Health*

"Never before have I read a book and shouted, 'Oh my God, that's ME!' every time I turned the page. It is no exaggeration to say that I think managing hormones is the single most important thing women my age are dealing with. I don't just want to read Sara Gottfried. I want her to be my doctor, my friend, and my sister."

—Ayelet Waldman, *New York Times* best-selling author of
*Bad Mother: A Chronicle of Maternal Crimes, Minor
Calamities, and Occasional Moments of Grace*

"If I could recommend just one book to women concerned about hormones, perimenopause, and menopause, *The Hormone Cure* would be it. Dr. Sara Gottfried is a genius, compassionate and wise, not to mention a first-class writer. You must read this book!"

—Jonny Bowden, the Rogue Nutritionist, author of *The Great
Cholesterol Myth: Why Lowering Your Cholesterol Won't Prevent Heart
Disease and the Statin-Free Plan That Will*

"Finally, a cogent, hilarious, and wise explanation about why women feel the way they do at different times in their hormonal cycles—and some sensible advice about what to do about it. Dr. Gottfried is Dr. Weil and Dr. Christiane Northrup's love child—she is part of the new conversation about hormones."

—Adair Lara, author of *Naked, Drunk, and Writing*

"*The Hormone Cure* is a breakthrough hormone guide for women everywhere—an entertaining, persuasive, and hilarious biography of your hormones, why they're off, and most importantly, how to cure hormone imbalance naturally (and in most cases, without a doctor's prescription). Dr. Sara Gottfried is the most cutting edge and brainy physician I know, and she has stellar credentials. She's applied her decades of clinical experience taking care of women, and her keen mind to get to the root of your issues, from low energy and fatigue, low sex drive, anxiety to weight gain. This book is gold."

—Marci Shimoff, *New York Times* best-selling
author of *Love for No Reason*

"*The Hormone Cure* is the playbook for your mojo, mind, and bootie. With every chapter I thought, 'So THAT's how that works.' Then I wanted to call every girlfriend and give them the goods on how to glow, now and always. Gottfried's done something beautiful here—she's putting the knowledge in our hands. Pick it up."

—Danielle LaPorte, author of
The Fire Starter Sessions and *The Desire Map*

"Occasionally a health-related book comes along that is perfect for its time—the right topic, the right information, from the right authority. Such is the book by Sara Gottfried, MD, *The Hormone Cure*. So much has been written about how women should manage their hormonal health during and after menopause, much of it not by someone with the background, training and clinical skills that Dr. Gottfried has as a specialist in gynecology and women's health. Her book is a definitive integration of safe and effective approaches to the management of issues of the brain, breast, bones, and heart that come with the onset of menopause. This is a book of our time that will help women navigate successfully through the challenging neurohormonal changes that come with menopause."

—Jeffrey Bland, PhD, founder of
the Institute of Functional Medicine

"This wonderful book transforms the approach we take to addressing women's health issues. The 'mindmap' is an amazingly easy way to understand how to achieve hormonal equilibrium for women who suffer from fatigue, depression, and other endocrine-based neuropsychiatric symptoms."

—Jay Lombard, DO, author of *Balance Your Brain, Balance Your Life:
28 Days to Feeling Better Than You Ever Have*

"Thoughtful, poignant, and devilishly irreverent, Dr. Sara's *The Hormone Cure* is the only book you will need for lasting health from head to toe. Dr. Sara turns your hormones and heart into allies that create the life you want to live. If you are a woman or know a woman, get this book! Half yogini, half hardcore hormone healer, Dr. Sara combines Eastern modalities with Western science to give women what they so desperately deserve: a sexy, satisfying, and all-together awesome hormone cure to last a lifetime."

—Jamie Dougherty, nutritionist

"How many years did I suffer in hormone hell? If only I had Sara's wisdom sooner. This book is going to help save the world—because too many women's gifts are smothered by hormone imbalances, preventing us from doing our great work."

—Jennifer Louden, author of *The Life Organizer:
A Woman's Guide to a Mindful Year*

"Dr. Sara is bridging the chasm between the woman who wants to take action to feel better and the encapsulated medical body of knowledge. Dr. Sara hunts the core issues women are wrestling with and answers the essential question 'What the hell is wrong with me and what can I do about it?' I am making this book required reading for my yoga-teacher training."

—Ana T. Forrest, founder of Forrest Yoga and author of
*Fierce Medicine: Breakthrough Practices to Heal
the Body and Ignite the Spirit*

THE
HORMONE CURE

RECLAIM BALANCE, SLEEP, AND SEX
DRIVE; LOSE WEIGHT; FEEL FOCUSED,
VITAL, AND ENERGIZED NATURALLY
WITH THE GOTTFRIED PROTOCOL

SARA GOTTFRIED, MD

SCRIBNER
New York   London   Toronto   Sydney   New Delhi

SCRIBNER
A Division of Simon & Schuster, Inc.
1230 Avenue of the Americas
New York, NY 10020

First Scribner trade paperback edition March 2014

SCRIBNER and design are registered trademarks of
The Gale Group, Inc., used under license by Simon & Schuster, Inc.,
the publisher of this work.

For information about special discounts for bulk purchases,
please contact Simon & Schuster Special Sales at 1-866-506-1949
or business@simonandschuster.com.

The Simon & Schuster Speakers Bureau can bring authors to your live event.
For more information or to book an event contact the Simon & Schuster
Speakers Bureau at 1-866-248-3049 or
visit our website at www.simonspeakers.com.

Designed by Julie Schroeder

Manufactured in the United States of America

1   3   5   7   9   10   8   6   4   2

Library of Congress Control Number: 2012031931

ISBN 978-1-4516-6694-6
ISBN 978-1-4516-6695-3 (pbk)
ISBN 978-1-4516-6696-0 (ebook)

In memory of my grandfather,
GENERAL H. C. TEUBNER
(1919–2012)
a great man and kindred spirit, whose curiosity about the
natural world and zeal for education helped him rise from
poverty to become a brilliant MIT engineer
(and courageous World War II B29 bomber pilot).

Grandpa didn't practice yoga but believed strongly in lifestyle
management for radical prevention, and taught me the
virtues of fish oil and vitamin E more than forty years ago.
He got how my mind works and that it mattered.

CONTENTS

FOREWORD

Christiane Northrup, MD

I first "met" Sara Gottfried, MD, when I was sent a copy of *Yoga Woman*, a beautiful film documenting the amazing health benefits of yoga. And there she was, on screen in all her beauty and health—a board-certified gynecologist and renowned yoga teacher—embodying the best of both East and West, talking about the incredible power of yoga to heal mind, body, and spirit. Sara Gottfried is a modern-day healer-goddess if ever there was one, and she also happens to be a Harvard Medical School graduate and rigorous physician-scientist. I later learned that my work in women's health had been a beacon of light and hope during her medical training and obstetrics/gynecology residency years. How delightful to discover that she was following the path I had so painstakingly blazed years before—and now making it wider and easier for others to follow!

Like me, Dr. Gottfried had some early role models that defied the stereotypes of midlife women and aging that we too often see as the "norm" in both medical school and later in our practices. Her great-grandmother Mud, who danced at her wedding, displayed the vitality and health well into her nineties that we associate with much younger women. My own mother and her best friend, Anne, when three years Mud's senior, completed the Appalachian Trail while in their seventies and climbed the hundred highest peaks in New England shortly thereafter. Then my mother trekked a hundred miles to a Mount Everest base camp at the age of eighty-four—with no oxygen, despite the fact that there is 50 percent less of this precious substance at those altitudes. Her oxygen saturation levels remained normal, a testament to her health and fitness.

Clearly Dr. Gottfried and I are kindred spirits. And if you are reading this book, chances are that you are too! We both started our conventional training already immunized against the "doom and gloom" approach to aging that is part and parcel of medical training. We already knew that the best years of life don't actually begin until age fifty or so. We already knew that midlife does not have to be the beginning of an inevitable downhill slide into disease and disability that ends in a painful, disease-ridden death. We both hold a vision for all women about what's possible at midlife and beyond. But the kind of joy, vitality, and pleasure that are our birthrights cannot become reality unless we know exactly what to do to balance our hormones, keep our weight at healthy levels, and quell cellular inflammation before it leads to chronic degenerative disease.

Modern conventional medicine—with its focus on pathology, drugs, and surgery—functions largely by using drugs to mask symptoms. But that still-small voice in each of us knows that depression is not a Prozac deficiency and that a headache is not an aspirin deficiency. Taking symptom-masking drugs can be likened to shooting out the indicator lights on the dashboard of your car to reassure yourself that all is well. A much wiser approach is to look under the hood and see where the problem lies in the first place. Believe it or not, most problems, including hormone imbalance, can be largely relieved through lifestyle changes alone.

Happily, we now have far more sophisticated methods for identifying and testing for hormone and energy imbalances than were available even ten years ago. The science of psychoneuroimmunology and epigenetics has advanced light-years in a short time. And Dr. Gottfried is on the leading edge of all of this. She practices what is known as "functional" or integrative medicine, which works to optimize the minute-to-minute processes and functions of the body before diagnosable diseases develop. Since most symptoms are the end result of cellular inflammation left unchecked for years, we now know it is possible to short-circuit most chronic degenerative disease in its early stages or prevent it altogether.

Be assured that the kind of medicine in *The Hormone Cure* is the medicine of the future—now. Dr. Gottfried's approach will require you to be an active participant in your own health care. She doesn't suggest a quick-fix magic-bullet approach. That is not sustainable. As both a skilled yoga teacher and gynecologist, Dr. Gottfried knows in her own body and mind the incredibly satisfying results you can get from consciously and mindfully working with the wisdom of your body. And she will help you to do just that.

If you want to regain the lost sense of optimism and vitality that you had in your youth—or attain even more optimism and vitality than you ever had—your answers are here. Or if you simply want to continue to stay as vital and youthful as possible for as long as possible, your answers are also here. In *The Wisdom of Menopause* (Bantam 2012), I referred to the perimenopausal years as the big wake-up call—a time when we reach a crossroads in our lives. Everything that is no longer working has to be addressed and left behind! One road says Die; the other says Grow. In *The Hormone Cure*, Dr. Gottfried will take you by the hand and show you exactly how to follow the path that says Grow!

PREFACE

Modern women face an unacknowledged epidemic of hormonal imbalance. Unremitting stress, superwoman expectations, and misinformation about hormones have led to a full-blown crisis. We are offered crash diets, sleeping pills, or anxiety medication. Now, one in four women in the United States takes a prescription medication for mental health reasons, the majority of which are women aged forty and older. Doctors lead us to believe that this is just what it's like to get older. We're told that it's normal to feel fatigued, anxiety ridden, unsexy, fat, and cranky.

That's not true. It's not normal.

If you're reading this book, you are most likely one of these suffering women. Maybe you are struggling with moodiness, focus, sleeplessness, brain fog, excess weight, or waning sex drive. Or maybe you just don't feel like your old self. You should know that there's a different way to live: You can feel delicious, vital, and genuinely content. I'm here to show you that you can live an extraordinary life and that you can feel great—regardless of your age, even if it sounds unlikely or unimaginable.

I've helped many women transform hormonal problems using simple yet powerful techniques. The good news: *It's easier to rebalance your hormones than to live with the misery of hormonal imbalance.* In fact, it's totally realistic to feel better in middle age than you did in your twenties as a perfect hormonal specimen. I'll guide you. You no longer need to be disappointed in the medical system—and you don't need to settle for anything less than feeling fully alive and joyous before, during, and after middle age.

Not convinced? Let's start with one real-life example. When I first met Diane, age forty-six, in my integrative medicine practice, she was overweight and drinking two glasses of wine a night to cope with her stress-crazed emotions, amped-up hormonal system, and marital discord. She had gained 20 pounds over the previous six months. She had always been a runner, she told me, but now she felt depleted after each run, rather than brimming with feel-good endorphins as she used to. She often felt cold, her hair fell out in chunks, and she was extremely irritable. Sex drive? On a scale of 1 to 10 (10 being sex of the dreamy/creamy variety), she gave herself a 1.

"I feel as if something has taken over my body," Diane confided, arranging her long skirt over her thickened belly and legs, adding, "I have a chronic dialogue with myself about all the ways in which I fall short: I'm not sexy, I'm not fit, I'm not a good mom, I'm not fun anymore." She had asked her male gynecologist for help and was advised to eat less and exercise more. As we talked, I gained insight into her symptoms and overall lifestyle. My hunch was that Diane was suffering from high cortisol. We tested her for that stress hormone, and *whammo*: proof that Diane wasn't crazy. She didn't have to accept that her sex life was over, that she was destined to have a muffin top forever, or that collapsing in bed after dinner each night was the new "normal."

Together, she and I worked out a lifestyle and supplement plan that would turbocharge her metabolism, boost her mojo, and help her hit the "pause" button. Based on The Gottfried Protocol—my step-by-step, integrative approach to hormonal balance—Diane began a new way of eating (no gluten or sugar for three months) and targeted exercise that lowered her cortisol rather than raised it (studies show that running raises cortisol levels). She set aside fifteen minutes each day for conscious de-stressing, in this case relaxing yoga, and we mended her hormonal imbalance with three supplements: fish oil, phosphatidylserine, and rhodiola.

When I saw Diane again, three months later, the change was remarkable: Her energy was clear and focused. She had a sparkle in her eyes. She told me that she had easily lost the 20 pounds and felt comfortable in her body once more. And, in that riveting woman-to-woman way, she described passionately how she felt sensual again and desired attractive men, particularly the one she had been married to for ten years.

You may not have exactly Diane's problems—that is, your symptoms and your story may be different—but the final goal is the same. It is possible to reset your hormones and to reclaim a satisfying and *downright enchanting* life—as an individual and as a woman—and it can be done without synthetic drugs or expensive therapies. Your progress through all stages of your life, and especially premenopause and perimenopause, doesn't have to be a tortuous slog through hormonal hell. With natural hormone balancing, these years can be fun, enlivening, and sexy. Your body deserves and prefers to be in hormonal homeostasis—a state of equilibrium.

You just have to know how to get there and make a commitment to a different path. Sometimes it's just a few tweaks; sometimes return to homeostasis entails major changes. But you have to understand the underlying causes first. My approach is to target what is causing the imbalance, and then to systematically fix it. I've written this book so that you will become an educated consumer and *partner* in your health optimization, able to work with (and even sometimes direct) your own doctor to create positive change. I will lead and encourage you, and teach you how to bring the most potent and effective methods into your life that I've honed in my practice for more than twenty years, so that we can transform your own health and well-being.

This calling to help women has been cultivated in me since childhood. When I was a little girl, my great-grandmother Mud (a family nickname—the abbreviated version of the German word for *mother*—that stuck) often traveled from California to Maryland to visit us. We were a typical American family of the '70s, living in suburbia, watching *Charlie's Angels,* eating the occasional Pop-Tart and Girl Scout cookie.

Mud had other ideas. She showed up at our house not with a box of See's candies like my best friend's grandma, but with wheat berries, fish oil, carob chips, wheat germ, and Meyer lemons. Needless to say, I thought she was weird.

But my embarrassment soon turned to curiosity. Mud looked twenty-five years younger than her seventy-something peers. Wiry and outspoken, she walked as erect as a queen, had perfect teeth, and regaled us with stories of multiple husbands and suitors. Rarely without a glass of warm water and fresh lemon in her hand, Mud moved with vitality and grace unusual for her years. Her skin glowed. She avoided sugar decades before Oprah made the *no-white-stuff diet* trendy. She literally slept on a board. Years prior to Lilias, Bikram, and Lululemon, Mud practiced yoga and could effortlessly raise her foot behind her head. She used to tell us at the dinner table, "I like wine, but it doesn't like me."

My eccentric great-grandmother captivated me. Through her actions and words, I grew to understand that an entire world of prevention, healing, and repair exists through nutrition and lifestyle; that the answers to health challenges cannot be found solely in a bottle of prescription pills; that eating whole foods is the foundation of robust health; that regular exercise and contemplative practice can keep your body humming.

As I absorbed the wisdom of brilliant professors at Harvard Medical School, Massachusetts Institute of Technology, and the University of California at San Francisco—for a grand total of twelve years of training to become a board-certified gynecologist—Mud's ideas about health still permeated the way I wanted to practice medicine. Her example motivated me to practice yoga to cope with the stress of med school and to question the fact that in all those years of education, only thirty minutes had been devoted to the topic of nutrition. Mud planted seeds that would grow into my life's work. My determination grew with the rigor of my conventional medical training and its encouragement to think creatively and to question dogma.

At ninety-six years old, Mud danced at my wedding. She had outlived four husbands and was flirting with my thirty-something male colleagues on the dance floor. At that time, I was in the midst of residency training, working in a disease-based and ailing healthcare system in which old people go to a hospital to die an undignified death. In contrast, Mud later died peacefully in her sleep at ninety-seven, still living independently, still able to lift her foot somewhere near her head.

Even as I trained in the mainstream medical system, it occurred to me that something was terribly wrong. On one hand, U.S. healthcare offers unparalleled innovation and scientific advances. On the other, the United States has the highest rate of obesity in the world: 36 percent of the population is considered obese (and another 34 percent are overweight), which leads to serious, costly, and *largely preventable* diseases such as diabetes, high blood pressure, gallstones, stroke, sleep apnea, heart disease, and cancer. Clearly, mainstream choices are not improving our overall health.

WHAT I DO LACKS AN APPROPRIATE NAME

Because of Mud, I learned the power and importance of looking beyond the symptoms of illness to the health of the whole person, and from my education, to apply the systems-based approach that I learned as a bioengineer at MIT. Studying hormone imbalance from this perspective, I often find there's not just one isolated reason for a problem. Yes, sometimes hormonal problems are a consequence of aging. But a hormone imbalance can also be caused, or worsened, by lifestyle and nutritional choices.

Mud taught me to see the body as a cohesive entity. This is also known as *holistic health*. Yet that's not a perfect term for what I do. Drs. Andrew Weil, Tieraona Low Dog, Victoria Maizes, and their colleagues at the University of Arizona popularized the phrase *integrative medicine*. Others call what I practice *functional medicine*, a term coined by nutritional biochemist Dr. Jeffrey Bland, who founded the Institute for Functional Medicine. Most recently, Dr. Mark Hyman applied the term *4P Medicine: Predictive, Participatory, Preventive, and Personalized*. My work was inspired by the pioneering achievements of Dr. Christiane Northrup; some label it *holistic gynecology*, or *natural hormone balancing*, to borrow a phrase from Dr. Uzzi Reiss. Colleagues of mine in Silicon Valley refer to it as *biohacking*, or Do-It-Yourself biology, outside the confines of traditional environments of universities and industry. For a while, I called what I do *evidence-based integration*, and occasionally *organic gynecology*. But the truth is that no one seems to understand what all these terms mean, nor whether one moniker is a better fit than another for the new, systems-based, and integrative approach to medical care. What's clear is that we need a completely new paradigm that encompasses a quantum shift toward being preventive, proactive, and lifestyle-based, with emphasis on the role and responsibility of the individual in daily choices, habits, and long-term consequences.

Here's how I understand it: I partner with women to mend their broken hormones, brains, and brain chemicals. I assess if a woman is getting enough of the essential building blocks, or precursors, to make the brain chemicals and hormones she needs. I find that Mud's vision is a valuable frame of reference: how you eat, move, supplement, and think governs most of how you feel. They are choices that exert powerful effects on your biology, but they don't have to be as extreme as sleeping on a board or doing pretzely yoga poses. I want to show you how to make the best choices each day based on your individual hormonal vulnerabilities.

The visionary medical practitioners I've mentioned are my mentors, and I owe them buckets of gratitude. Yet to me, each of these terms and the associated practices fall short. Hormones bring a woman into my integrative medical office, but it's the alliance we form that generates something new. We assess her hormones and how they relate to the body's neurotransmitters and mood. We move outward to her relationships and satisfaction with her work. We consider her diet, exercise, contemplative practice, if any, and how she manages stress (or not). This partnership yields something entirely different: repair, healing, harmony, and hope.

CHANGE IS SUSTAINED WHEN PACED, MINDFUL, AND NATURAL

For most of us, *change is hard,* and the path isn't always well defined in the mainstream, disease-oriented model. We all dream of a magic pill to improve things or return us to our youth. At one extreme, many people in the United States choose a risky surgery such as gastric bypass instead of changing the way they manage their lifestyle. There are countless people who think that a prescription pill or medical procedure will solve their problems, and that anything less is a waste of time. At the other extreme, there are people like my great-grandmother, who relentlessly pursue robust health and empower everyone around them to do the same.

In my experience, most of us inhabit the middle ground. We make changes when the pain of staying the same (same weight, same mood, same stress-crazed schedule) is greater than the perceived pain of change. I discovered (as have my patients) that there is a way to make those changes that is safe, proven, effective, easy, and even fun.

The best time to get and stay healthy is before you face annoying and inconvenient problems, such as weight gain and mood swings, and before you develop a serious health condition, such as depression or breast cancer. Why not create lasting change *now,* before you find yourself in a doctor's office, holding a prescription for meds because you've developed an illness—or worse, being rolled on a hospital gurney for an invasive surgery?

I hope this book will persuade you to take action to find the root causes of your symptoms. If you do, I believe you'll see significant, even dramatic, improvement: more blissful and productive days, more decades spent in your prime. Graceful, decelerated aging, with no need for the latest plumping serum to bring back the skin you were born with. A more relaxed relationship with your body, your diet, and your weight. Superb working memory. Restorative sleep. More zest, more spring in your step and joie de vivre. Who knows, maybe you too will dance at your great-granddaughter's wedding.

Sara Gottfried, MD
Berkeley, California
2013

PART I

EDUCATE AND ILLUMINATE: UNDERSTANDING THE NEW HORMONAL LANDSCAPE

INTRODUCTION:

WHY HORMONES MATTER

I'm a doctor who treats women's hormones. I use the best evidence to discover the root causes of hormone imbalance. Then I apply a science-based correction for hormone balance. Every woman has unique hormonal needs, and I meet these needs by leveraging whatever it takes: nutrition, botanical remedies, critical precursors (essential ingredients to make brain chemicals and hormones) such as amino acids and B vitamins, ancient methodology, and bioidentical hormones. I believe that weight gain, mood swings, fatigue, and low libido aren't diseases that can be "cured" with a quick injection or a pharmaceutical. Most of these problems can't be permanently solved by eating less or exercising more. *They are hormonal problems. They mean our bodies are trying to tell us that something is wrong.* And with a rigorous strategy—methodical, repeatable, scientifically supported—those problems can be resolved.

That's why I've designed a system I call The Gottfried Protocol, a step-by-step, integrative approach to natural hormone healing that emphasizes lifestyle design first and foremost. It's based on decades of research, my education at Harvard Medical School, my own experiences with hormonal imbalances, my belief in peer-reviewed, well-performed randomized trials to support my recommendations, and what I've learned from patients over the past twenty-plus years of practicing medicine. The Gottfried Protocol engages only the top hierarchy of scientific evidence and has been proven in scores of women in my practice.

I've spent my career taking care not to overpromise. After all, I'm a physician, bioengineer, and scientist. In fact, I'm rather conservative medically. Unlike most books on hormones that come from the alternative-health world, this book takes a data-driven approach to integrative medicine. But because I'm also a yoga teacher, The Gottfried Protocol integrates the new brain science that proves how ancient methods such as mindfulness and herbology provide lasting change. Add to that what I've gleaned from more than two decades of caring for thousands of women, listening carefully to their stories, and observing and *continuously tweaking* how they respond to our work together. I'm confident that if you follow the advice in this book, you will feel better, reclaim the bounce in your step, and bloom as you were intended.

The Unfair Truth

Many women don't know that hormonal imbalances cause them to feel crummy. My patients come to me distraught, complaining of relentless irritability, fatigue, poor stress resilience, irregular or painful menstrual cycles, dried-out vaginas, lackluster orgasms, and low libido. Many women feel their bodies have turned against them. In my years of clinical practice, I've seen it all: Women who would rather mop the floor than have sex with their husbands. Women who worry they can't perform as well as they used to on the job because of brain fog. Husbands who plead with me: "Help me find the woman I married." Women who are tired, unhappy, and perpetually overwhelmed.

It's not fair but it's a fact: women are much more vulnerable to hormonal imbalance than men. An underactive thyroid affects women up to fifteen times more often than men. According to national polls, women feel more stressed than men: 26 percent of women in the United States are on a pill for anxiety, depression, or a general feeling of being unable to cope, compared with 15 percent of men.

Why such a gender difference? For one thing, women have babies. Pregnancy amplifies the demands on the endocrine glands, which release hormones such as estrogen, testosterone, cortisol, thyroid, leptin, growth hormone, and insulin. If you lack the organ reserves to keep up with amplified need, you may suffer; in fact, organ decline is measurable before symptoms begin to show. It's not just pregnancy, as evidenced by the childless women I see in my practice. Women are exquisitely sensitive to hormonal changes. And they're susceptible to the stresses of juggling multiple roles.

Never heard of organ reserve? Here's the skinny: Your organ reserve is an individual organ's inherent ability to withstand demands (such as grueling schedules, trauma, and surgery) and to restore homeostasis, or balance. As you age, reserve declines: healthy young people have a reserve capacity that is ten times greater than demand. After age thirty, organ reserve decreases by 1 percent per year, so that by age eighty-five, organ reserve is a fraction of the original capacity.

———ORGAN RESERVE AND WHY IT MATTERS———

Organ reserve is the capacity of an organ, such as your ovaries, thyroid, or liver, to function beyond its baseline needs. For example, take your adrenal organs. You can test your adrenal (or stress) reserve by injecting a hormone to see if you can double or triple your adrenal gland's output of cortisol when needed, such as in an emergency. If your adrenal organ reserve is low, your cortisol may not go up as high as needed. Your output is depleted and subnormal. You can do a similar test for your thyroid. Don't worry about injecting hormones! Depending on your responses to the questionnaires in this book, I'll guide you through sensible change.

You'll find that if your organ reserve is full when you get pregnant, your postpartum hormonal roller-coaster ride will likely be a lot smoother. As you age, the same is true: your body bounces back more readily from the stressors of everyday life. However, accelerated aging is associated with low organ reserve and hormone imbalance.

Bottom line: organ reserve is a crucial aspect of longevity—the more you protect *and enhance* your functional capacity, the more able you are to bounce back from stresses such as illness, environmental toxins, and injury.

Hormonal Crosstalk

Food choices, environment, attitude, aging, stress, genetics, even the chemicals in our clothes and mattresses can affect our hormone levels. Another important influence is how our hormones interact. Remember Diane? Her problem was high cortisol, but the high cortisol blocked the function of other key hormones, such as her thyroid, the queen of metabolism, and her progesterone, the main antibloating hormone that also soothes the female brain. When you target and adjust several hormones simultaneously—the adrenal, thyroid, and sex hormones—you get better results. Many of these root causes, such as the primary role of the stress hormone cortisol in Diane's case, are simply overlooked by mainstream medicine. Hormonal problems are the top reason I find for accelerated aging, which occurs when the hormones that build muscle and bone decline more quickly than the hormones that break down tissue to provide energy. The result: our cells experience more wear and tear, less repair, and we feel and look older than our age. The goal is to have your breakdown in proportion to your repair, or even better, more repair than breakdown.

Untreated hormone imbalances can have serious consequences, including osteoporosis, obesity, and breast cancer. Clearly, it's important to tune the body's hormones to their optimal levels, both individually and in relation to each other.

My Hormonal Story

When I was in my thirties, I worked at a Health Maintenance Organization (HMO) and was preparing to launch an integrative medical practice. My busy husband traveled frequently (he is a green visionary who founded the U.S. and World Green Building Councils). I had two young kids and a mortgage to pay. As if this weren't stressful enough, monthly PMS made my life miserable. In the week before my period, I had night sweats that disrupted my sleep. My heavy, painful periods came every twenty-two to twenty-three days—and when you combine that with PMS, I had only *one good week* per month. Throughout the month, I suffered from low energy, a nonexistent libido, and a less-than-sunny attitude. As you might imagine, this was a truly terrible experience, and my entire family suffered.

I was too young to feel so bad. Antidepressants didn't seem like the right solution. I didn't want to dampen my dynamic range or mute the texture of my life. I just wanted to feel more alive and charged.

I was lucky. Because of my medical training, I knew what to do. I formed a hypothesis: my hormones were off balance. In med school, I was taught that measuring hormone levels is a waste of time and money, because hormone levels vary too much. But when I thought about how we track hormones such as estrogen, progesterone, thyroid, and testosterone when women are trying to conceive or are in the early months of pregnancy, I wondered why those numbers would be important indications of a woman's health in one situation but not another? Wouldn't my hormone levels be as reliable an indicator of my health after my pregnancies as before them? So I drew some blood and tested my blood-serum levels of thyroid, sex hormones including estrogen and progesterone, and cortisol, the main stress hormone. And I discovered what millions of other women face: my hormones were seriously off kilter. I was a frazzled new mom, harried wife, and busy doctor, with significant imbalances in my estrogen, progesterone, thyroid, and cortisol levels.

Despite the lack of nutrition and lifestyle education in the hallowed halls of Preparation H (our nickname for Harvard Medical School), I did learn how to approach a problem systematically. I was taught how to assess evidence and to distrust dogma. But rather than masking the symptoms of my hormone issues, as I had been taught to do (usually with a birth control pill or antidepressant), I wanted to seek the root causes. I sought to uncover *what* was wrong, as well as *why* things went sideways for me hormonally. As I struggled with PMS, habitual stress, attention problems, disordered eating, and accelerated aging, I slowly developed a progressive, step-by-step, lifestyle-driven approach to treat my hormone imbalance naturally—that is, without prescription drugs.

Eventually, I got religious about fish oil, vitamin D, and important precursors to hormones and neurotransmitters (including amino acids such as 5-HTP, a precursor to serotonin, one of the "feel-good" neurotransmitters, or brain chemicals). For the first time in my life, I faithfully practiced what I preached: I ate seven to nine servings of fresh fruits and vegetables per day. I stopped exercising so hard, in an obsessive attempt to burn calories, and exercised smarter. I began meditating regularly. My weight dropped 25 pounds. I was happier. I didn't yell at the kids so much. I could find my keys. My energy improved greatly. I was even more open to sex. I knew that I was on to something.

A Word About Evidence

Not long ago, the *New York Times* ran an article about women injecting themselves with the pregnancy hormone hCG in order to lose weight. As a gynecologist and a woman, I'm fully aware of people trying to inject themselves to thinness. But it stunned me to see the fad had reached a fever pitch—that women will pay thousands of dollars to "treat" symptoms of what are, in truth, hormone imbalances, emotional eating patterns, and nutritional gaps with a shot of pregnancy hormone. In my humble medical opinion, this is absurd.

I've pored over the literature on human chorionic gonadotropin (hCG). Since 1954, twelve randomized research studies have shown *no benefit for weight loss from hCG.* It's bad enough that the advantages of injecting hCG to lose weight have proven nonexistent, but it's truly frightening that there are no studies that guarantee the safety of injecting this hormone for this purpose. Yet significant numbers of women are trying it.

Evidence matters. In medical school, I was taught to prescribe Prempro to women over forty who were suffering from hot flashes, night sweats, sleepless nights, anxiety, and/or depression. Prempro is a combination of two drugs containing synthetic sex hormones: Premarin and Provera. (Premarin is a synthetic concoction of ten estrogens—none of which are similar to the estrogens you make in your own body—extracted from the urine of pregnant horses. Provera, a synthetic form of progesterone, can cause depression.) Conventional wisdom claimed this was the miracle combo for hormone-replacement therapy, because it had been shown to reduce heart disease in observational studies, such as one known as the Nurses' Health Study.

But observational studies are not what I consider best evidence, because the information is gathered from people who are *already using a drug,* rather than participants chosen at random to take it in a controlled environment, with another group, also selected at random, that is given a placebo instead of the drug. Here is what I believe is the best evidence: the randomized, placebo-controlled trial—one that is designed well, with a large enough sample size to show the effect, *if there is one,* and ideally more than one trial showing benefit. (If there are three randomized trials showing the same result, then I do the happy dance.)

When randomized, placebo-controlled trials of Prempro finally took place in 1999, the results showed that Prempro *increased* heart disease. In 2002, another large randomized trial, the Women's Health Initiative, confirmed these findings. Huge wakeup call: for fifty-seven years, the mainstream medical community had been prescribing synthetic hormones before understanding their true effect on women's health. Like thousands of other obstetricians, gynecologists, internists, and family-practice physicians, I had been doling out the wrong advice. It was a dramatic turn of events for me: I had to reconcile my belief in "best evidence" with the fact that the method for best evidence was neither *taught to* nor *practiced by* most doctors in the United States. The truth is that most prescriptions for hormone problems are not supported by hard science, and that the criteria for best evidence are not evenly applied. The experience taught me to be far more skeptical of hormone therapy and to demand the best evidence before prescribing any hormone, as well as to engage lifestyle changes first. In my practice, as a last resort, I do sometimes recommend hormone therapy in the smallest yet most effective doses and for the shortest duration, as you will see in chapters 4 through 9.

Since 2002, 80 percent of women stopped their hormone therapy. Yet the damage had already been done—women became fearful and suspicious of hormone therapy, as well as the doctors who urged them to take it. This was a very unfortunate outcome for several reasons, including the following: first, women faced far fewer options to manage the hormonal bedlam of perimenopause and menopause; second, the media oversimplified and distorted the results—there was little room to discuss the nuances of the data and how they applied to an older subset of women (average age sixty-six and older); third, a few bad eggs (synthetic hormones) ruined the reputation of all hormones, both synthetic and natural or bioidentical; and fourth, hormones could not have become a more polarized topic. Restriction in choice is never a good thing, above all when it comes to a woman who is feeling mildly or moderately insane from lack of sleep and progesterone in middle age.

Short version: *randomized, placebo-controlled trials produce better data.* I have robust evidence, based on the best quality of scientific investigation, including validated questionnaires and randomized, placebo-controlled trials, that I can't wait to share with you. Even today, just 15 percent of the drugs prescribed in mainstream medicine are supported by these studies. In my practice, 85 percent of my recommendations are supported by such trials—and the other 15 percent are sufficiently low risk (such as a vitamin or a shift in mind-set) that they are unlikely to cause any problems.

A New Paradigm

Mainstream medicine is marvelous for broken bones and works wonders with a life-threatening bacterial infection or heart attack, but we've lost something as we've become increasingly technical, specialized, and downright vocational. In this country, the average appointment with a doctor is seven minutes long. *Seven minutes.* But I believe that women's health issues, lifestyle choices, and symptoms are complex and take time to decode. That's why an appointment in my medical practice is fifty minutes or longer.

As you probably know, the problem in mainstream medicine isn't lack of spending. U.S. healthcare costs are a whopping $2.5 trillion per year and rising. Yet 70 percent of costs are spent on diagnostic procedures and treatments that could be avoided through better lifestyle choices. Increasingly, our population is hormonally imbalanced and overweight, and the root cause is tied to how we eat, how we move, missing nutrients, age-related changes, and, increasingly, exposure to environmental toxins called endocrine disruptors. Nevertheless, a lifestyle-based approach has been unsung and undervalued by most mainstream health practitioners, which is particularly shocking when you review the science and realize just how effective lifestyle design can be when applied to hormones, mood, longevity, stress-related problems, and prevention of disease.

Most prescriptions are not a "cure." In my opinion, most conventionally trained doctors haven't a clue about how hormones wreak havoc on a woman's physical and emotional state; the effects of these imbalances fly beneath their radar. The inclination is to write a prescription—too often for the antidepressant du jour. Not only can antidepressants cause weight gain, stroke, low sex drive, preterm labor, and infant convulsions, but recent data link antidepressants with breast and ovarian cancer. As if these adverse effects weren't enough, I see no evidence that prescriptions for mental-health maladies offer a *cure*. Yes, there is a time and a place for prescription medication, and some people urgently need such medication. But I find that mental-health prescriptions are handed over too readily, when the root cause and contributing factors, such as neuroendocrine imbalance, have not been fully explored. A *cure* restores health, but most prescriptions are not a cure—they merely mask symptoms. When you address original causes of poor health and neuroendocrine imbalance, you are far closer to a cure than at the bottom of an expensive pill bottle.

There must be a better way. Ten years ago, when I still worked in the trenches of conventional medicine, before I spun off to start my own integrative medicine practice, I figured there had to be a better way to fill the gaps that women encounter between what we struggle with and what mainstream medicine offers. I discovered that the most important gap was *adrenal function*. Your adrenals are the tiny little endocrine glands on top of your kidneys that secrete several stress hormones, including cortisol and DHEA. In my medical training, I learned about tumors of the adrenal glands, and what to do if a patient had an extreme excess of cortisol (Cushing's syndrome) or complete failure of the adrenals (Addison's disease). I had been trained to identify the weeds and dead plants, but not to look for the early and subtle signs of ailing to come. Your adrenals may just be the most important plants in your garden for us to nurture and help bloom.

You see, in mainstream medicine, we tend to have either/or thinking. Either your liver is working or you have liver disease. Either your thyroid is working or you have thyroid insufficiency. Either your adrenals are working or you have adrenal failure. There is rarely a "middle ground." The truth is that most of us exist in a wide space between those two extremes, which I call dysfunction or dysregulation. I believe it's not only worthwhile but ultimately your responsibility (along with the help of a trusted clinician) to intervene *before* your organs become diseased. Intervention before failure, before insufficiency, is proven to contribute to lasting health and longevity.

How could conventional medicine benefit from ancient traditions? Conventional medicine tends to focus on what's *not* working, rather than on what *is* working. Conventional doctors are trained to fix what's broken in the body; they focus on removing the bad, whether that's a diseased appendix or cancer cells. Sometimes the singular focus on "fixing the bad" becomes a self-defeating cycle in which we see only *what's not working.* If we widen our lens to see also what is working, we can understand how to best nurture the good, and thereby amplify the beneficial effect. This larger view allows us to work smarter rather than harder. Leveraging your strengths rather than concentrating on your weaknesses creates the most profound and lasting change. A significant body of research supports this kind of strength-based approach.

Pareto's Principle, applied to hormones. What I've observed in my practice is that 80 percent of righting your hormonal balance comes from 20 percent of your efforts. This is an application of Pareto's Principle, or the 80/20 Rule: a general notion that 20 percent of effort is responsible for 80 percent of the results. In my office, the 80/20 Rule leads to one basic question: what are the most efficient ways to harness your resources and optimize your hormones? Rather than randomly seeking every possible cause for a neurohormonal problem, we first identify the small changes that will have the largest impact.

Many women wind up in my office looking for answers they intuitively know exist but cannot seem to find within the limited scope of conventional medicine. They identify me through a referral from their own puzzled gynecologist; a friend who lost 30 pounds following one of my protocols; an interview I've performed on the radio, a speech, or from my blog at http://www.saragottfriedmd.com; or after a despairing online search for information on how to rekindle their sex drive. Once we talk, they often exclaim that they've had an epiphany: they've finally found a mentor and a partner in health, someone who actually listens and presents them with enlivening, safe, and proven choices.

Use this book as your personal appointment with me to decode your hormonal DNA so you'll feel and look gorgeous, radically prevent degenerative aging, and rock your middle age, whether that's several years away or where you are right now. We'll create a new hormonal roadmap, just for you.

Women Desperately Seeking Answers

I recently worked with a professor of sociology to come up with a quantitative survey of my clients. The survey polled my female patients: 26 percent under the age of forty, 57 percent between forty and fifty-four, and 17 percent fifty-five or older.

Here's what we found:

- Spare beach floatie? 64 percent of my clients have one.
- Hair loss? Yikes, 40 percent struggle with this.
- Half of my clients feel they're *constantly* running from task to task (like a chicken with its head cut off).
- Poor sleep? 80 percent struggle with it at least once per week, and 20 percent every night.
- More than half feel there's not enough time in the day to accomplish the things they need to accomplish.
- Headaches? Yep, in 48 percent, either menstrual or non-cyclic.
- Of my clients, 48 percent have skin problems, ranging from eczema to excessive thinning or prematurely aging skin.

- More than half felt they *couldn't get going* at least three or more days of the past week.
- Vaginal dryness (or as inhumanely coined in medical parlance: *atrophic vaginitis!*) is experienced by 37 percent.
- Fortunately, only 9 percent have high blood pressure.

The numbers don't end there. These figures reflect the percent of my clients desperately seeking particular results they cannot get from conventional medicine: 91 percent want more energy; 80 percent want a better sex drive; 69 percent wish for better mood; and 26 percent yearn for the end of hot flashes or night sweats.

These metrics show the epidemic plaguing modern women. It's not just looking good that interests women. It's feeling good from cells to souls. In my practice, I find that many women initially believe anything short of a prescription drug is a waste of time. Mention the word *holistic* and they run for cover. But I urge you to stay. Ultimately, you and your family will be glad you did.

Dr. Sara's Mindmap: Principles of Hormone Balancing

- Recognize the inherent wisdom of the body. Natural order, particularly as it applies to the control of hormone metabolism, prefers equilibrium. When we remove obstacles, we move toward balance. Balance is often a matter of identifying and then removing obstacles rather than prescribing medications. Plus, learning what the obstacles are for you and how to work with them are an essential part of healing.
- Identify the root causes of the imbalance. Sustained health results from treating underlying causes, rather than suppressing symptoms.
- Be systems oriented, proactive, and intelligent about replacing hormones. Work with the control system, located

in the brain, rather than replacing every hormone that is low. Focus on what is working as well as on what isn't.

- Do no harm. Using best evidence, including the gold standard of randomized trials, provides treatments that are proven safe and effective.
- Be an active partner. Make sure you become actively involved in the quest for balanced hormones. The more you invest as an equal partner and participant with your practitioner, the better you will sustain the changes you create together.

The Gottfried Protocol

Science has proven that while your genes control your biology, a rather simple, nondrug formula of nutrient-rich food, targeted supplements to address missing precursors, and lifestyle changes can keep your genes in perpetual "repair" mode. Even if you're genetically programmed to develop depression or cancer, *the way you eat, move, and supplement* can alter the expression of your genetic code. This emerging field of epigenomics examines the influence of environmental inputs on genetic expression. Catalyzed by the revelation of the human genome, epigenomics is a fascinating area that informs how genes are modified without changing the DNA sequence—that is, how a gene for obesity, for instance, is modified by eating nonstarchy vegetables versus cupcakes. You'll read more about how you can leverage epigenomics to overrule genetic predispositions.

Your genes are merely a template. In other words, your body is full of natural mechanisms for repair and healing. When you nourish and augment these built-in mechanisms, you may prevent and even reverse disease.

This is the foundation of The Gottfried Protocol. No matter what the hormonal problem is, the solution starts with lifestyle design, including a nutritious food plan, identifying and filling in the missing precursors to your proper neurohormonal communication, and targeted exercise. Creating a methodology to assess, support, and maintain hormonal balance for myself and my clients took more than ten years. I defined, tested, and refined a progressive, systematic approach that is reproducible and proven.

When I dealt with my own hormone imbalances, my goal was to discover the root causes, to formulate a customized and rigorous fix, and to track my progress. I drew upon many sources, including traditional Chinese and Indian (Ayurvedic) medicine. In The Gottfried Protocol, I combine the latest medical advances and cutting-edge techniques with ancient treatments validated by modern research.

The recommendations in this book are based on this evidence-based integrative approach. This three-step strategy is a sequential system that includes

1. lifestyle design: food, nutraceutical, and targeted exercise
2. herbal therapies
3. bioidentical hormones

Most of my recommendations are available without prescription. When women put an earnest effort into Step 1 of The Gottfried Protocol—and implement a customized food plan; specific supplements that include missing vitamins, minerals, and amino acids; and targeted exercise—they find most of their symptoms of hormone imbalance disappear. If they don't, we shift to Step 2—proven botanical therapies. After completing Steps 1 and 2, few women need bioidentical hormones (Step 3), but for those who do, the doses and duration of treatment are often lower than if they'd skipped the lifestyle design and herbal therapies.

Sometimes it just takes a small adjustment to induce big changes: I relish the moment a patient realizes that her presumed life sentence of low sex drive can be altered with a particular form of meditation and a *maca* smoothie.

The Hormone Cure

This book will change your life for the better. By nature I am a skeptical person, but I've seen the benefits of The Gottfried Protocol over and over in my own practice. We are conditioned as women to live in such a way that *gets our hormones to work against us,* and I want to help you adjust your hormones naturally so they are allies. As I've witnessed the healing that women experience when their hormones are reproportioned, as I've documented both the results and the transformation that occur in everyday lives, I've come to believe that The Gottfried Protocol is far more likely to succeed than a prescription medication—particularly a medication that is completely foreign to your body.

The Hormone Cure is divided into two parts. *Part I: Educate and Illuminate* provides the foundational elements. Chapter 1 offers several questionnaires—checklists to help you identify your main hormonal imbalances. After responding to these questions, you will have a good idea if you are high or low in any of the targeted hormones, and then know which chapters you should read first. Chapter 2 offers an overview of what hormones are, what they do, and how they interact. Chapter 3 describes when it all starts to go awry: perimenopause, which typically begins between the ages of thirty-five and fifty (menopause, on average, occurs at age fifty-one in the United States).

Part II: Assess, Diagnose, Treat describes what you need to know about individual hormones. Based on exhaustive research and drawing on my years of clinical experience (plus forty-five years in a female body with seemingly every hormonal symptom possible), I describe the common causes of specific hormonal imbalances and what to do about them.

Part III: The Appendix, offers important reference materials for hormonal balance. I've included a summary of The Gottfried Protocol according to root cause, a glossary of terms, a table of hormones described in this book and their jobs, how to find and work collaboratively with clinicians, recommended laboratories for home testing, and the food plan that I recommend to my patients and follow myself.

In reading each chapter, you'll refer to the questionnaires at the beginning of this book to help you assess your symptoms and perhaps even identify issues that you didn't know could be related to hormones. I focus on a specific hormone in each chapter: cortisol, estrogen, progesterone, androgens (including testosterone and DHEA), and thyroid. Along the way, you'll also meet other hormonal characters, including insulin, pregnenolone, vitamin D, leptin, and growth hormone.

You'll learn what each hormone is, what its job is, what you feel like when it's functioning properly—and when it is not—and what might have caused the imbalance in the first place. After introducing you to the hormone in question, I dive deeper into the science behind what's happening in your body to cause that hormone to become imbalanced. Understanding the science is important to some of my patients, while others feel they don't care about it and just want to know how to feel better now. In this book, you can decide how much science you want to know, or skip past it.

Once we've defined your hormonal problem, you'll find a strategy for what to do. That's where The Gottfried Protocol comes in; we make a plan instead of taking a shot in the dark. (I'll let you know when you need to visit a doctor.) Finally, to help you feel that you're not alone, each chapter contains a few case studies from my files, true stories of real patients: their symptoms, our treatment protocol, and the results.

The Ideal Hormonal Specimen

Picture the Ideal Hormonal Specimen. Her hormones perfectly balanced, she has high energy throughout the day, stable moods, and no food cravings. Her full head of hair is glossy and her skin is clear. She easily maintains her weight and her sexual energy. Colleagues never worry that she'll weep in the middle of a big meeting or start sweating profusely. Well-intentioned friends don't gently suggest "seeing someone, a therapist, maybe?"

The Hormone Cure is for the rest of us, the women who haven't quite reached the status of Ideal Hormonal Specimen—but we aspire to it. I believe the majority of women want to look better, feel better, and age more gracefully. They want to become Ideal Hormonal Specimens.

This book is for women of all ages. A common myth about hormones is that you don't need to worry about them until menopause. The truth is, many hormone levels, such as estrogen and testosterone, start to drift downward when you're in your twenties. Some hormones, such as cortisol, may spike too high and pull other hormones offline. Women younger than thirty may not yet feel affected by the aging process, but perhaps they want to get pregnant or avoid the diagnosis of breast cancer their mom just received.

Those in their thirties may feel increasingly tense and overwhelmed, in need of better strategies on how to relax. They may want to prevent the high blood pressure, prediabetes, and accelerated aging that come with chronically high stress levels. Women in their forties and fifties may want to regain some of the buoyancy of their youth. Perhaps they want to wake up feeling restored again, without the brain fog from disrupted sleep. Women in their sixties, seventies, and eighties may want to optimize their cognitive and executive functioning—to improve their thinking, memory, and competitive edge.

The Hormone Cure was born of my passion to help women, one hormone at a time. I don't want women to suffer; I don't want them to be underserved by their doctors, miseducated by the media, tired, frazzled, and ashamed. I'm not a magician who can turn back the hands of time and make you twenty-five again, nor do I believe that's best for you. What I can do is return something you've lost: the properly proportioned hormonal organization that provides clarity, confidence, and longevity.

The human body has an innate ability to repair and self-regulate, but that ability often gets bulldozed by the enduring stressors, distractions, and interruptions of modern life. Once you rediscover your body's ability to shift toward balance, informed by the new science of integrative women's health and aided by The Gottfried Protocol, you'll find that it's easier to move toward balance than to stay imbalanced. Attend to your hormones today, and the process will serve your mood, weight, energy, sex drive, sleep, and resilience for decades to come.

CHAPTER 1

GETTING STARTED:
FILL OUT THE QUESTIONNAIRES

If you have this book in your hands, I imagine you want to get started on your hormone cure. Answering some key questions is the first step. I designed several questionnaires, which I use in my practice, to identify the most common hormonal problems that can occur during premenopause, perimenopause, and menopause. By responding to these questions, you will discover which problems may be yours. Then I'll guide you toward the chapters that can best help you in your quest for hormonal balance. (Please note, it is important for everyone to read Part 1, regardless of your questionnaire results.)

The Quest for Optimal Health

Balance. It's the province of an elite gymnast on a beam or a yogini posing on one leg. It's the basis of a nourishing meal (like those we're often too busy to prepare or enjoy). It's work *and* life, self *and* family. It's a soul-infused pie chart, where all the pieces complement one another and feed our spirit. Balance is the means *and* the end. Balance is the holy grail, something all of us seek. Balance is stable and sustainable. Balance is health. And balance is elusive.

We *know* that balance can help us run the gauntlet of working, child rearing, grocery shopping, caregiving, errand running, and juggling our other interests while keeping our health and sanity intact. Balance enables us to take on those tasks in a less harried, frantic, and fragile way. Needless to say, our never-ending pursuit of balance can be stressful in itself. Often, we're frustrated with ourselves for not attaining balance.

However, the reason it's so hard to find balance might not be *you*. It might be instead that your hormones are off, and that's what's making you *feel* off balance. When your hormones are disordered, you can feel lethargic, irritable, weepy, grumpy, unappreciated, anxious, depressed. And then you have even more trouble running the daily gauntlet. How do you know if your hormones are off kilter? That's where my questionnaires come in.

Health is a complex ecosystem. The biological processes of our bodies, whether they're functioning ideally or are disordered, affect our mood, psyche, and the way we live. So your hormones might be affecting more than you could possibly imagine.

Never underestimate the power of stress. The stresses in our lives can alter the biochemical machinations of our bodies. This isn't *woo-woo*; it's medical fact. Stress is the top reason behind most visits to the doctor, and it contributes to all the big causes of death, including heart disease, diabetes, stroke, and cancer. A robust medical inquiry ensures that we consider all the variables. If any one of them is left out, we might not find the root cause of the hormone imbalance.

My questionnaires are loosely modeled on the theories of Dr. John Lee, a well-known physician who worked in the field of hormonal balance. My questions have been adjusted over the years through my own study and experience with the women in my medical practice, and integrated with a hefty dose of evidence. I encourage my patients to see the path toward hormone balance as an epic journey—a womanly version of an odyssey. Every epic, life-altering quest begins with a task. That's what these questionnaires are: the journey-starting, readiness-testing task for balance-seeking *she*roes. Your answers to these questions become the map to the rest of the journey. Your tools will be the treatments described in The Gottfried Protocol.

Quest(ionnaires) for Hormonal Balance

The following questionnaires, similar to the ones I administer in my practice, are designed to identify correctly the undiagnosed hormone problems you may face. I use the results to find the sweet spot between mainstream medicine's tendency to underdiagnose without the tendency to overdiagnose that I sometimes observe in alternative medicine.

Read carefully through the list of symptoms, put a checkmark next to any you experience, and add up the checks within each grouping. Note that each part should be answered separately. Just like a Venn diagram of overlapping circles, you may have symptoms that fit into more than one part (such as infertility and mood issues). In other words, some of your answers may be repeated—but usually one or two areas will stand out as your key hormonal challenges. Don't fret! At the end, we'll work through what your answers mean.

DO YOU HAVE OR HAVE YOU EXPERIENCED IN THE PAST SIX MONTHS . . .

— PART A —

- A feeling you're constantly racing from one task to the next?

- Feeling wired yet tired?

- A struggle calming down before bedtime, or a second wind that keeps you up late?

- Difficulty falling asleep or disrupted sleep?

- A feeling of anxiety or nervousness—can't stop worrying about things beyond your control?

- A quickness to feel anger or rage—frequent screaming or yelling?

- Memory lapses or feeling distracted, especially under duress?

- Sugar cravings (you need "a little something" after each meal, usually of the chocolate variety)?

- Increased abdominal circumference, greater than 35 inches (the dreaded abdominal fat, or muffin top—not bloating)?

- Skin conditions such as eczema or thin skin (sometimes physiologically *and* psychologically)?

- Bone loss (perhaps your doctor uses scarier terms, such as *osteopenia* or *osteoporosis*)?

- High blood pressure or rapid heartbeat unrelated to those cute red shoes in the store window?

- High blood sugar (maybe your clinician has mentioned the words *prediabetes* or even *diabetes* or *insulin resistance*)? Shakiness between meals, also known as *blood sugar instability*?

- Indigestion, ulcers, or GERD (gastroesophageal reflux disease)?

- More difficulty recovering from physical injury than in the past?

- Unexplained pink to purple stretch marks on your belly or back?

- Irregular menstrual cycles?

- Decreased fertility?

— PART B —

- Fatigue or burnout (you use caffeine to bolster your energy, or fall asleep while reading or watching a movie)?

- Loss of stamina, particularly in the afternoon, from two to five?

- An atypical addiction to a negative point of view?

- Crying jags for no particular reason?

- Decreased problem-solving ability?

- Feeling stressed most of the time (everything seems harder than before, and you have trouble coping)? Decreased stress tolerance?

- Insomnia or difficulty staying asleep, especially between one and four in the morning?

- Low blood pressure (not always a good thing, since your blood pressure determines the correct amount of oxygen to send through your body, especially into your brain)?

- Postural hypotension (you stand up from lying down and feel dizzy)?

- Difficulty fighting infection (you catch every virus you meet, particularly respiratory)? Difficulty recovering from illness or surgery or healing wounds?

- Asthma? Bronchitis? Chronic cough? Allergies?

- Low or unstable blood sugar?

- Salt cravings?

- Excess sweating?

- Nausea, vomiting, or diarrhea? Or loose stool alternating with constipation?

- Muscle weakness, especially around the knee? Muscle or joint pain?

- Hemorrhoids or varicose veins?

- Your blood seems to pool easily, or your skin bruises easily?

- A thyroid problem that's been treated, you feel better, and suddenly you feel palpitations or have rapid or irregular heartbeats (a sign of a low cortisol/low thyroid combo)?

— PART C —

- Agitation or PMS?

- Cyclical headaches (particularly menstrual or hormonal migraines)?

- Painful and/or swollen breasts?

- Irregular menstrual cycles, or cycles becoming more frequent as you age?

- Heavy or painful periods (heavy: going through a superpad or tampon every two hours or less; painful: you can't function without ibuprofen)?

- Bloating, particularly in the ankles and belly, and/or fluid retention (in other words, you gain 3 to 5 pounds or more before your period)?

- Ovarian cysts, breast cysts, or endometrial cysts (polyps)?

- Easily disrupted sleep?

- Itchy or restless legs, especially at night?

- Increased clumsiness or poor coordination?

- Infertility or subfertility (you've been trying hard to conceive but haven't hit the official twelve-month mark of no conception—six months if you're thirty-five or older)?

- Miscarriage in the first trimester?

  Keep going! We're halfway there!

— PART D —

- Bloating, puffiness, or water retention?

- Abnormal Pap smears?

- Heavy bleeding or postmenopausal bleeding?

- Rapid weight gain, particularly in the hips and butt?

- Increased bra-cup size or breast tenderness?

- Fibroids?

- Endometriosis, or painful periods? (Endometriosis is when pieces of the uterine lining grow outside of the uterine cavity, such as on the ovaries or bowel, and cause painful periods.)

- Mood swings, PMS, depression, or just irritability?

- Weepiness, sometimes over the most ridiculous things?

- Mini breakdowns? Anxiety?

- Migraines or other headaches?

- Insomnia?

- Brain fog?

- A red flush on your face (or a diagnosis of rosacea)?

- Gallbladder problems (or removal)?

— PART E —

- Poor memory (you walk into a room to do something, then wonder what it was, or draw a blank midsentence)?

- Emotional fragility, especially compared with how you felt ten years ago?

- Depression, perhaps with anxiety or lethargy (or, more commonly, dysthymia: low-grade depression that lasts more than two weeks)?

- Wrinkles (your favorite skin cream no longer works miracles)?

- Night sweats or hot flashes?

- Trouble sleeping, waking up in the middle of the night?

- A leaky or overactive bladder?

- Bladder infections?

- Droopy breasts, or breasts lessening in volume?

- Sun damage more obvious, even glaring, on your chest, face, and shoulders?

- Achy joints (you feel positively geriatric at times)?

- Recent injuries, particularly to wrists, shoulders, lower back, or knees?

- Loss of interest in exercise?

- Bone loss?

- Vaginal dryness, irritation, or loss of feeling (as if there were layers of blankets between you and the now-elusive toe-curling orgasm)?

- Lack of juiciness elsewhere (dry eyes, dry skin, dry clitoris)?

- Low libido (it's been dwindling for a while, and now you realize it's half or less than what it used to be)?

- Painful sex?

— PART F —

- Excess hair on your face, chest, or arms?

- Acne?

- Greasy skin and/or hair?

- Thinning head hair (which makes you question the justice of it all if you're also experiencing excess hair growth elsewhere)?

- Discoloration of your armpits (darker and thicker than your normal skin)?

- Skin tags, especially on your neck and upper torso? (Skin tags are small, flesh-colored growths on the skin surface, usually a few millimeters in size, and smooth. They are usually noncancerous and develop from friction, such as around bra straps. They do not change or grow over time.)

- Hyperglycemia or hypoglycemia and/or unstable blood sugar?

- Reactivity and/or irritability, or excessively aggressive or authoritarian episodes (also known as 'roid rage)?

- Depression? Anxiety?

- Menstrual cycles occurring more than every thirty-five days?

- Ovarian cysts?

- Midcycle pain?

- Infertility? Or subfertility?

- Polycystic ovary syndrome?

— PART G —

- Hair loss, including of the outer third of your eyebrows and/or eyelashes?

- Dry skin?

- Dry, strawlike hair that tangles easily?

- Thin, brittle fingernails?

- Fluid retention or swollen ankles?

- An additional few pounds, or 20, that you just can't lose?

- High cholesterol?

- Bowel movements less often than once a day, or you feel you don't completely evacuate?

- Recurrent headaches?

- Decreased sweating?

- Muscle or joint aches or poor muscle tone (you became an old lady *overnight*)?

- Tingling in your hands or feet?

- Cold hands and feet? Cold intolerance? Heat intolerance?

- A sensitivity to cold (you shiver more easily than others and are always wearing layers)?

- Slow speech, perhaps with a hoarse or halting voice?

- A slow heart rate, or bradycardia (fewer than 60 beats per minute, and not because you're an elite athlete)?

- Lethargy (you feel like you're moving through molasses)?

- Fatigue, particularly in the morning?

- Slow brain, slow thoughts? Difficulty concentrating?

Sluggish reflexes, diminished reaction time, even a bit of apathy?

Low sex drive, and you're not sure why?

Depression or moodiness (the world is not as rosy as it used to be)?

A prescription for the latest antidepressant but you're still not feeling like yourself?

Heavy periods or other menstrual problems?

Infertility or miscarriage? Preterm birth?

An enlarged thyroid/goiter? Difficulty swallowing? Enlarged tongue?

A family history of thyroid problems?

Interpreting the Questionnaires

Said yes to three or more questions in one category? News flash: you have a hormonal imbalance. Dear Reader, you are not alone. I've seen women literally jumping up and down after answering these questions, because somebody finally acknowledged and named their daily struggles something other than "crazy" or "PMS." Help is on the way. I created this test to distill the latest medical research into an actionable plan for you to get back into hormonal balance. Each questionnaire is designed to mirror what you're thinking, feeling, and experiencing, regardless of your age. Thousands of women in my medical practice have found these questionnaires helpful in identifying the next steps to correcting their hormones.

If you have more than three checks in one grouping of symptoms (for instance, Part A and Part C), move to the suggested chapter(s) after reading the following information. If you have more than five symptoms in one grouping and your symptoms are worsening or you feel moderately distressed (or worse) about it, you may need to work with your local and trusted doctor in order to tailor the treatment for you. Please understand that the questionnaires are signposts, helpful hints, designed as tools to clarify how you can most efficiently balance your hormones. The questionnaires are just the beginning of *The Hormone Cure* process, and by no means an end point. You'll also find the latest version on my website (go to http://thehormonecurebook.com/quiz). In any case, your next mission is to start seeking answers, and my protocol will definitely help. Here's the roadmap.

Part A: High Cortisol

This is by far the most common hormone imbalance affecting modern women.

Five or more of these symptoms: Red alert! *Chances are* that you are high in cortisol. You need to read chapter 4 ASAP and get cortisol back to its correct level—not too high and not too low.

Three or four: You *may need* to address this hormone imbalance.

Fewer than three or unsure: I recommend asking your physician to test your blood (serum) cortisol level in the morning, before nine. Ideally, the level should be 10 to 15 mcg/dL. You can also test yourself at home with salivary cortisol levels at four points throughout the day, in a method called the diurnal cortisol panel. (*Diurnal* simply means periodic alteration of a condition with day and night— similar to how flowers open by day and close by night). Often, diurnal cortisol levels are more helpful because you can monitor your cortisol over the course of a day, rather than basing your findings on a single data point of a blood test. Please see the Appendix for more information.

For more information: Read "Part A: The Nitty-Gritty on High Cortisol" in chapter 4 (page 75).

Part B: Low Cortisol

Remember, you can have both high and low cortisol—even on the same day, within a twenty-four-hour period.

Five or more symptoms: You are *likely* low in cortisol.

Fewer than five symptoms: Consider checking your cortisol level, in either your blood or your saliva. Most mainstream doctors don't look for gradations in adrenal problems, which is what low cortisol is. As described in Part A, your cortisol should be greater than 10 mcg/dL in the morning, but as mentioned previously, a twenty-four-hour cortisol level is more useful than a single data point. See the Appendix for more information.

Regardless of how many symptoms you have: Read "Part B: The Nitty-Gritty on Low Cortisol" in chapter 4 (page 88).

Part C: Low Progesterone and Progesterone Resistance 6

Low or slow progesterone is the second most common hormone imbalance experienced by women over thirty-five.

Five or more of these symptoms: You are *probably* low in progesterone.

Three or four: You *may* need to address this hormone imbalance.

Fewer than three or unsure: I recommend asking your doctor to test your blood (serum) progesterone level on Day 21 of your menstrual cycle. Ideally, the level should be more than 10 ng/mL; optimally, 15 to 25 ng/mL.

Right now: Read chapter 5, "Low-Progesterone Blues and Progesterone Resistance."

Part D: Excess Estrogen 6

Wherever you fall on the spectrum, I encourage you to become more aware of your possible exposure to xenoestrogens discussed elsewhere in this book.

Five or more of these symptoms: Probably high in estrogen. Estrogen dominance affects 80 percent of women over thirty-five.

Three or more symptoms: High estrogen is a *significant possibility*.

Required reading: Proceed directly to chapter 6, "Excess Estrogen."

Part E: Low Estrogen 10

Most women don't notice a significant drop in estrogen until their forties or even fifties.

Five or more of these symptoms: You are *probably* low in estrogen.

Three or more: There's *a good chance* you are low in estrogen.

Either way, the best next step: Read chapter 7, "Low Estrogen."

Part F: Excess Androgens

This is the most common endocrine reason for infertility in women.

Five or more of these symptoms: You are *very likely* high in androgens.

Three or four: You *might* have excess androgens, and I urge you to address this hormone imbalance, since it puts you at significant risk for infertility and possibly diabetes.

Fewer than three of these symptoms or are unsure: I recommend asking your doctor for a blood (serum) test of your free-testosterone level or Free Androgen Index (FAI).

To find out more: Read chapter 8, "Excess Androgens."

Part G: Low Thyroid

Many doctors view women who are concerned about their thyroid as if they're suffering from mild hysteria. Stand your ground.

Five or more symptoms: You *likely* have a thyroid problem. I recommend asking your doctor to test your thyroid, particularly with the most sensitive tests that measure Thyroid-Stimulating Hormone (TSH), free triiodothyronine (T3), and reverse T3.

Between three and five symptoms: You might have a problem.

Next action: Read chapter 9, "Low Thyroid," to become an educated consumer.

Symptoms in More Than One Category

Hormones don't exist in a vacuum. As much as I like to put items in their distinctive categories (you should see my spice drawer!), this doesn't work with the intricate and interrelated systems of the body. Some symptoms mask others: adrenal and sex-hormone issues can mask thyroid symptoms, and vice versa. Sometimes age plays a factor: thyroid issues of weight gain, lousy mood, and fatigue are more common after thirty-five, a trend that has been labeled *thyropause*. Occasionally symptoms change over time, even hour by hour: some women have symptoms of high and low cortisol within the very same day. If you have fewer than five symptoms but see some overlapping symptoms from other chapters—such as estrogen dominance or high or low cortisol—read more in chapter 10 about the most common combinations of hormonal imbalance. In chapters 2 and 10, I describe in more detail the chain reactions among these hormones and how to deal with them.

Choosing Supplements

Many of us have been there. We go to the supplements aisle at the health food store with the idea we'll get something natural to fix a symptom. Standing in the aisles, however, we are confronted with a solid wall of choices, brands, and doses. It can be overwhelming even to the most savvy person. What's a consumer to do? As you may know, there is minimal mandatory regulation for nutritional supplements, which means "buyer beware." Quality of a product is left to the manufacturer, which means that you must take great care as you choose your supplements, ideally with a knowledgeable clinician who has no conflict of interest.

By the way, if your doctor (or other health practitioner) asks for evidence of the supplements that I recommend in The Gottfried Protocol, suggest he or she read the scientific review (with hundreds of citations) on my website, available at http://thehormonecurebook .com/practitioners.

Even with minimal regulatory oversight, there are several strategies that I find helpful to navigate the overwhelming number of supplements available, many of which are not worth your money and time.

Please keep in mind that supplements are not for everyone, but most of us, as we become middle aged (that's forty or fifty, depending on your perspective), begin to lack key nutrients such as vitamin B_{12}. Yet supplements, including herbal therapies (also known as botanicals), often lack the scientific scrutiny that the Federal Drug Administration requires prescription medications to have. That puts additional pressure on you to become a knowledgeable consumer. When I was a kid watching my great-grandmother pop fish oil, I had no idea that I'd work for decades to educate myself about which supplements truly move the needle for my patients and myself, but I'm glad I did, so that I can share my hard-won knowledge with you. (Additionally, please see the sidebar "How to Approach Herbal Remedies," page 39, for more information.) Here's how I advise my patients to select a good supplement:

- **Start with research.** I advise my patients to assess supplements first on the National Center for Complementary and Alternative Medicine (NCCAM) database, which is part of the National Institutes of Health. Two other options, which are fee-based, are Consumer Lab and Natural Medicines Comprehensive Database. All three services, described below, are thorough and educate the public with integrity.
  - NCCAM keeps an unbiased evidence-based list of supplements, including what they're used for, what the science tells us, safety, and adverse effects at http://nccam.nih.gov/health/. You can also call them at 1-888-644-6226. It's not as current as the options below (for instance, the information on chasteberry, an herb for PMS and infertility, was last updated in July 2010).
  - Check out Consumer Lab at http://www.consumer lab.com, an independent testing organization that offers online reviews of more than nine hundred supplements. Membership in Consumer Lab is about $2 per month, but you can subscribe to a free newsletter. Check first for a product review, includ-

ing quality ratings and product comparisons, then look for warnings, price checks on popular brands, expert tips, and recalled products.

- Finally, consider Natural Medicines Comprehensive Database, which is run by Therapeutic Research Faculty (http://naturaldatabase.therapeuticresearch .com). Mostly run by pharmacists, the company has been around for more than twenty-five years and is respected for shunning advertisers and pharmaceutical influence.

- **Look for proof.** When possible, choose a supplement that has been proven in a randomized trial. Usually it will declare this on the label. Sometimes you need to resort to an Internet search to find the randomized trials, such as Pubmed, available to the public at: http://www.ncbi.nlm .nih.gov/pubmed/.

- **Be aware of labels, which are often restricted from mentioning specific diagnoses.** Because of FDA rules, supplement manufacturers cannot claim on a label any preventive or therapeutic qualities. For instance, magnesium, vitamin B$_6$, and the herbal treatment chasteberry (*Vitex agnus-castus*) are proven to help premenstrual syndrome (PMS), but the labels cannot claim this effect. Instead, a label for magnesium might read "helps nerve and muscle function" but not mention PMS, even if that's the reason you're purchasing it.

- **Seek third-party validation.** Some supplements have been vetted by an objective third party, such as the International Fish Oil Standards (IFOS), which tests and provides in the public domain a list of fish oil supplements and the levels of mercury and other toxins they contain. IFOS studies omega-3 products using the international standards of the World Health Organization and the Council for Responsible Nutrition to assess purity and concentration of toxins that are known to affect your hormone levels. Another third-party certification is GMP (Good Manufacturing Practices), which ensures minimum quality standards, freedom from contamination, and accurate labeling. However, GMP does not address the safety of ingredients (look to Consumer Labs Natural Medicines Comprehensive Database and Pubmed, mentioned above, for guidance), or the effects of ingredients on your health once the appropriate manufacturing practices are in place. A more stringent form of regulation is offered by Australia's Therapeutic Goods Administration (TGA), which is considered to be the most rigorous regulatory agency in the world. Only a handful of supplement manufacturers in the United States are certified by TGA.

- **Check for regulation.** Supplements that have voluntary registration with the FDA are more highly regulated than supplements that are not. Also look for "USP" or "NF," plus a lot number and expiration date, indicating the supplement meets U.S. Pharmacopoeia-quality standards.

- **Clean? Read labels.** Make sure your supplement is free of preservatives, fillers, dyes, gluten, yeast, and other common allergens. Labels contain valuable information about the extras that you don't want in your supplement. This is particularly true if you have one of the common food intolerances or allergies, such as to gluten or dairy.

- **Remember price is only one variable.** More expensive doesn't mean higher quality. Don't be fooled by the idea that the more costly supplements are better. Sometimes this is true, but other times you are paying for the packaging or marketing.

- **Ask the experts.** Some, though not all, people working in the supplements department are highly educated about different brands and quality. Use them as a resource and ask them specific questions, or ask to talk to the buyers who work directly with the companies. However, employees may have a conflict of interest, and I find the reports on NCCAM, Consumer Lab, and Natural Medicines Comprehensive Database to be more consistent in quality and objectivity.

Note: Pay attention also to which supplements you should take on an empty stomach (such as amino acids) versus with food (such as vitamins and fish oil).

HOW TO APPROACH HERBAL REMEDIES

In many parts of the world, herbal remedies are a first line of defense, according to the World Health Organization. In Germany, where doctors are taught to prescribe herbs and to integrate conventional with alternative medicine, one out of every three prescriptions is for an herb. Herbal remedies are a safe and effective approach to resolving many neuroendocrine problems, from insomnia to anxiety and PMS.

However, just as you must be aware of the risks, benefits, and interactions of prescriptions in conventional medicine, you also must be aware of these issues when it comes to natural therapies. In addition to the considerations I've provided when selecting supplements, I recommend the following guidelines when approaching herbal remedies.

• **Consult first.** Start with the lifestyle design first, and talk to your doctor (or other practitioner) and pharmacist before taking herbal therapies so that any drug or herbal or other supplement interactions can be assessed. I offer questionnaires to help you assess the root cause of your symptoms, and offer a step-by-step method to "cure" the root cause, but this process works best when you collaborate closely with a clinician. Your safest option is to obtain an accurate medical diagnosis before taking an herb. Herbs work best when the diagnosis is extremely precise, and a medical diagnosis cannot be from a book—you need a thorough medical history and examination to exclude other causes of your symptoms. I'm well aware that most conventional doctors don't think highly of herbs, and believe that anything less than a prescription is not worthwhile, but that's when you can refer them to my website for the proof of effectiveness.

• **One herb at a time, at least initially.** When choosing an herbal approach, start with a single herbal remedy. In The Gottfried Protocol, several herbs may be suggested. Try one at a time for at least six weeks to give the herb the necessary time to take effect. If you need the herb, it will help you return to homeostasis, and the process usually takes between six and twelve weeks. If it isn't working, move on to the next.

• **Record any adverse effects.** Report any problems with herbal remedies immediately to your clinician.

• **For adults only.** I do not advise, nor am I trained, to offer herbal therapies to children. The information and education in this book apply only to adult women who are not pregnant or breastfeeding.

Please consider my questionnaires an invitation to initiate the hormonal turnaround. I understand how intimidating hormones can be, particularly if one of your hormones is out of whack. When that happens, you can feel overwhelmed, especially at the prospect of starting a new endeavor.

How to Use This Book

I've designed *The Hormone Cure* to be used in one of two ways.

• *Streamlined.* If you want to streamline your reading, go from the questionnaire in chapter 1 directly to the corresponding problem that you've identified. If you have multiple hormone imbalances, go to each related chapter, plus read chapter 10, "Common Combinations of Hormonal Imbalances." For a real cheat sheet, in each chapter you can read the introduction, skip *The Science,* and go directly to *The Solution,* which is The Gottfried Protocol for that particular hormone imbalance.

- **Comprehensive.** For those of you who may want to know the details, who love to learn about the body, or for clinicians who may want to check the citations, please read *The Science* of each relevant chapter. You will find the best evidence to support my details about each hormone, how it interacts with other hormones, and, most important, what's proven to make you feel your best. I've synthesized hundreds of citations that document The Gottfried Protocol to the book's website, http://www.thehormonecure book.com.

It's good to know the foundations before you start a dialogue with your endocrine system and begin your evidence-based hormone cure. After all, the goal for you is to experience full hormonal optimization, not just the quick fix. I hope that you, like the many women I've treated in my practice, can find hormonal repair and deep healing within these next chapters.

You can do this! Let's get started with a primer on these hormones, and then we'll discover how to get them back in balance, so you can regain your verve.

CHAPTER 2

A HORMONAL PRIMER: EVERYTHING YOU NEED TO KNOW ABOUT HORMONES

The journey of a hormone starts with a dozen endocrine glands: your adrenal glands, pituitary gland, hypothalamus, thyroid, pancreas, and ovaries, among others. These glands control important physiological functions by releasing hormones into the blood, through which they travel to distant organs and cells. In other words, hormones are chemical messengers, like snail mail in the body. They influence behavior, emotion, brain chemicals, the immune system, and how you turn food into fuel.

For instance, the adrenal glands produce cortisol, one of the most powerful stress hormones. Cortisol, in turn, directs your body on how to react in times of stress—more on this later. The ovaries, which are mostly silos of eggs, produce many hormones, including estrogen, progesterone, and testosterone. (These are referred to as sex hormones because they determine features such as fertility, menstruation, facial hair, and muscle mass.) The pancreas secretes insulin, which has the primary job of moving glucose into your cells, thereby lowering the glucose in your blood. Fat cells are the largest endocrine gland in the body: fat secretes hormones such as leptin, which regulates appetite, and adiponectin, which adjusts how you burn fat.

Hormonal Job Descriptions

Each hormone has a job. Figure 1 (page 44) shows the top three hormones for women: estrogen, thyroid, and cortisol—the major hormones that affect your brain, body, stress, and weight. *Cortisol* is your main source of focus and function when you are under acute stress—but when you're chronically stressed, your levels may rico-chet from too high to too low. *Thyroid* affects your metabolism, keep-ing you energized, comfortably warm, and at a manageable weight. *Estrogen* is actually a group of sex hormones responsible for keeping women juicy, joyous, and jonesin' for sex.

——HORMONES AND THEIR JOB DESCRIPTIONS——

I've listed the most important jobs for your top three hormones, but keep in mind that there are many more. For instance, estrogen has more than three hundred jobs or biological tasks in the female body, and influences more than nine thousand genetic messages that your body sends out to regulate itself.

In addition to the three primary hormones in Figure 1, sev-eral other hormones play important roles in driving your interests, mood, libido, and appetite. *Progesterone* counterbalances estro-gen by helping regulate the uterine lining (i.e., keeps the lining from getting too thick), emotions, and sleep. *Testosterone* is the hormone of vitality and self-confidence—and producing too much is the main reason for female infertility in this country. *Pregneno-lone,* the lesser-known matriarch of the sex-hormone system, is responsible for maintaining a facile memory and vision in vivid Technicolor. *Leptin* controls your hunger, determining whether you use food as fuel or store it in your midsection; it cross-reacts with the thyroid and most of the other hormones. *Insulin* regulates how your body uses fuel from your food, and directs your muscle, liver, and fat cells to take up glucose from the blood and store it.

Some hormones multitask. *Oxytocin* is both a hormone and a neurotransmitter, which means it acts as a brain chemical that trans-mits information from nerve to nerve. Some call oxytocin "the love hormone" because it rises in the blood with orgasm in both men and women. Oxytocin is also released when the cervix dilates, thereby augmenting labor, and when a woman's nipples are stimulated, which facilitates breastfeeding and promotes bonding between mother and baby. *Vitamin D* is a hormone synthesized from cholesterol and exposure to sunlight. It can also be ingested from food, but it is not officially an essential vitamin because it can be made by all mammals exposed to the sun. (A molecule is considered an "essential dietary vitamin" when it is necessary for the body to function but cannot be produced sufficiently by an individual and must be consumed from food or taken as a supplement.)

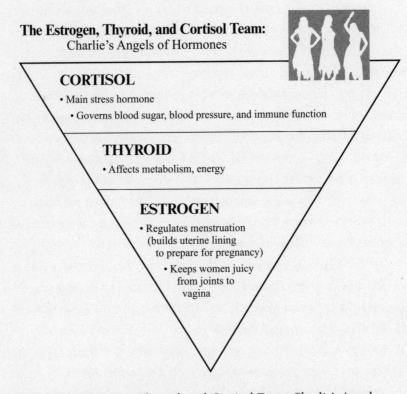

The Estrogen, Thyroid, and Cortisol Team:
Charlie's Angels of Hormones

CORTISOL
• Main stress hormone
  • Governs blood sugar, blood pressure, and immune function

THYROID
• Affects metabolism, energy

ESTROGEN
• Regulates menstruation
(builds uterine lining
to prepare for pregnancy)
  • Keeps women juicy
from joints to
vagina

Figure 1. The Estrogen, Thyroid, and Cortisol Team: Charlie's Angels of Hormones. Your most essential hormone is cortisol, the main stress hormone, which will be produced in your adrenal glands under most conditions, stressful or not. Thyroid is the next most important hormone, and of the three, estrogen is considered less essential than the cortisol or thyroid hormones, since you don't need to ovulate to survive.

The Hormonal Control Systems

Your brain is the locus of control; it is in charge of when and how these hormones get released. As you will learn in future chapters, feedback loops between the brain and hormones are involved in this process to help your body stay in balance. Additionally, several hormones influence one another with cross talk.

Your cells are perpetually bathing in a broth of various hormones. In women, the broth changes on a daily, and even minute-by-minute, basis, depending on factors such as whether you are menstruating, how long it's been since your last period, the amount of stress you sense in your environment, what you eat, how much you exercise, and whether you are pregnant. Your cells have receptors, which respond to specific hormones. Receptors are like locks on a door. The hormone fits into the lock to open the door. For example, when you face danger, the main stress hormone, cortisol, fits into the lock in a cell and opens the door to generate a burst of glucose, which enables you to run faster and stronger. If the cell is not designed to interact with a particular hormone, its receptor (lock on the door) will not fit the hormone's key. Scientist Candace Pert aptly calls this process "molecular sex." If the lock is broken—such as with insulin or cortisol resistance—likewise, the door will not open and blood levels of the hormone will rise.

Most hormones are made in the endocrine glands from a precursor hormone, also known as a prehormone. Prehormones are the body's efficient way of producing the hormones you most need on the fly, without starting from scratch.

Many of the common sex hormones in the human body are originally derived from cholesterol, which your body turns into pregnenolone. Pregnenolone is the "mother" hormone (or "prehormone") from which other hormones are made. Under normal and calm circumstances in your adrenal glands, pregnenolone is converted either into progesterone or DHEA, another stress hormone and a precursor to testosterone. When you are chronically stressed, you make more cortisol—it gets stolen from pregnenolone and other hormone levels may fall—a process called *Pregnenolone Steal*. Of course, not all hormones are derived from cholesterol (more on that later!).

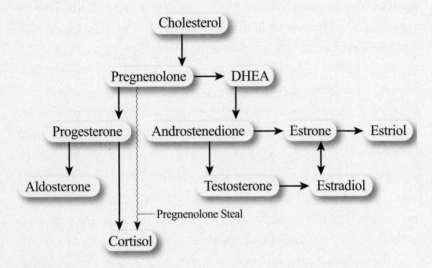

Figure 2. Hormone Tree: Pathways of Selected Hormones (How Sex Hormones Are Made in Your Body). In your adrenals and ovaries (and fetus/placenta when pregnant), cholesterol is converted into several hormones. The hormones listed in this figure are called sex steroid hormones because they are derived from cholesterol's characteristic chemical structure and influence your sex organs (note that other hormones, such as thyroid and insulin, are not sex steroid hormones and are produced elsewhere). Further subclassification or *families* of hormones that you may encounter include the following. Progesterone is part of the *mineralcorticoid* family (affects salt—mineral—and water balance in the body), whereas cortisol is a member of the *glucocorticoid* family (*gluc*ose + *cort*ex + ster*oid*; made in the cortex of the adrenal glands, binds the glucocorticoid receptor, and raises glucose, among other tasks). Testosterone is a member of the *androgen* family (made by men and women; responsible for hair growth, confidence, and sex drive); and estradiol, estriol, and estrone are members of the *estrogen* family (sex steroid hormones produced primarily in the ovaries to promote female characteristics such as breast growth and menstruation).

Greatest Hits: Top Hormone Imbalances

When your hormones are in balance, neither too high nor too low, you look and feel your best. But when they are imbalanced, they become the mean girls in high school, making your life miserable. Here's the good news: realigning your hormones is a lot easier than running around like a crazy person, depleted and anxious about the little things in life.

Here are the top hormone imbalances I see in my practice:

- High cortisol causes you to feel tired but wired, and prompts your body to store fuel in places it can be used easily, as fat, such as at your waist.
- Low cortisol (the long-term consequence of high cortisol, or you might have high and low simultaneously) makes you feel exhausted and drained, like a car trying to run on an empty gas tank.
- Low pregnenolone causes anomia: trouble finding . . . what's that again? Oh, the right word. Low levels are linked to attention deficit, anxiety, mild depression, brain fog, dysthymia (chronic depression), and social phobia.
- Low progesterone causes infertility, night sweats, sleeplessness, and irregular menstrual cycles.
- High estrogen makes you more likely to develop breast tenderness, cysts, fibroids, endometriosis, and breast cancer.
- Low estrogen causes your mood and libido to tank and makes your vagina less moist, joints less flexible, mental state less focused and alive.
- High androgens, such as testosterone, are the top reason for infertility, rogue hairs on the chin and elsewhere, and acne.
- Low thyroid causes decreased mental acuity, fatigue, weight gain, and constipation; long-term low levels are

associated with delayed reflexes and a greater risk of Alzheimer's disease.

Common Combinations of Hormone Imbalances

More often than not, I care for women who have more than one hormonal imbalance. Here are the most common combinations of hormone imbalances I see in my practice. (Read more about these and other common hormonal combinations in chapter 10.)

- Dysregulated (high and/or low) cortisol with low thyroid function. (Here I define *dysregulated* to mean that the body's response to chronic stress is poorly modulated, or regulated, such that cortisol is not kept within an optimal range for the body and is either too high or too low, usually at different times within the same twenty-four-hour period.)
- Dysregulated cortisol with dysregulated sex hormones (estrogen and progesterone).
- Women in their thirties will often have symptoms of low progesterone and high androgens, and wonder why it's taking so long to get pregnant.
- Women in perimenopause, which starts sometime between ages thirty-five and fifty, have low progesterone, and in the final year before their final period, low estrogen. They experience low progesterone as anxiety, sleep disruption, night sweats, and shortened menstrual cycles—and fret over work and field trip permission slips in the middle of the night. Low estrogen may add mild depression to the mix.
- Women in menopause commonly have low cortisol during the day (which makes them feel tired) and high cortisol at night, which makes them worry about everything from the stock market to whether their children are

exposing themselves to sexually transmitted diseases or finding their dream job.

In addition to pregnancy, the most common, and often overlooked, causes of any hormone imbalance include:

- aging
- genetics
- poor nutrition and/or inadequate "precursors" to make hormones
- environmental exposure to toxins
- excess stress
- lifestyle choices

Everything Is Interrelated

The main thing you need to know is this: a hormone does not exist in a vacuum. Some hormones dramatically affect other hormones; high levels of one can interfere with the action of another. When you're chronically stressed, for instance, your levels of cortisol go up, and if they rise too high, they can block cells from getting progesterone, which calms you down. As described above, hormones fit into the receptor on a cell like a lock into a key, in a process that we identified earlier as *molecular sex*. If cortisol is busy having molecular sex with the progesterone receptor, the lock is occupied and unavailable to another hormone, and the progesterone molecule can't get into its own receptor. Even if your blood progesterone levels are normal, you may *feel* progesterone deficient, which means you might have trouble becoming calm or getting pregnant. Because of these interrelationships, it's crucial to treat multiple symptoms at the same time.

Many hormones, including cortisol and thyroid, are controlled by a feedback loop that shuts off production when levels get high. In addition to interaction with one another, the hormones interact with and depend on the light/dark cycle in the natural world. For instance, cortisol levels peak after the sun comes up (after seven a.m.), and melatonin gets suppressed. Conversely, at nine p.m., ideally you make more melatonin as cortisol levels decrease.

Why do these things matter? When you understand how your hormones interact with one another, it's easier to find hormonal harmony. When you assess and treat multiple hormonal systems—the adrenal, thyroid, and sex hormones, in particular—at the same time, you get better and faster results.

The Solution Is Nuanced

One word of caution: the "solution" with wayward hormones is more nuanced than simply slapping more hormones on the problem in order to effect a cure. This is because of hormone resistance (including cortisol, progesterone, and thyroid resistance, which I'll explain later); genetic predispositions; and the complexity of downstream chemicals made from the major hormones considered in this book.

For instance, PMS is related to a problem with progesterone, but frosting yourself in progesterone cream does not automatically fix the symptoms in all women. Our best science shows that PMS is the result of the poorly synchronized interplay among four entities: progesterone, allopregnenolone (a derivative of progesterone), and in the brain, the GABA and serotonin pathways. It's a complicated neurohormonal mix that results in progesterone "resistance," which is why topping off your progesterone may not be the answer. Your body may respond better to a "cure" that addresses upstream causes—including precursors, such as vitamin B_6, that help you make serotonin, or perhaps an herb that alters progesterone sensitivity, such as chasteberry, as well as lifestyle techniques to calm your brain.

Meet Your Hormonal Charlie's Angels

Remember Charlie's Angels—Sabrina, Jill, and Kelly, the TV trio of crime-fighting, bad-guy-busting women with brains, brawn, and physical agility? Seeing the three of them working in sync was poetry. It was empowering. So it is with your hormonal system. When the hormones work together, the team is powerful, graceful, and effective.

Bear with me as I pursue this analogy. Sabrina is cortisol. She stands up to Charlie more than the other angels do, and she's less inclined to manipulate men with her feminine wiles. She's the smart angel, the no-nonsense, strategic-thinking one. Just as Sabrina is the one who rescues the "angel in danger," cortisol, coursing through your bloodstream, alerts your nervous system to threats, whether it's an imminent car accident or a toddler heading toward a wall socket. Cortisol helps you respond to the scary effects of your everyday adventures by regulating the levels of other hormones, such as thyroid and estrogen.

Jill is thyroid. She is the sporty angel, lithe, athletic, and adventurous. Thyroid keeps you energetic, slender, and happy; it is the Jill of hormones. Without enough thyroid, you feel fatigued, gain weight, go through life in a low mood . . . and libido? Fagettabout it.

Kelly is estrogen. She is the sensitive angel: soft and voluptuous, but also street-wise and tough. She can be powerful and in control one minute, a seductress the next. This is like estrogen, which keeps you flush with serotonin, the feel-good neurotransmitter. Estrogen keeps your orgasms toe-curling, your mood stable, your joints lubricated, your sleep and appetite right, your face relatively wrinkle-free. Estrogen keeps the other angels, cortisol and thyroid, in balance.

To bust the bad guys—depression, slow metabolism, lack of energy—you need your hormonal angels working in sync. That's absolutely pivotal for a feeling that all is right with the world. Get each in the proper proportion, and you will feel more balanced and aligned. Each hormone is important, useful, and essential on its own. But when they work together at the height of their individual powers, *magic happens.* Health. Happiness. Vitality. Libidic lusciousness.

Your Vigilance Centers: The "Reptilian" and Limbic Brain

A key feature of women's hormones is that some tend to get more out of control than others. Take cortisol, for example. At chronically high levels, cortisol often behaves like a runaway train. That is, as you rush from task to task, your cortisol levels climb even higher (similar to a runaway train that picks up speed over time), causing cravings for sugar or wine, depositing more fat around your belly, and giving you a false sense of energy or a second wind. Before you know it, you're still surfing the Internet and you have to get up for work in six hours, yet you're so wired you can't sleep.

When this happens, cortisol is running roughshod over your other hormones. Cortisol is the alpha hormone, and couldn't care less about its long-term relationship with your ovaries and thyroid. So your thyroid steps in and tries to fix the problem, which results in less thyroid hormone production. When cortisol is high, it blocks the progesterone receptor, making it difficult for progesterone to perform its calming duty. Less thyroid hormone slows down your metabolism, which is the rate at which you burn calories. Now you're tired, wired, and gaining weight.

Unfortunately, cortisol is primarily controlled by the most ancient and, we might say, *less flexible* parts of your brain. Some call it the *reptilian brain*, which developed earlier than the *limbic brain* and the *cortex* ("thinking" brain). The connections between these three aspects of the brain overlap. Structurally, the reptilian, or lower, brain includes the brain stem and cerebellum. (I prefer the term *lower* brain because it is more descriptive and the term *reptilian* gives me the creeps.) This innate, deep part of our brain biochemically controls such instinctual behaviors as aggression and dominance. It developed many ages ago, before other parts of your brain, when survival depended on running from predators such as lions and tigers. In other words, your reptilian brain is reliable but rigid, and sometimes that's good. If someone throws a rock at your head, your lower brain will cause you to duck rapidly.

Your lower brain also shares many tasks with your limbic brain, which is the seat of emotion, learning, and memory. Limbic structures include the amygdala, hypothalamus, and hippocampus, plus several others. Your amygdala decodes emotions, including threat, which trips the body's alarm circuits. Beyond fight or flight, the limbic brain governs mating (particularly ovulation and the sex drive). Together with the lower brain, the amygdala provides vigilance. With the help of your limbic brain, your lower brain manages such important tasks as breathing, digestion, elimination, circulation (as in, send more blood to the leg muscles so this body can run!), and reproduction.

Your thinking brain works too slowly for fight-or-flight tasks such as dodging flying objects. The problem is that your lower brain and amygdala often run the show—perpetually searching your environment, your e-mail, and your marriage for potential threats, perhaps filling in the details when the threat is vague or unclear. The vigilance centers often behave like street-wise punks, and they run the show based on thousands of years of evolution, unless you consciously change the manner in which you respond to stress. Blame it on the cortisol that surges under stress and leaves us reacting instead of reasoning.

Calm Down the Vigilance Centers

To get our hormones balanced, we've got to calm down the overactive lower and limbic brain. Ultimately, hormones are far more likely to be in proportion if we are able to learn how to tolerate emotions with more equanimity, and not feel like we're constantly dodging bullets.

Your hormones are designed to work for you, not against you. With nature's preference for hormonal harmony, it's easier to be in balance than to remain out of balance. But an interloper—your lower brain—keeps getting in the way. Fortunately, there are ways of calming down: meditation, yoga, exercise, walking in nature, therapy, and orgasm. Each person needs to find what calms her best. Yoga, meditation, hot baths, and targeted exercise, such as Pilates or power walking with girlfriends (not running, because it raises cortisol), work best for me.

Circadian Congruence

You also want your circadian rhythms to be working properly and aligned to the light/dark rhythm outdoors. Nearly every hormone is released in response to your circadian clock and the sleep/wake cycle. Some of us are morning people; some are night owls. When we do shift work at night, the natural rhythms are disrupted. But the basic rule is, to the extent you can, go to bed each night at the same time, wake up at the same time, and get out in the sunshine. This creates circadian congruence, which optimizes your hormone balance naturally.

Numbers, Numbers, Numbers Versus Other Ways to Optimize Hormones

Many of my patients want to check their hormone levels first thing at a laboratory or at home, and sometimes this is helpful. Nevertheless, there are several reasons why I use questionnaires to identify your hormonal issues rather than immediately checking levels in the blood, urine, or saliva.

- Most hormones vary according to time of day, similar to a flower that opens by day and closes by night.
- Due to hormone resistance, sometimes *what you feel* is not reflected in the blood, urine, or saliva level of a hormone. Your felt experience correlates with the hormone levels *inside your cells,* and especially inside the nucleus of your cells, which is where your hormones interact with your DNA (your genetic code). You see, most hormones have receptors on the cell nucleus, and if your hormone receptors are jammed, it doesn't really matter what your hormone levels are outside of the nucleus or outside of the cell (in the blood, urine, or saliva). Hormone resistance has been documented for multiple hormones, such as insulin, cortisol, progesterone, and thyroid.

For these two reasons, I recommend that you start with the questionnaires (rather than checking your levels and getting focused on your numbers rather than on what you are feeling), which will guide you to the appropriate chapter containing your hormonal issue. Once you identify the root cause of your hormonal symptoms, move on to the lifestyle reset in Step 1 of The Gottfried Protocol of the corresponding chapter to get your hormones back in balance again.

CHAPTER 3

PERIMENOPAUSE: YOUR OWN PERSONAL GLOBAL WARMING CRISIS, HYPERVIGILANCE, AND TIGHTER JEANS

Perimenopause refers to the years of hormonal upheaval before your final menstrual period. It can begin in your midthirties or your forties. However, perimenopause is a state of body and mind, not a chronological destination. It begins with dropping progesterone levels and ends with dropping estrogen levels. For some women, it is a time when mood becomes unpredictable, weight climbs, and energy wanes—and most commonly, women experience a conflation of all three. Other women may feel free of the hormonal straitjacket of the fertile years and start speaking the truth about what they want and need. Which camp you join may be determined by how you prepare to navigate these subtle, and at times *dramatic,* hormonal changes.

Here's the bottom line: perimenopause is not well understood by most women, and certainly not by their doctors. Most women don't realize that perimenopause is much rockier and more difficult than menopause, because hormones fluctuate month to month, sometimes mildly and sometimes fiercely. In my midthirties, I figured menopause was some future cliff I'd fall from, around age fifty or so, in the distant future. *Not so.* Your body has been preparing for this cliff for years, and it will pay future dividends for you to understand the "perfect storm" of perimenopausal hormone imbalances. I had signs of imbalance already—and my more frequent periods, PMS, deteriorating libido, and growing waistline were the clues. You may find that old methods of coping (occasional exercise, yoga a few days per week, chocolate, a glass of wine most nights) don't seem to work as well. Metabolism becomes less forgiving. You may feel more stressed out. Sleep erodes. Amygdala hijack can occur almost daily—meaning your "reptilian" brain and amygdala, not your rational being, take over, and overreaction may become the norm. Sometimes your spouse or partner feels like the enemy.

Perimenopause doesn't have one particular hormonal root cause. Rather, it's an expression of hormonal interdependence. In other words, you are not experiencing increased neurotic tendencies, but instead, the interplay of your major hormones at a time of great neuroendocrine chaos. This life stage need not be a death march through middle age; perimenopause is simply a period of biological rough waters that can be navigated optimally with a smart captain at the helm of the ship. That means you, with the help of this book and, if necessary, a trusted clinician.

Here are some signs that might indicate you're suffering from perimenopause, not that you've suddenly lost your mind.

DO YOU HAVE, OR HAVE YOU EXPERIENCED, IN THE PAST SIX MONTHS . . .

- Feeling far less jolly about doing the grocery shopping, laundry, dishes, and cooking than you did, say, ten years ago?

- A preference for social isolation combined with wardrobe malfunction (you're newly introverted, reluctant to wear anything *other than your yoga pants* if you have to leave the house)?

- A need to unbutton your jeans to make room for the roll around your waist, which seemed to arrive overnight?

- Emotional instability—for the first time in your life, you burst into tears at work when in a crucial meeting and your kid calls with an adolescent crisis?

- A lack of satisfaction with exercise, since it doesn't seem to affect your weight?

- A general feeling of blah or reclusiveness; do you find yourself watching the clock and wondering when it might be socially acceptable to extricate yourself from normal activities and retire for the evening?

- A problem sleeping (indiscriminant debates and ruminations awakening you in the middle of the night)?

- A habit of waking up so sweaty that you need to change your nightgown and sheets, and perhaps even your husband (or partner)?

- A face with crow's feet and a permanently furrowed brow?

- A lack of attention to personal grooming habits (you really don't care how attractive you look)?

- An attitude toward your children that's less gung-ho and more ambivalent than it once was?

- A menstrual period so unpredictable that you don't know whether you're in for spotting or flooding or some weird combination of the two?

- Sudden forgetfulness when walking into a room (knowing you had a purpose but searching for clues as to what it was)?

- A continual doubting of your own instincts and insights?

- More frequent announcements to the family that "Mom's going to take a nap now" or "Mom needs a time-out"?

- A preference for chocolate or a glass of wine over sex (which, frankly, may just be your lowest priority)?

- A notion that Zoloft or a little Prozac sounds increasingly appealing?

- An opinion that addressing your mood issues by giving up sugar, alcohol, and flour, taking various supplements, and hormonal tweaking sounds like *way too much work*?

How to Evaluate Yourself

If you have five or more of these thoughts or feelings most of the time—whether you've yet to reach middle age (ages forty to sixty-five) or are staring at it through the rearview mirror—*welcome to perimenopause.* This means your ovaries have started to sputter and are no longer manufacturing the same, predictable, and consistent levels of the sex hormones—estrogen and progesterone—that they used to. To make matters worse, your brain is less responsive to the hormones your ovaries still do produce—a phenomenon of the middle-aged female brain—and the happy brain chemicals such as serotonin may head south. Some women sail through perimenopause with nary a worry; others believe they are going crazy. Both are a normal reaction to the midlife hormonal flux known as perimenopause.

You may be saying to yourself: *Yes! Yes! That's me! Now what?* If you address your hormonal imbalances identified in the questionnaires of chapter 1, you will calm the storm of perimenopause. Chapter 10, on the most common combinations of hormone imbalances, provides additional counsel.

When women hit forty, they're often shocked by dramatic hormonal changes that affect everything from memory to sex. These changes didn't sneak up on them overnight. That's right: your estrogen, testosterone, and growth hormone started to fade, albeit slowly, up to two decades before you started feeling forgetful, sleepy, and sick of sex. When you're in your twenties, these changes are often imperceptible—but they signal the body's first steps toward what most women experience in their fourth decade, perimenopause: the stage of life, usually lasting a decade, that heralds the shift from regular menstrual cycles to utter hormonal chaos.

The main change is that your ovaries no longer stay on task with monthly ovulation. They start to go intermittently offline, and ultimately stop producing eggs altogether. As this happens, many women feel as if they've fallen into an episode of the TV show *24.*

Remember that action-packed drama in which each episode covered a single day and *a lot* happened to the main character? Jack Bauer got kidnapped, got duped by the girl, became a good guy, then a bad guy, then a good guy who saves the day. Women in perimenopause often feel like Jack: each day, each hour, sometimes each minute feels like an increasingly challenging game of survival.

The Science of Perimenopause

In medical school, we were taught that menstrual bleeding is the defining characteristic of a woman's transition from her fertile years—classically, monthly ovulation or release of eggs and the production of fertility hormones (estradiol and progesterone)—to her infertile years and menopause. The word *menopause* is derived from the Greek *pausis* (cessation) and the root *men* (month)—the end of the monthly cycle.

The formal medical definition suggests that you plan *your menopause party* a year after your final menstrual period. The implication is that menopause is a one-day event, and the one-year anniversary represents the official retirement of a woman's ovaries. But the truth is, just as modern retirement doesn't mean zero activity, at menopause the ovaries still make certain hormones, such as testosterone and estrone. It's just that they no longer produce the high levels of estradiol and progesterone associated with ovulation.

In my years of clinical practice, I have found a long list of perimenopause-related symptoms that arise between the ages of around thirty-five and forty-five and predate the changes in your period. Those symptoms are hormonal clues, signals from your ovaries that you are entering a new life stage. Typically, those symptoms or clues involve your mood, sleep, weight, sex drive, and willingness to accommodate the people in your life.

In many ways, menopause is the opposite of puberty, the stage of life when females become fertile. Perimenopause, then, is similar to the years leading up to puberty. Just as in the years prior to your first period, hormone levels are once again chaotic. During perimenopause, you need your ovaries, thyroid, and adrenal glands working at their best to feel your best—but several things conspire against you.

First, you have the aging process unfolding in the *ovaries*. You're no longer ovulating every month, so your periods get shorter in frequency, or longer, or altogether unpredictable. Since your body is no longer producing as many ripe eggs, the pituitary gland cranks up production of the control hormones—what we call follicle-stimulating hormone (FSH) and luteinizing hormone (LH)—to stimulate the ovaries to do more. The ovaries hang a "semiretired" sign in response, which only leads to harder-working control hormones and higher FSH numbers. In the midst of all this, you may start to have magical thinking that having another baby—*quick! before you can't!*—is somehow a good idea. Remember: this is just your hormones talking and not a logical response to your current reality. Soon your FSH numbers are reaching fifty, and you're hot-flashing and sweaty, officially and chemically menopausal, and you choose to get a dog instead of another child.

Next, your *thyroid* becomes sluggish. Your metabolism slows. Your weight climbs even if you eat less and exercise more. You start to feel depleted, and your mood becomes erratic.

Simultaneously, the *adrenal glands* get into the act. With all these hormonal changes, your stress response becomes heightened. You just can't roll with the punches the way you used to. You can't focus or concentrate. You don't have the energy to get anything done after the kids go to bed, and before you know it, it's midnight. You go to bed, but you wake up constantly, because you're hot, or you need to pee, or your husband is snoring.

Put it all together, and you have a perfect neuroendocrine storm: all three hormonal systems—ovaries, thyroid, adrenals—working together to pull the rug out from under you. Your new mantra is that life is unpredictable. You have three beautiful days of bliss followed by losing your mind completely when the school calls to report your child has lice. Irritability becomes a dominant state. Sex drive could use improvement, but meeting your husband in the middle feels too huge. Sugar, alcohol, and chocolate become a daily salve. Bear with me. We'll work together to help you reclaim hormonal balance so you feel like your old self.

OVERWHELMED? MIGHT BE YOUR GENES

Several genes may conspire against you in perimenopause, specifically during the last year when estrogen levels dwindle. Lower estrogen levels may affect genes involving serotonin, dopamine, and brain-derived neurotrophic factor. While there's nothing you can do about your genes, knowing these risks occur may help mobilize you to learn to take better care of yourself, consider adjusting your hormone levels, and take supplements proven to help.

• **Serotonin-transporter gene (SLC6A4).** Up to 40 percent of Caucasians have a genetic variant in the way serotonin is transported cell to cell in the brain, resulting in an increased susceptibility to depression, particularly after stress. Normally you carry two copies of the *long serotonin transporter gene*. Women who have one or two copies of the *short serotonin transporter gene* are less stress resilient, demonstrate cortisol resistance (your brain becomes numb to cortisol, the main stress hormone), and have a diminished response to depression medication belonging to a class of medications called the selective serotonin reuptake inhibitors (SSRIs) than women without the short gene. In other words, women with short serotonin transporters show greater amygdala hypervigilance—and it may get even worse *when estrogen declines*. Although normal levels of estrogen can override the effect of the gene, in perimenopause, low estrogen may cause a woman with the short serotonin transporter to become suddenly stressed out and depressed, seemingly overnight.

• **Catechol-O-methyltransferase (COMT).** COMT is one of the enzymes that helps your brain process brain chemicals called catecholamines, which include dopamine, epinephrine, and nor-epinephrine. The normal COMT gene is "Met/Val," which refers to the type of amino acids in the DNA. Women with the "Met/Met" genetic variant have problems processing estrogen.

• **Brain-derived neurotrophic factor (BDNF).** BDNF is a brain chemical that encourages growth of nerve cells and neuroplasticity, particularly in the parts of the brain associated with learning, long-term memory, and higher thinking. The level of BDNF is controlled by the BDNF gene. Estrogen increases BDNF, as does exercise. Not surprisingly, cortisol reduces production of BDNF. Here is another example of cross talk between hormones, neurotransmitters, and your genes: in perimenopause, as cortisol rises and estrogen drops, BDNF can become diminished.

—————IS THE PROBLEM MOTHERHOOD?—————

I had to wonder if my flagging energy in my late thirties was related to having two kids. I rallied through 120-hour weeks of med school and residency, but found the years following childbirth to be even more grueling. It seemed like a zero-sum game, in which I constantly sacrificed one beloved aspect of my life for another. I never seemed able to fully recharge my batteries, and the result was that my productivity and patience withered. This isn't only my experience; collectively, Americans report the worst psychological well-being occurs between the ages of thirty-five and fifty, mostly linked to increased worry and sadness.

Was the problem motherhood? No, it was hormonal. How do I know? Because 20 percent of my clients in their forties do not have children, and they struggle with the same issues. They consistently don't sleep well, they worry about extra pounds, they wonder why they don't feel or look as vital as they once did.

The Forty-Something Seeker

In *The Tree of Yoga,* yoga master B. K. S. Iyengar describes the four developmental stages in the Hindu scheme of the Ashramas: student, householder, forest dweller, renunciate. (These are not unlike life stages described by Carl Jung and Erik Erikson.) Iyengar says that this system allows the middle-aged (the forest dweller) to be free of familial and social obligations in order to pursue yogic contemplation. In other words, you bloom best if, starting around age forty-two, you gradually withdraw from the external world, and its constraints, to turn inward.

Sounds good, but it took me forever to get on with the childbearing. Now I'm in my midforties, and I'd love to be a forest dweller, but I've got these cute kids (ages eight and thirteen) to attend to. I'd like to be 100 percent behind my responsibility to my family, but often it feels as if my brain and body would prefer me to be a seeker, with a side order of detachment from immediate concerns.

I'm not alone in feeling this way. Women in their forties are wired hormonally to be seekers, free of domestic responsibility, but many of us had kids later in life. At the time our bodies want us to be forest dwellers, we're stuck feeling frustrated and burdened by the householder's to-do lists.

Dr. Louann Brizendine is a psychiatrist at the University of California at San Francisco who studies hormones, women, and mood. She's concluded that, in the service of the householder tasks— securing a mate and having children—the predictable hormonal changes of our fertile years drive women to be accommodating and nurturing. Some call this attitude the hormonal cloud or veil. Then we wake up in our forties (probably around two a.m.), convinced we want a divorce. We're sick of all the needy, self-absorbed narcissists in our life; we're tired as hell, and we need a break. We are primed and ready, anciently wired, to be forest dwellers.

It's not all bad. Remember, perimenopause is a natural life stage, not a disease. Here's the cool thing. Once past the householder years, you become less interested in what other people think. You care less about your clothes and makeup, about your mother's opinions on your hair, about offending others. Why? Your ovaries are making less estrogen, and estrogen is what makes you want to have babies, look pretty, and please people. Less estrogen means you stop accommodating people indiscriminately and perhaps finally blurt out what you've been meaning to say since you were twenty-five.

The Chinese character for crisis (危机) has two meanings: danger and opportunity. Women in perimenopause are dangerous because we stop sucking on the selfless pipe of being all things to all people. We start to say, "That's fine, but respectfully, *I do not care.*" No longer oppressed by the "let me please you" hormonal veil of our twenties and thirties, we become ignited, wiser, more creative. We come fully into our own power.

And the craziness does cease, believe me. In *The Wisdom of Menopause,* Dr. Christiane Northrup reminds us that in perimenopause we are shifting from the hormonally fluctuating years to a time of life with a more even current, when we once again (as in prepuberty) have the same level of hormones from day to day. Ultimately, having the same hormones daily after menopause means more stability in your life. I promise.

Finding the Middle Way

I've noticed two ways of approaching perimenopause. On one side of the spectrum is mainstream medicine, where women see a doctor who offers them the same treatment regardless of their symptoms. Generally, this means birth control pills for the younger patients and hormone therapy for women in their midforties and older. Or, since 2002, when women got scared silly about taking hormones, more mainstream doctors have been prescribing an antidepressant for anything ailing their middle-aged female patients—from anxiety to obsessive compulsive disorder to just feeling overwhelmed.

Here's the catch: have you read the warning label that comes with your prescription? On average, antidepressants come with seventy possible adverse reactions, and for some, as many as five hundred. Occasionally they conflict: one drug causes drowsiness, but read a bit further and it also causes insomnia.

The other end of the spectrum disavows medication, enamored with the idea that extreme lifestyle vigilance can get a woman through perimenopause. Stop drinking alcohol! Drink only filtered water, 65 ounces a day! Restrict your calories! Exercise harder! Never drink caffeine or diet soda again! Consume more fiber! No sugar, ever! One bite of chocolate, but after breakfast only! Eat flaxseeds! Eat many small meals! Scratch that: Eat only three meals, no snacks, and certainly no food after seven p.m.! Sleep eight hours per night! Spend as much time as you can with girlfriends but don't neglect your husband! In fact, have sex a minimum of three times a week—preferably more, because it burns 200 calories in thirty minutes! I read the same *more sex* recommendation from most of the prominent male doctor/authors advising women on how to cope with low libido—this advice is plain wrong, patronizing, and inaccurate. Don't tell a woman with low sex drive to just buck up and have more sex. Low sex drive is a *couple's issue*. Blaming the woman and bypassing the root causes without considering the relationship issues leaves women cold and misses the point.

Dear Reader, I'm exhausted just writing this—all the prescriptions and proscriptions by well-intended people do not address the root of the problem, which is hormonal impairment. More willpower isn't the solution; rather, the solution is understanding and then fine-tuning your hormones.

My mission is to recommend the important lifestyle choices—such as exercise, nutrient-dense food, proven contemplative practice, and nutraceuticals—as part of a way of life that can be relaxed, without excess tension or stress, and specific to your hormonal needs. Neither of the aforementioned options—medicine bottle or daily deprivation—appeals to me, nor have I seen them help women in the long term.

Let's define what hormonal balance looks like for you (preferably before you hit perimenopause, but I'll help you regroup if you're there). This process starts with understanding what's happening physiologically. We hunt for root causes and implement needle-moving changes, rather than settle for the superficial symptom smooshers your doctor may try to persuade you to take. It's a journey to feeling your best, most authentic self. Are you in?

PART II

ASSESS, DIAGNOSE, TREAT: FROM IMBALANCE TO IDEAL HORMONAL SPECIMEN

CHAPTER 4

HIGH AND/OR LOW CORTISOL: STRESS CASE? IS LIFE WITHOUT CAFFEINE NOT WORTH LIVING?

S tress can be good or bad. Some folks thrive on a moderate level of stress while others crumple. Your response to stress is mediated primarily by glucocorticoids, including cortisol, combined with your genetics, the status of your ovaries and thyroid, and how adeptly you manage what's on your plate. Cortisol, the "stress hormone," is the most complex and misunderstood hormone in my practice. Stress causes high cortisol. But in later stages of long-standing stress, cortisol can swing too high *and* too low, and everything in between, sometimes within a matter of hours in the same day. That's why I've included both extremes in this chapter as well as the proven lifestyle management that helps regardless of your cortisol level. Ultimately, if stress is unaddressed and unremitting, the adrenal glands, which produce cortisol and the stress neurotransmitters epinephrine (also known as adrenaline) and norepinephrine, cannot keep up, and cortisol becomes persistently low. Although I'm necessarily simplifying complex information, here's the main point: you may experience several of the high-cortisol symptoms, plus low-cortisol symptoms. Optimally, you want the Goldilocks experience of getting your cortisol just right: not too high and not too low. If you recognize your symptoms in the questionnaires of Part A and/or Part B of chapter 1, *I urge you to manage your cortisol as if your life depended on it (it does), because most mainstream doctors don't look for gradations in adrenal problems,* which is a characteristic of both high and low cortisol. Even if you have fewer than five symptoms in

Part A or Part B, but five or more when the two parts are combined, consider getting your cortisol level checked. (See Appendix E for appropriate testing and recommended laboratories.) In this chapter, Part A discusses excess cortisol; Part B covers low cortisol.

Cortisol 101

Cortisol is the hormone that governs your hunger cravings, digestion, blood pressure, sleep/wake patterns, physical activity, and capacity to cope with stress. It belongs to the *glucocorticoid* family—a fancy name for substances that can raise your glucose. This is cortisol's main job: to increase your glucose and store the excess in the liver, through a process called glycogen storage. Glucose gives you energy. If your cells don't get enough, you wilt. Perhaps when exercising hard, you've had the experience of "bonking." Suddenly, you feel light-headed, irritable, and downright hypoglycemic, clues you've used up your main energy supply.

As the most potent of the glucocorticoids, cortisol keeps us alive via three key properties. It

- raises blood sugar
- increases blood pressure
- modulates inflammation

The Pendulum of Stress and Cortisol: Short Version

Stress is unavoidable, rampant, and growing. It's part of life, and if anyone knows how to live without it, please phone me immediately. It's not a bad thing in itself: under normal conditions, your body produces a brief surge of cortisol—the hormone released when you're under stress—that is beneficial and protective and, ideally, *infrequent*. The stress reaction is an appropriate alarm; perhaps a friend has a medical emergency or your house was burglarized. Once you respond and cope with the situation, your cortisol should return to normal levels, similar to the rise and fall of a tide. When your cortisol is functioning properly and proportionally, so is your alarm system, and vice versa.

However, for many women, the alarm—*that cortisol surge*—never turns off. The pendulum, which is designed to gently sway, gets stuck on the "alarm" side. Far too many of us struggle with symptoms of unrelenting stress and hypervigilance that are listed in Part A of the questionnaire in chapter 1 (such as chocolate cravings, lousy sleep, belly fat, anxiety). If you're reading this chapter, chances are you're feeling the ravages of unremitting stress. I've got good news for you. I've been there, and I know what to do. I've waded through the proof of what works and I'll share it with you. You may think you can't make radical changes to your lifestyle in the pursuit of good health, but I am here to tell you that *small shifts in how you approach the many roles you're juggling* can start you on a path to a revitalized you.

My Slamming Pendulum of Stress

In my thirties, I was a textbook example of a chronically stressed woman—and as a result, I experienced the collateral damage of high cortisol. I sweated the small stuff, like traffic and laundry, even making my kids' lunches. I'd forget to pick up my kids from school, or I'd remember and would have been on time, really, if I could have found my keys. One cup of coffee made my heart beat like a jungle drum. I'd look forward to a glass of wine at the end of the day, but if one glass led to two, my sleep suffered.

Despite exercise and a healthy diet, my blood sugar was high, and my sugar cravings overwhelmed my self-control. My waist got thicker, and when the clerk at Whole Foods asked if I was pregnant (when I wasn't), I nearly went into a rage. My stress-coping mechanisms were faltering. I discovered that my perception of stress was the true problem—in other words, *I'm responsible for manufacturing much of the stress I feel.* Everyone has demands and problems; when

I stopped blaming external circumstances for how I felt and improved my mental flexibility, a whole new, hormonally supportive space opened for me.

How Women Respond to Stress: Men Fight, Women Talk

When men feel stressed, they tend to react in the classic manner, with the fight-or-flight response.[1] Men are more likely than women to lash out or withdraw; in particular, men use methods of "avoidance coping," such as substance abuse. Men's response to stress is thought to be at the root of their poor health relative to women and their lower life expectancy.

The original data on stress response was gathered from men by Walter Cannon, the doctor who coined the term *fight or flight*. The assumption was that it would apply equally to women. Newer data shows that stress elicits a different reaction in women—what Professor Shelley Taylor of the University of California at Los Angeles calls *tend and befriend*. When under stress, women seek out the company of others while most men do not.[2]

That's what I like to do as part of my de-stressing program. When I'm socializing with other moms, and we dish about our lives or trouble-shoot behavioral problems in our kids and husbands, we form a network of stress-reducing, protective females and leverage oxytocin, the "love" hormone that also acts as a neurotransmitter (brain chemical). The whole feels much greater than the sum of the parts, as Aristotle famously said, and oxytocin rises in our blood and brains, which lowers cortisol.

We used to think men and women released different amounts of cortisol in response to stress, which led to all sorts of speculation about women, high cortisol, and emotionality. What appears to be the case, however, is that rather than just producing more cortisol than men do, women make far more oxytocin as a way of buffering stress. Levels of this powerful hormone rise when we kiss or hug, have sex, give birth, or breast-feed. Women's neurocircuitry relies more heavily on oxytocin than does men's. Since women have boat-loads more estrogen than men, and estrogen enhances the bonding effects of oxytocin, women are more likely than men to opt for the tend-and-befriend response. Certainly women also run or take flight when a threat is severe, but taking off is not the first or primary instinct, as it is with men.

Marriage, Stress, and Cortisol

Marriage favors men more than women when it comes to health.[3] Compared with women, married men have lower blood pressure when at home versus at work.[4] Among heterosexual married couples with young children, the cortisol levels of the women rise dramatically when they worry about work (whether their own or their husband's), while the men's cortisol levels correlate only with their own work worries.[5]

Sometimes the responses of men and women to stress are remarkably similar. Among dual-earning couples with at least one kid under the age of five, working longer hours, for instance, raises the total daily levels of cortisol similarly in men and women.[6] Both wives and husbands who devote time to housecleaning after work had higher levels of evening cortisol. Not surprisingly, husbands who focused on leisure activities after work had lower evening cortisol levels. When husbands helped with the housework, their wives had stronger evening-cortisol recovery. In a nutshell, division of labor within couples improves your health, so make sure your partner pitches in with the housework.[7]

Part A: The Nitty-Gritty on High Cortisol

Stress and release of glucocorticoids are inextricably linked, and often your stress response does more harm than good. When we are startled or feel threatened, an ancient communication system responds, and hormones from the brain tell the adrenal glands to start pumping more cortisol. Almost all the cortisol is released by the cortex—the outer portion or perimeter—of the adrenal glands, little endocrine glands that sit atop each kidney like a cap. (Tiny amounts are also made in the brain and the gut.) Our bodies were designed to respond to a crisis, like the sudden arrival of a tiger, with a burst of cortisol. There are two reasons for this: first, to put glucose into your muscles so that you can fight or run. Secondly, to raise your blood pressure, so that plenty of fresh oxygen gets to your brain and you can think clearly. This is the process behind fight or flight.

The scientific term for stressed out is *hyperarousal,* which means that the body's alarm system never shuts off. In 2011, the American Psychological Association found three-quarters of Americans claimed they have an unhealthy amount of stress to bear. When asked what they do when they feel stressed, here's what they replied (some gave more than one response): 39 percent overeat; 29 percent skip meals; 44 percent lie awake at night. Women reported higher levels of stress than men.

As Dr. Mark Hyman, family physician and five-time *New York Times* best-selling author, notes, "Ninety-five percent of disease is either caused by or worsened by stress."[8] The American Institute of Stress reports that 75 to 90 percent of all visits to healthcare providers are connected to stress-related conditions. Clearly, our current methods of handling stress are not working for us.

The Science of High Cortisol

Jump ahead to "Part A: The Gottfried Protocol for High Cortisol" (page 100) if you are not interested in the scientific background.

Stress enters your body via certain parts of your brain, including the hypothalamus, amygdala, hippocampus, plus a few other structures that modulate emotion and behavior. You respond to stress via a hormonal-control system called the hypothalamic-pituitary-adrenal (HPA) axis, which sets off a chain reaction of fear and response.

The HPA axis is like the public announcement (PA) system in high school. The principal (your hypothalamus) tells the assistant principal (your pituitary, the boss of your adrenals) to make an announcement through the PA system (your adrenals) that goes out to all the students (your cells, which interact with the cortisol and other mediators of stress). Yes, this clunky, antiquated system determines how you deal with stress. Indeed, it's a bit of a shocker to learn that such an old-school method regulates such crucial tasks as digestion, immune function, sex drive, energy use, and storage, and how you cope with emotions and moods—both your own and that of others.

"A" Is for Allostasis

This system is designed to help your body master the important process of *allostasis,* which literally means maintaining stability (homeostasis) through change. In the normal sequence of events, the HPA induces the adrenal glands to increase cortisol production, and then, via a feedback loop, the increased cortisol inhibits the HPA, which settles down until the next alert. Basically the cortisol tells the HPA, "Don't worry, we've got this," so the HPA calms down and returns to normal. But with overexposure to stress, the cortisol is so busy flooding the bloodstream that it doesn't remind the HPA to calm down. As a result, the HPA keeps signaling your adrenals to keep churning out more and more cortisol. This leads to high blood pressure, high blood sugar, and a poorly working immune system. These changes are temporary if the stressors subside and you perceive that you are free from imminent danger. However, over time, if these temporary conditions persist, they may lead to hypertension, diabetes, perhaps even cancer and stroke.

Running Low on the Happy Brain Chemicals

It's as if your HPA is the boy who cried wolf, and the adrenals no longer believe in the threat. Researchers call this phenomenon a *blunted response:* you can't deal appropriately with stress anymore because your feel-good neurotransmitters, such as serotonin, nor-epinephrine, and dopamine, are depleted. This deserves attention, Dear Reader. You're running ragged. You don't get the hit of joy from your usual sources. When you think of things that usually make you happy, you now feel a global "*meh.*" You feel mildly apathetic.

The problem is this: HPA controls our response to actual, anticipated, and *perceived* danger. Many of us are so accustomed to unremitting stress—whether from long work hours, or a difficult marriage, or demanding children—that we've actually rewired our brains to perceive danger when it's no longer a threat, or when it's relatively minor. Remember my problem with packing lunch for my kids? It was just lunch, but my hormones didn't know the difference. There's a significant cost to unskillfully managing stress, which is a problem for at least 75 percent of the adults in the United States.

Perpetual activation of the HPA leads to overactivity, followed over time by underactivity. It makes sense that once you've burned through your adrenal reserve, your once-hyperactive HPA would become sluggish—like an athlete who's given her all and now feels *spent.* You can see how this could lead to exhaustion, a greater susceptibility to contagious illness, decreased sex drive, low blood pressure, and orthostatic hypotension (you can't keep your blood pressure normal when you stand up, and feel like lying down again, literally and figuratively).

Cortisol and Aging

Women in their twenties are the hormonal gold standard, and under normal conditions, produce a tidy 15 to 25 mg of cortisol per day.

(Men make 25 to 35 mg per day at the same age.) Our understanding of how cortisol production changes with age has been unclear until recently; it turns out that cortisol levels tend to rise as we get older.[9] In fact, between ages fifty and eighty-nine, cortisol levels increase by 20 percent, in both women and men.[10] One theory is that higher cortisol is related to the decrease in sleep quality that for most begins in middle age.[11]

It is also possible that the process of aging, rather than stress, may be the primary factor behind higher cortisol after age fifty—especially when we take into account the studies that show people are generally more satisfied with their lives, and *feel less stressed,* as they hit fifty and beyond. When you're between ages eighteen and fifty, the opposite seems to be true. In a survey of more than 300,000 Americans, those with the worst mental health scores were between ages thirty-five and fifty.[12]

Another subtle shift with age is that our cells become more resistant to cortisol. High cortisol generates the long list of maladies associated with too much of this hormone. When we age, however, we don't absorb cortisol into the cells the way we used to in our twenties and thirties (not to mention that high cortisol itself accelerates aging). This means more cortisol in our blood as we age, and less in our cells. These two imbalances—in the blood and in the cells—means that we feel tired (low cortisol) and wired (high cortisol).

How High Cortisol Accelerates Aging

Recall that cortisol's main job is to normalize your blood-sugar levels. When you make too much cortisol, you raise your blood sugar excessively. This may lead to prediabetes (as measured by a fasting glucose level between 100 and 125 mg/dL) or diabetes (fasting glucose > 125). Both are common causes of accelerated aging. (To slow the aging process, we must prevent overly taxed adrenal glands and persistently elevated cortisol.) Newer data suggest you should keep fasting glucose less than 87 mg/dL. Here's a pop quiz: who ages faster, a marathon runner or a Tibetan monk? You guessed it. The marathon runner has far higher cortisol levels from running, gets more injuries, and ages faster.

Not only that, prolonged elevation of cortisol causes a domino effect: when your adrenals are monomaniacally producing cortisol, the rest of the hormone cascade falls into neglect. It's not a pretty picture. Your skin sags. Your muscles droop. Even worse, your confidence and resilience erode. Life and body are not as lively as they once were.

Here's what concerns me most: extensive research demonstrates that prolonged exposure to high cortisol constricts blood flow to the brain. That adversely affects brain function, decreases your emotional intelligence, and accelerates age-related cognitive function. To sum things up: *your memory begins to suck, and then you become demented. Yes, Alzheimer's disease becomes established more than thirty years prior to symptoms. Unmanaged stress is bad for the brain, and wayward cortisol is a warning sign.*

—DIURNAL CYCLES: DON'T LOSE WHEN YOU SNOOZE—

Our bodies are designed to produce cortisol in different amounts depending on the time of day. Ideally we make a lot in the morning, less during the day, very little at bedtime, and a minimal amount while we sleep. Referred to as diurnal variation—*diurnal* simply means a recognizable daily cycle, similar to how a flower opens and closes during a twenty-four-hour cycle—the process can be documented in a "diurnal cortisol" measurement at four points between about six a.m. and ten p.m.: when we awaken, before lunch, before dinner, and at bedtime. There should be a gentle downhill slope over the course of the day.

The burst of cortisol in the morning, generally between six and eight, is known as the cortisol awakening response (CAR). Under normal circumstances, your CAR gets you out of bed feeling restored. It also sets up one of your most important *circadian rhythms*, another crucial aspect of hormonal control. Operating on a twenty-four-hour cycle, circadian rhythms establish your bio-chemical and physiological peaks and valleys, almost like a tide within the body. When the cortisol tide is out, around midnight, and your cortisol is at its lowest, your cells perform their greatest repair and healing. If your cortisol is still high at night, your body can't do the repair work it needs.

Sometimes, when you should be winding down, you get a second wind. That's no good: when you are most in need of rest, the high cortisol makes you feel you don't need it—which only depletes your adrenals further, because your adrenals heal at night. Furthermore, depleting your adrenals will cause you to start running low on important feel-good neurotransmitters, including serotonin, dopamine, norepinephrine, and epinephrine.

In addition, nighttime is when your hormones get a chance to harmonize and resync with one another. Melatonin and growth hormone, for instance, which help you fall asleep and stay asleep, are mainly secreted at night. If you are low in one or both, your cortisol may become inappropriately high at night; over time, the lack of sleep may make it harder to sleep because of higher cortisol. Then it becomes an endless cycle.

In older, traditional cultures, you'd start to unwind with the loss of light as the sun went down. Artificial light allows us to catch up on e-mail, finally listen to that webinar, sign our kid's field-trip permission slip, and order a birthday gift, all while getting dinner together. With high evening cortisol, it's no wonder you have trouble falling asleep, staying asleep, or sleeping deeply. I've had hundreds of women tell me they simply can't understand why they feel tired in the morning after they've slept eight hours. I just ask them what they do before going to bed. More times than not, they're checking e-mail, reviewing the next day's to-do list, or catching up on a crime show. It doesn't take a Harvard-educated gynecologist to understand why these women can't get some decent shut-eye.

Most folks with symptoms of overwhelming stress have low

cortisol in the morning and high cortisol at night—the opposite of what it's supposed to be. You don't want to develop this inversion. What you want is that diurnal variation: a steep, downward slope to your cortisol levels.

Find Out If You Have High Cortisol

In mainstream medicine, you don't often find a doctor who is interested in checking your cortisol levels unless you're a textbook case of Cushing's syndrome, a rare cause of excess cortisol found in just one out of 500,000 people. People with Cushing's have a long list of symptoms, some of which overlap with those in my questionnaire, but most of which are more extreme. Most doctors will screen for this with a urine cortisol test, but even the best screening test for Cushing's is subject to debate.[13] Because Cushing's is a very serious health condition, if you are diagnosed with it, you should follow your doctor's advice.

Another reason to test your cortisol is a relatively new hormonal condition that is garnering more attention among conventional doctors: *subclinical hypercortisolism,* which lacks clear diagnostic criteria.[14] People with subclinical hypercortisolism have a peculiar cluster of characteristics: high blood pressure, high cholesterol, central obesity (more than a muffin top), bone fractures, and increased risk of diabetes. The rate of hypertension, or high blood pressure, is 48 to 92 percent—a consequence of excess cortisol.[15] Their cortisol levels are not quite high enough to warrant a diagnosis of Cushing's. But there's no clear diagnostic criteria for how high is too high when it comes to cortisol, which makes distinguishing between stress-related excess cortisol and Cushing's syndrome difficult.

Bottom line: test yourself before starting supplements. If you find you have five or more of the problems in the questionnaires of Part A and/or Part B of chapter 1, I recommend starting The Gottfried Protocol with the lifestyle adjustments, but test before going further and trying the botanical or bioidentical therapies. You can easily and inexpensively measure your cortisol level using the labs listed in Appendix E. I check cortisol in the blood, saliva, or urine; you can even check it in your hair.

If you are still menstruating, there is one important variable, and that's where you are in your menstrual cycle. Your cortisol awakening response (CAR) appears to rise at ovulation.[16] When I have a menstruating patient measure her cortisol level, I suggest checking around Day 21 or 22 of her cycle, so that we'll have a level of consistency when we compare one result to another.

VIGILANCE AND ITS REMEDY

Novelist Meg Wolitzer has described the way she sleeps since becoming a mother: "Waking up in the middle of the night is the problem of every woman I know. I don't know if men are less vigilant but my husband doesn't wake up in the middle of the night. He could sleep in a dunking booth" (*The New York Times*, November 6, 2011).

In my practice, I find such hypervigilance common. Vigilance and fear are mediated by the amygdala, which in turn is regulated by the prefrontal cortex, the area of the brain that controls temperament, flexibility, and joy.

For women, vigilance seems to relax only in one particular circumstance: orgasm.[17] This can be seen with another type of brain imaging, positron emission tomography (PET). We know that female climax and release of oxytocin reduce activity in the parts of the brain responsible for anxiety and fear. As a result of decreased activity, specifically in the vigilance centers, the brain looks dark (that is, brain activity shuts down) during orgasm, and women enter a trancelike state. The brains of men at orgasm also indicate a decline in vigilance, but most of the female brain goes dark—significantly darker than the male brain—at orgasm. Female orgasm also lasts significantly longer than male orgasm.

These data make sense to me. Women can't be in a fear state and simultaneously have an orgasm. And after an orgasm, it's nearly impossible to feel fear or anxiety. I think of fear and orgasm as a toggle switch; for women, the two sides can't be on at the same time. Boiled down: orgasm lowers cortisol and reduces vigilance.

ARE YOUR TELOMERES SHRINKING?

Elizabeth Blackburn, PhD, a professor at the University of California at San Francisco, garnered the world's attention for her research on telomeres: stretches of DNA at the end of our chromosomes that protect our genetic data. Like the plastic tips on shoelaces, they keep the chromosome ends from fraying. Without telomeres, the chromosome would get shorter each time a cell divides; instead, the telomeres become shorter when cells divide. Excessive shortening of telomeres is associated with developing cancer and experiencing a higher risk of death, as well as with aging. Blackburn won the Nobel Prize in Medicine in 2009 for her telomere research.

Indeed, telomeres are considered the best marker of biological, as opposed to chronological, aging. You want long telomeres; shortened telomeres indicate premature or accelerated aging.

Dr. Blackburn and her colleagues first got my attention when they found that women with children in intensive care had shorter telomeres than the control groups.[18] Since then, researchers have documented several connections between short telomeres and stress, attitude, sleep, and mood issues.

A case of shrinking telomeres is not irreversible, however, at least not until closer to the end of your life. You want to increase your telomerase, the enzyme that lengthens telomeres. How to do this? Meditation and exercise appear to be the most effective at keeping you young. Fortunately, you don't have to exercise excessively: one study found optimal telomere length in moderate exercisers. Meditation has been shown to contribute to a more positive cognitive-stress cycle, meaning that you feel you have more control, appraise challenges more realistically, and feel more balanced.[19]

FROM THE FILES OF SARA GOTTFRIED, MD

Patient: Charlotte

Age: Sixty-two

Plea for help: "*Help me find balance. I want to explore what to do now that I don't have an insane work schedule.*"

Charlotte is an editor and former journalist who rose through the ranks of the Associated Press, became a bureau chief, and ran a newsroom for several decades. She has a blended family and keeps track of eleven children. When she came to see me, she described her mood as optimistic and upbeat; her main symptoms were mild fatigue, intermittent insomnia, and occasional brain fog. Charlotte exercises regularly, mostly walking briskly with her husband in the Elmwood district of Berkeley. While she no longer has the grueling deadlines of her journalism days, she loves to work as an editor and tends to drive herself hard. When I looked at her diurnal cortisol, measured in saliva four times throughout the day, I found her cortisol was too high in the morning.

Treatment protocol: We started a program of tyrosine, an amino acid that has been shown in a randomized trial to reduce the response to stress (although it may cause anxiety in some people).[20] I prescribed a nightly supplement that contained vitamins B_6 and B_{12} plus taurine. In addition, Charlotte took on her insomnia like a breaking story and became a scholar of Dr. Gregg D. Jacobs's *Say Good Night to Insomnia*.[21] In his book, Jacobs challenges long-held assumptions about sleep. Even though it may seem counterintuitive, reducing your time in bed can work wonders in triggering your body to consolidate sleep. No more waking in the middle of the night! Then you gradually add hours to get the amount of sleep you need.

Results: After three months, Charlotte reported that her sleep and energy had significantly improved. Not all people are able to tolerate tyrosine and B vitamins because they can be too activating for the nervous system and cause anxiety, but this protocol worked well for Charlotte. Several months later, we measured her telomeres and found that she was twenty years younger than her chronological age. Charlotte is remarkably resourceful and resilient, and I think these traits have kept her telomeres long despite a stressful career.

DR. SARA'S TOP 7 HEALTH RISKS LINKED TO HIGH CORTISOL

1. Abnormal blood sugar, diabetes, and prediabetes. Cortisol's main job is to raise glucose levels. Even small increases in cortisol, such as those experienced when drinking caffeine, can raise blood sugar and increase insulin resistance.[22]

2. Obesity, increased body fat, and metabolic syndrome in women. Too much stress makes you fat, especially at your belly, where fat cells have four times more cortisol receptors than fat located elsewhere.[23] Metabolic syndrome, present in 24 percent of the U.S. population, is a cluster of signs, including high blood pressure; high triglycerides, low HDL (or good cholesterol), thick waist (greater than 35 inches in women, 40 in men), and elevated fasting glucose.[24]

3. Mood and brain problems, including depression, Alzheimer's disease, and multiple sclerosis (MS). Patients with high cortisol have problems with emotion perception, processing, and regulation, similar to the mood symptoms found in depression.[25] Hypercortisolism and an overactive set point of the HPA system are linked to depression and suicide, and half of people diagnosed with depression have high cortisol.[26] Excess cortisol shrinks your brain, causes cognitive impairment, decreases brain activity, and is associated with Alzheimer's disease.[27] An overactive, stressed-out nervous system has been linked to neurodegeneration (breakdown of the nerves) and increased disability; both developmental and progression of MS are linked to stress and HPA reactivity, and at all stages, MS patients show high cortisol levels.[28]

4. Delayed wound healing. Among men who volunteered to receive a 4mm biopsy, cortisol levels predicted speed of wound healing, whereas alcohol consumption, exercise, healthy eating, and sleep did not.[29]

5. Infertility and polycystic ovarian syndrome. PCOS, the top reason for infertility in the United States (see chapter 8), has been linked to an overactive HPA axis, which makes sense since high levels of androgens, such as DHEAS (member of the androgen family, and a precursor to testosterone), are associated with early adrenal dysregulation.[30]

6. Worsening sleep. Insomniacs have higher twenty-four-hour cortisol levels.[31]

7. Bone loss in menopausal women and a higher rate of vertebral or spinal fractures are also associated with higher cortisol levels.[32]

─────DR. SARA'S TOP 5 WAYS TO LOWER─────
CORTISOL WITH YOGA

People practice yoga for various reasons—flexibility, weight loss, healing of one type or another—yet I believe that yoga is the best tonic for stress and getting your cortisol to a sweet spot. When you do yoga, here's where you should focus your attention:

1. Chant. Light up your memory and reduce vigilance by a simple chant, such as OM, pronounced *ah-ohhh-ummm*. Start with a deep inhalation, and chant on the exhale. Repeat slowly, synched with your breath.

2. Deep breathe, through the nose. When we breathe shallowly all day, similar to a rabbit, emergency "sensors" alert the body that we're under attack and need a constant flow of adrenaline and cortisol. Instead, when you breathe into the lower lobes of the lungs, calming sensors tell your body to settle down. Breathing through the nose, slowly and deeply, is especially effective in triggering the calm response.

3. Cultivate presence, and release those clenched muscles. Getting into the present moment is your ticket to normalizing cortisol (assuming you're not exchanging gunfire at this moment and require sharp focus). Most women I know unconsciously grip their muscles, whether in the jaw, neck, shoulders, or lower back. Yoga teaches how to release muscle tension, and this helps to lower cortisol.

4. Invert. Any time you put your feet above the level of your heart, even with your legs straight up against the wall, you activate your parasympathetic nervous system, the *rest-and-digest* counterbalance to *fight or flight* (or *tend and befriend* in women) of the sympathetic nervous system.

5. Be sure to do corpse pose (Savasana). The final pose of a yoga practice, called Savasana in Sanskrit, which means "corpse pose," is considered the most important, and most difficult, pose because it is where you integrate the key stress-relieving practices. While lying flat on your back, close your eyes, breathe deeply, and tune in to a clear state of mind and subtle shifts of energy in your body.

Part B: The Nitty-Gritty on Low Cortisol

It may sound counterintuitive, but after you've had continuous high cortisol, low cortisol often follows. In fact, low cortisol is the end game of an overtaxed stress-regulating system. Irritability, burnout, and depression are common symptoms, along with low blood pressure, orthostatic hypotension (which is when your blood pressure drops when you stand and you feel light-headed), and uncharacteristic pessimism. You feel out of sorts and out of sync with the natural rhythm that you once had.

It wasn't long ago that I was addicted to all the things that I preach against—sugar, adrenaline, and caffeine. At Harvard Medical School, I was taught (and blithely internalized) the message that *the ruthless and dogged pursuit of medical knowledge was noble,* even if it meant denying basic needs. I gladly worked 120 hours per week for many years. I denied myself sleep, food, exercise, and even going to the bathroom. I delivered a thousand babies. I removed ovaries with minimally invasive surgery. I performed five hundred hysterectomies. I saw thirty patients per day in the office for ten years. In the process, I burned out my adrenal glands. It took me years to recognize my problem with cortisol, mostly because I never learned about it in medical school, and neither had the mainstream doctors whom I saw due to my symptoms. I discovered that *the only doctors who are aware of adrenal dysregulation are the ones who developed the problem themselves.* Otherwise, I find that mainstream health providers don't believe in the existence of adrenal burnout.

After my self-diagnosis, it took months to heal myself. I want you to care about this because it may be happening to you right now, as you multitask and read this book. I want you to prevent the potential crash of your health because of persistent stress, and if you're already experiencing the symptoms of adrenal anarchy, the good news is that I came back to normal and you can too. I'll show you how in "The Solution," later in this chapter.

Mind the Gap: You're Not Crazy Even If Your Doctor Ignores Your Symptoms

Low cortisol is an issue that you won't hear about from a mainstream medical doctor unless you are flat on your back, in adrenal crisis, with blood pressure so low that you can't send oxygen to your brain. I love mainstream, or allopathic, medicine—I'm board certified in it, and many of my closest friends are mainstream physicians. But there are certain problems that allopathic doctors are not educated to treat. Low-grade symptoms such as fatigue, anxiety, and stress plague most of my clients, yet they were not well addressed in my own allopathic medical training, so it's not surprising that women with these issues have trouble finding solutions in mainstream medicine.

Hypocortisolism, Explained

Hypocortisolism, or low cortisol, occurs when your adrenal glands are unable to make a normal amount of the main stress hormone, cortisol. Second only to *hyper*cortisolism, or high cortisol, *hypo*cortisolism is the next most common hormonal imbalance I find in my patients. Hypercortisolism is the precursor to *hypo*cortisolism.

In the normal sequence of events, the HPA axis induces the adrenal glands to increase cortisol production, and then the increased cortisol inhibits the HPA, which settles down until the next alert: nature's perfect feedback loop. Perpetual activation of the HPA, however, leads to overactivity—or persistently high cortisol—followed over time by underactivity. In most people, the HPA can work overtime only a limited number of years before it starts to erode. Eventually, it waves the white flag of surrender, exhausted; that's when you have low cortisol.

In addition to cortisol, the adrenals release other hormones and neurotransmitters, including the following:

- Pregnenolone is made from cholesterol and serves to reduce your anxiety. It's considered the "mother" hormone because all other sex steroids—such as estrogens, progesterone, cortisol, testosterone, and aldosterone—are made from it.
- Dehydroepiandrosterone (DHEA, also made in the outer layer of the adrenal glands along with cortisol) is the most abundant circulating steroid hormone in the body. DHEA plays important roles in mood, immunity, and cardiovascular health.

- Epinephrine and norepinephrine (made in the inner core of the adrenals), which help you focus, rock your mission, start a nonprofit, chase your toddler or a new lover, and solve problems.

The Science of Low Cortisol

Warning: If you are an overachiever and want more information, this section is for you, but please know this is a trait that puts you at greater risk for adrenal dysregulation. If all this talk is actually wigging you out a bit, feel free to skip this section, and go directly to "Part B: The Gottfried Protocol for Low Cortisol" (page 116).

Causes of Low Cortisol

The following conditions are causes of low cortisol, all of which are documented in mainstream medicine.

1. **Primary adrenal insufficiency (Addison's disease).** This occurs when the adrenal glands fail to make enough cortisol, typically caused by the body's own immune system attacking the adrenal glands and ultimately destroying them. John F. Kennedy was the most famous person to have Addison's, although his handlers concealed his diagnosis from the public.

2. **Congenital adrenal hyperplasia (CAH).** The second official reason (that is, not "stress related") for low cortisol is CAH, a rare condition in which you inherit from a parent the tendency to make an insufficient amount of cortisol and too much of one of the other sex hormones (such as 17-hydroxy-progesterone, which is a screening test for CAH) because you lack the enzyme that helps keep these hormone levels normal. There are several types of CAH, and not all are associated with low cortisol.

3. **Secondary adrenal insufficiency.** This occurs when the pituitary gland fails to produce enough of the hormone adrenocorticotropin (ACTH) to stimulate the adrenal glands to produce cortisol. This can occur when the pituitary, the boss of the adrenals, is wiped out, usually suppressed by an outside source of cortisol, such as the medication Prednisone, or even hydrocortisone, a hormone that some antiaging physicians prescribe. Eventually, the adrenal glands can shrink and stop making cortisol.

4. **Hypopituitarism.** This condition is when the pituitary does not make normal amounts of some or all of its hormones—including the hormones that control the ovaries, thyroid, and adrenals—as a result of head injury, brain surgery, radiation, stroke, or a problem called Sheehan's syndrome, which is when a woman bleeds severely with childbirth (an obstetrician's worst, cortisol-raising nightmare). Symptoms of Sheehan's syndrome include fatigue, inability to breast-feed, lack of menstrual periods, and low blood pressure.

5. **Hypothyroidism.** I describe this condition in chapter 9, but I want to remind you of the interdependent relationship of the adrenal glands with the thyroid. Both low and high cortisol can exacerbate the symptoms of an underactive thyroid, or hypothyroidism, which include fatigue, weight gain, and mood problems.

6. **Trauma.** I find low cortisol in some people who experienced a traumatic event early in their lives. However, for reasons not yet understood, not everyone with severe trauma develops low cortisol.

7. **Late stage of stress.** As I've described, low cortisol follows periods of unremitting stress, when you've entered the exhaustion phase of adrenal function. This is a consequence of low organ reserve in the adrenal glands.

From Adrenal Health to Adrenal Dysregulation

Adrenal health is the key difference between my approach to wellness and that of the traditional medical establishment, which holds that the adrenals are unimportant unless they completely fail, or are extremely overactive (that is, you have Cushing's Disease). I regard stress resilience and adrenal wellness as the foundation of health and vitality, and I believe that it is largely unrecognized and under-addressed in conventional medicine.

Time and again I have seen that the healthiest, most vibrant individuals cope successfully with stress and have found ways to keep their adrenals in top form. Those are the ideal hormonal specimens who experience the smart function of their glucocorticoids. That is, they experience an external stressor—a true physical threat—such as a car accident or robbery, and stress hormones such as cortisol help them focus and problem solve, and shunt blood to their legs and away from nonessential activities such as getting pregnant and digestion. They adapt to the stressor, recover swiftly, and then blood and energy can be directed once again to digesting lunch, reproduction, growth, and repair. Their cavewoman tendencies to constantly scan the environment for threats are contained and mostly dismissed.

I don't know many of these women.

Wondering how things go south? Most women I know respond the same way almost daily to the emotional stress of financial worries or traffic tie-ups or the state of their marriage as they would to an immediate physical stress. When psychosocial stress is incessant, or when you perceive that life is incessantly stressful, you move progressively from healthy adaptation to toxic, stress-related harm to your body. I call this *adrenal dysregulation*.

What happens? You develop nutritional gaps, such as in B vitamins. You run low on certain amino acids, and it's harder for your brain to make serotonin, norepinephrine, and dopamine. You deplete your happy neurotransmitters. Over time, your problem may evolve beyond a minor issue to a serious health threat—you start to experience blood pressure problems or unstable blood sugar—and you need to intervene, even though your mainstream doctor may not agree.

Ultimately, when mired in habitual psychosocial stress, your body starts to show signs of maladaptation. Your adrenal cells can no longer keep up with demand. Perhaps your cortisol slope, which should show a daily downhill pattern—high in the morning and low at night—becomes flattened. I notice that women in my practice develop low DHEA first and then low cortisol. Or in some cases perhaps they had severe childhood trauma, have been diagnosed with posttraumatic stress disorder (PTSD), and arrive on my doorstep low in all of the stress hormones.

Stress-induced secretion of glucocorticoids such as cortisol evolved to help us respond to physical threats in our external environment. Ironically, the same stress response is mostly triggered in our modern lives by emotional stress and causes damage. Understanding what happens during adrenal dysregulation is helpful when you're exploring what integrative treatments may be most appropriate and effective, as described later in *The Solution* section for high and low cortisol.

DR. SARA'S TOP 5 CONSEQUENCES OF HYPOCORTISOLISM

There are several troublesome consequences of low cortisol. Some examples include the following:

1. **Electrolyte problems.** Low sodium and potassium may occur if production of aldosterone, another hormone made in the outer shell or cortex of the adrenal gland, is low from adrenal dysregulation. Aldosterone controls the level of electrolytes in your blood and urine, mediating water retention and blood pressure. Symptoms include a fast pulse, palpitations, light-headedness, fatigue, frequent urination, thirst, and salt cravings.

2. Fibromyalgia. Symptoms of this medical disorder include widespread and protracted pain, a heightened sensitivity to pressure, joint stiffness, debilitating fatigue, and difficulty sleeping. It can be caused by stress and is often coupled with anxiety, depression, and post-traumatic stress disorder (PTSD).

3. Chronic fatigue syndrome. Chronic fatigue syndrome (CFS) is a serious and complicated disorder defined by profound fatigue that is unimproved by rest and worsens with activity; it is associated with low cortisol. Symptoms may include weakness, muscle pain, sleep problems, and impaired memory and concentration, and they may result in reduced participation in daily activities.

4. Bone loss and possible fracture. Women with low cortisol have higher rates of hip fracture.[33]

5. Burnout. When allostatic load is more than you can tolerate, you are at significant risk for burnout. See the sidebar "Diagnosis: Burnout" for more information.

HYPOCORTISOLISM AND THYROID

Sometimes I see low cortisol in women who are suffering from low thyroid. (See chapters 9 and 10 for further details.) If the hypocortisolism is undiagnosed or inadequately treated, thyroid medication may work only temporarily or completely fail to help with symptoms. It can even start causing heart symptoms like rapid heartbeat.

Take my patient Amy, forty-eight. She had thyroid problems for ten years. "Just when things started getting a bit better on a new thyroid medication," she says, "I'd get palpitations." Before she came to see me, she tried adding various constitutional homeopathic remedies, such as ozone, to different versions of her prescription thyroid medication. But she never felt better in a sustained way. When I started working with her, I diagnosed her with hypocortisolism. Amy needed an adrenal reset. She started taking licorice, which helps the adrenals produce more cortisol, and got on her proper dose of thyroid medicine. The results? She eliminated the heart palpitations. For more information, see chapter 10, "Common Combinations of Hormone Imbalances."

DIAGNOSIS: BURNOUT

While not recognized by most psychiatrists and other mainstream physicians as an official diagnosis, burnout is a late-stress state that I often see in the women who come to my office. Common symptoms include fatigue, headache, disturbed sleep, pain, attention deficit disorder, feelings of apathy and meaninglessness, and detachment from work. The International Labor Organization estimates that 10 percent of the workforce in North America and Europe experiences burnout. Allostatic load is a measure of biological strain on your body from poor stress response, and imbalanced cortisol is the primary marker. Recently, fifteen biological markers of stress reactivity were consolidated into an allostatic load index and shown to predict burnout. The best predictor of burnout was low salivary cortisol in the morning.[34]

Burnout can happen to anyone, but it's seen frequently in teachers, caregivers, nurses, doctors, and social service staff—professions in which people care directly for others and in which women predominate. A study of female teachers showed higher cortisol levels while they were teaching and lower to normal levels when not teaching.[35]

Some of my patients exit adrenal overdrive only when they go on vacation, and even then they take their cell phones and laptops. The parasympathetic nervous system never has a chance to calm their systems back to normal. Our penchant for smartphones and our endless availability, overwork, multitasking, and perhaps our addiction to excess have led to an allostatic load that's often more than we can bear.

Many mainstream doctors take the easy way and prescribe

an antidepressant, yet here's what concerns me: few women are tested for hormonal causes of their ennui (for instance, 20 percent are known to have thyroid problems associated with depression), and even fewer are informed about the increased risk of stroke, breast and ovarian cancer, low libido, preterm birth, infant convulsions, and weight gain associated with taking antidepressants. Even worse, very few of these women are told that antidepressants help only the most severe cases.[36] Given the list of adverse effects, *antidepressants are worse than placebo if depression is mild to moderate.* Don't get me wrong: I'm not suggesting that we discard antidepressants any time soon. I simply believe that they're overused, few patients get full informed consent, and the root cause—often neuroendocrine imbalance—is sometimes overlooked. We want to avoid the either/or thinking that polarizes women—that makes women feel damned if they do take an antidepressant given the risks and loss of sexual interest, and damned if they don't. Women need more choices, preferably choices that are natural and address the root cause of their discontent.

Some conventional clinicians might even be resistant to considering any other options, such as looking at your cortisol levels, despite the documentation I've provided in this chapter (and on my webpage specifically for practitioners: http://thehormone curebook.com/practitioners) and lifestyle reset. I believe that with a closer look, many burned-out women would show adrenal dysregulation, given the telltale signs of insulin resistance, decreased immunity, midsection weight gain, fatigue, tension, and low mood. This is when you need to find a doctor who will work with you, in a partnership that feels aligned with your goals and belief system. It's also important to develop tools to dance with stress and to deal with a frantic lifestyle. In Appendix D, I've included a checklist for how to find a practitioner who is an ally in your health goals.

——LOW PREGNENOLONE, ANOTHER PROBLEM—— CAUSED BY DEEP-ROOTED STRESS

Pregnenolone has long been the poor relation of hormones more familiar to us—the ones deserving of chapters in this book—such as cortisol, estrogen, progesterone, thyroid, and testosterone. But just because you might not recognize its name, pregnenolone is still important. In fact, pregnenolone is considered the mother of all the sex hormones, because it is the prehormone (the necessary precursor) to all the others.

SYMPTOMS OF LOW PREGNENOLONE

- moderate fatigue
- poor memory
- less interest in socializing
- fuzzy sleep/wake cycles
- PMS (mild or raging)
- moderate muscle or joint aches
- reduced joint mobility

While a genetic predisposition could cause you to make too little, aging and stress are the main causes for low pregnenolone. Women have a rapid decline of pregnenolone beginning in their thirties, while men reach their peak in their twenties, with only a minor decline through their sixties.[37] We all worry about high cholesterol, but a certain level of cholesterol is needed to create pregnenolone. If your cholesterol is too low, your pregnenolone level can drop. Ask your doctor to measure it in your blood. This could cause you to run low in cortisol and other hormones, as described in chapter 10.

So why haven't we heard more about pregnenolone? That's easy: it hasn't gotten the same research attention as the others, likely because there is no financial incentive for pharmaceutical manufacturers. Despite all my medical training, I knew nothing about it until I took an advanced hormonal seminar with a European endocrinologist. Indeed, pregnenolone is largely unknown in the United States, although that's beginning to change.

The Solution

Stress is your response to change, such as external or internal factors that knock us out of homeostasis. Negative stressors, especially the emotional type, lead to excess glucocorticoids. When it is dysregulated, cortisol can be very troubling for many women. As I mentioned, cortisol often starts out high and then over time becomes low. Or, you could have both high and low cortisol throughout the day. A common pattern in women after age thirty-five is to have low cortisol during the day and high cortisol at night, which may make it hard to fall asleep and/or stay asleep. Although The Gottfried Protocol solutions below are separated into algorithms for high and low cortisol, remember that balancing cortisol is related to stress reduction. So whether your cortisol is high or low, always start with the lifestyle changes that you can make to mitigate stress in your life, both real and perceived. Here's a recap of the aim of The Gottfried Protocol:

- Start with lifestyle redesign: optimize nutrition, exercise, and mental retraining. No need for testing or consulting with a practitioner before beginning these strategies.
- Assess environmental inputs objectively and prevent harm—including real and perceived stressors—as well as exposure to environmental toxins such as endocrine disruptors. Seek professional help for chronic emotional stressors.
- Provide adequate precursors for neuroendocrine balance, ideally with a doctor or other health practitioner as a partner. Testing may also be helpful to identify and

fix efficiently your missing vitamins, minerals, and amino acids (the building blocks of protein).

- Apply botanical therapies when the previous strategies do not reestablish hormone balance, but first make sure you have an accurate diagnosis by working with a knowledgeable practitioner.

- As a last resort, consider bioidentical hormones, at the lowest doses and for the shortest duration proven to be safe.

Part A: The Gottfried Protocol for High Cortisol

Although it may be appealing to treat excess stress with sugar and coffee, I consider these "fake" energy boosts that ultimately undermine your hormonal progress. Coffee, in particular, is similar to a high-interest loan, taken out against your HPA, with the payoff including substantial fees at a future date. My preference is that we make the necessary tweaks so that you wake up each morning feeling restored, and coffee is not necessary. Start with Step 1 and the interventions that are easiest to integrate into your life, since you'll be more likely to sustain habits that fit into your day. Of course, talk to your doctor about what supplements and dosages might be best for you.

Step 1: Targeted Lifestyle Changes and Nutraceuticals

Unremitting cortisol-raising stress tends to produce free radicals, which may cause mutations and other forms of DNA damage in your cells, and deplete certain micronutrients, including vitamins B_1, B_5, B_6, B_{12}, C, and tyrosine. Excess stress also can cause you to excrete magnesium, a mineral key to calcium absorption. Basic supplements can help lower cortisol. I'm often asked how many supplements to take, and the answer depends on severity. If you are suffering with five or more symptoms of low cortisol, and your low progesterone is confirmed through testing with your doctor, I recommend taking all of them. If you are suffering from fewer than three symptoms, and are a minimalist who wants to see how few supplements it takes to optimize your adrenal function, I recommend starting first with lifestyle adjustments. If you need more adrenal healing after four to six weeks, move on to the B vitamins.

Eat dark chocolate. In what may be the most popular study ever performed on cortisol, dark chocolate (40 grams per day for two weeks) lowered urine cortisol levels. But take the results with a grain of salt (perhaps combined with the square of chocolate)—the study was sponsored by Nestlé.[38]

Limit alcohol. Alcohol raises cortisol, and the effect persists for twenty-four hours in men—probably longer for women.[39] If your cortisol is high, I recommend avoiding alcohol, or at least keeping your consumption to less than three glasses per week. Alcoholics have heightened HPA reactivity, and according to one study, abstinence lowers cortisol.[40]

Wean from caffeine. Caffeine, the world's most popular psychoactive substance, directly induces the adrenocortical cells to produce more cortisol, as well as more epinephrine, norepinephrine, and insulin. Caffeine increases physiological arousal (duh! That's why we drink it!)—sometimes too much, leading to an overactive brain. Advocates of coffee point to the studies of the antioxidant benefits and longevity.[41] I believe there is a generous middle ground when it comes to your morning cup. If you suffer from insomnia, anxiety, or bruxism, which is clenching or grinding your teeth at night, I suggest you wean yourself off caffeine. If you lack these cortisol-driven problems, consider your dose response. What is the smallest dose of caffeine that supports your productivity yet doesn't undermine your health? Caffeine's effects are dose dependent.

Get a massage once a week to once a month. The vagus nerve wanders from your brain stem to your colon. Massage of the pressure receptors in and under the skin stimulates vagal activity, which is one reason massages are so relaxing. One study compared people who had a single forty-five-minute session of either Swedish "light" massage or deep tissue massage. The deep-tissue massage lowered cortisol and raised oxytocin, the hormone of affiliation and bonding.[42] The study also documented improved immune function. Sign me up!

Chanting daily. Perhaps you prefer something more active than meditation or massage. Chanting is great for those who love to sing. Don't think about the words; just learn them by heart and use them often. Chanting lights up particular regions of the brain, such as the hippocampus. (Remember what that does? Helps with memory. . . .) It deactivates the vigilance centers, such as the amygdala, and increases blood flow in the brain.[43]

Try acupuncture. A pilot study of traditional acupuncture, three times a week for twelve weeks, versus sham or no acupuncture, showed a decrease in hot flashes and night sweats, lower twenty-four-hour urinary-cortisol levels, and improved quality of life in menopausal women. Taken together, these outcomes indicate that acupuncture reduces HPA overactivity.[44]

Do a little HeartMath. Another way of observing yourself, if you need more external accountability, is to purchase a gizmo called an emWave HeartMath. Briefly, HeartMath methodology is based on the fact that the time between each beat of your heart varies according to emotional arousal, *heart-rate variability.* Loss of variability is a sign of inner emotional stress and waning adaptive suppleness, as well as of heart disease. If a patient rolls her eyes at my prescription of yoga or meditation, I whip out my emWave, which is smaller than a smartphone. HeartMath training has been shown to lower cortisol by 23 percent. This isn't some outlandish practice—Stanford Medical School, the U.S. military, and corporations such as Hewlett-Packard use HeartMath for helping employees rebalance mentally and emotionally.

Practice forgiveness. Harboring resentment ages you and raises cortisol. While this has been documented in healthy men, but not women, forgiveness training has been shown to lower stress and anger.[45] Among people with high blood pressure and anger, forgiveness training lowers blood pressure.[46] Even conditional forgiveness of others was identified as a major predictor of longevity.[47]

Have an orgasm. Here's a titillating approach! If you think it sounds fringy, consider that stroking of the clitoris was once used as therapy for women with hysteria, though the more sanitized term was "medical massage."[48] After the 1930s, medical massage was replaced with psychotherapy, but orgasm is still effective at relieving stress. How does it work? Within sixty seconds of orgasm, oxytocin, the hormone of love and bonding, floods your system. Oxytocin lowers cortisol, and women are designed, physiologically and neurologically, to generate far more oxytocin than men. Yet when faced with a choice between stress and pleasure, we often pick stress. Rethink that choice whenever you can.

Don't worry, be happy. Women with a greater tendency to use defeatist coping strategies, such as restraint, denial, and disengagement—what specialists call behavioral disengagement coping (BDC)—show more dysregulation of cortisol.[49]

Gratitude practices have actually been shown to help change traits such as pessimism and worry, as have support groups and individual psychotherapy. Direct your anxiety toward your health: use your concerns about your high cortisol and elevated blood pressure to motivate you to stay positive and appreciate what you do have, not what you lack.

Vitamin B₅. Pantethine (B_5) appears to reduce the hypersecretion of cortisol in humans under high stress.[50] I could not find this confirmed in any English-language peer-reviewed journals; however, vitamin B_5 is a low-risk treatment. If you're under prolonged stress, I recommend taking 500 mg/day.

Vitamin C. Shown to lower cortisol in surgical patients and children in stressful situations, vitamin C is a safe supplement to add to your regimen.[51] Adult doses shown to lower cortisol levels were 1,000 mg three times/day, for a total dose of 3,000 mg/day.[52] Exercise that pushes you to maximal capacity, such as ultramarathon running, also raises cortisol. Vitamin C at a dose of 1,500 mg per day has been shown to lower postrace blood cortisol in ultramara-thoners.[53] Note: In some people, this dose can cause loose stool.

Phosphatidylserine (PS). This supplement is an extract from the membrane of a cell, a portion called the *phospholipid component,* and has been shown to reduce cortisol levels when taken in pill form. Several older studies of men show that PS buffers stress-related rises in cortisol.[54] The optimal dose appears to be 400 to 800 mg/day. Another study, in which the subjects took 300 mg/day, showed that PS improves mood under stress.[55]

Fish oil, aka miracle drug! Men and women who took 4,000 mg (4 grams) of fish oil a day for six weeks lowered morning cortisol to healthier levels and increased lean body mass.[56] This study confirmed previous findings in men showing that fish oil lowered cortisol levels that were increased by mental stress.[57] I recommend choosing a form of fish oil that has been third-party tested and free of mercury and other endocrine disruptors.

L-theanine. A component of green tea, the amino acid L-theanine is thought to reduce stress without causing sedation. I could find no trials showing that it affects cortisol levels, although one study demonstrated reduced heart rate and salivary immunoglobulin A (SIgA) under acute stress (SIgA is an important biomarker of stress in the gastrointestinal tract). L-theanine's effects on heart-rate variability and SIgA are thought to be related to calming down the sympathetic nervous system.[58] One randomized trial showed L-theanine reduces anxiety and activation in patients with schizophrenia and schizoaffective disorder, when L-theanine is added to antipsychotic therapy.[59] Dosage of L-theanine is 250 to 400 mg per day.

L-lysine combined with L-arginine. Several studies, one randomized, of more than one hundred subjects who took 2.64 grams each of amino acids L-lysine and L-arginine for one week showed that the combo reduces salivary cortisol levels as well as anxiety.[60]

L-tyrosine. Another amino acid that serves as a precursor to important neurotransmitters that can be depleted by stress, such as norepinephrine and dopamine, L-tyrosine has been shown in a randomized trial to improve response to stress.[61] The dosage used was 100 mg/kg, which for a 135-pound woman would be approximately 5,000 mg per day, but I recommend trying 1,000 mg per day to start. Another study showed that in men and women, supplementation with L-tyrosine improved working memory in a multitasking environment and prevented rise of cortisol.[62] Take a dose on an empty stomach, first thing in the morning, and sometimes a second dose before lunch. Taken later, it may interfere with sleep.

FROM THE FILES OF SARA GOTTFRIED, MD

Patient: Gail

Age: Thirty-six

Plea for help: "*I become frustrated with my children too easily. I just go-go-go all day, then I feel overwhelmed and stressed, as though I'm not doing enough. I don't have the energy for sex, or to do other things with much energy. Physically and mentally, I feel tired all the time.*"

A mother of three, Gail enrolled in Mission Ignition, a four-week online teleseries that I teach twice per year. At the beginning of the teleseries, on a scale of 1 to 10 (10 means you feel like a superhero), she rated her energy as 2/6/4/3, or 2 when she awakens in the morning; 6 at lunch; 4 at dinner; 3 before going to bed. Her cortisol was borderline high first thing in the morning and remained high the rest of the day. Gail had a depressed secretory immunoglobulin A (SIgA), one of the stress biomarkers that doctors track to assess for adrenal dysregulation and decreased immune function. SIgA is the main immune defense of your gastrointestinal tract against foreign bacteria, parasites, viruses, and yeast. It can be measured in your blood and stool. Low SIgA makes you more likely to have infections and other problems in your gut.

Treatment protocol: Gail cut out caffeine and started taking 2,000 mg/day of fish oil and 2,000 mg/day of powdered vitamin C. She couldn't imagine integrating meditation into her life, but she had recently read

Buddha's Brain: The Practical Neuroscience of Happiness, Love, and Wisdom, by Rick Hanson, PhD, so we started with a commitment that felt manageable. She downloaded the *Buddha's Brain* app onto her iPhone and committed to a daily fifteen minutes of breathing, assisted by the exercises in the app, five days a week.[63] She thought she could walk four days a week if she got up with her kids and walked them to their bus stop. I told her she'd get extra credit if she walked with a girlfriend at least once a week, to support the tend-and-befriend method of coping with stress.

Within a few weeks, Gail felt more energy and strength, especially in the morning. I then suggested that she and her husband try Orgasmic Meditation (OM), a fifteen-minute practice devoted to female orgasm, three days a week for six weeks.

Results: Six weeks later, Gail was a changed person. She sat up straighter, her cheeks flushed with robust color. Asked where she'd rate her sex drive now, she replied, "I can't believe this, but I'm back to my old self, and it's 10/10!"

Five Proven Mind/Body Practices That Regulate Cortisol

There are a number of ways to address a cortisol imbalance, as I'll outline below. You may want to consider hitting the pause button as your first line of defense. Here are some techniques.

1. **Diaphragmatic breathing.** Diaphragmatic breathing, used in yoga, meditation, and tai chi, entails bringing air deeply into your lower and upper lungs. The relaxing and therapeutic form of breathing is also called abdominal breathing and has been shown to lower stress and cortisol and to raise melatonin.[64]

2. **The relaxation response.** The techniques described in *The Relaxation Response,* by Herbert Benson, MD, of Harvard's Mind/Body Medical Institute, have been adopted by scores of healthcare providers and others around the world. Based on meditation, the relaxation response is a

counter to the fight-or-flight response, moving the body from a state of physiological arousal (increased heart rate, blood pressure, and stress hormones) to physiological relaxation, which is your ideal normal state.[65] Practicing the relaxation response involves sitting quietly for ten to twenty minutes at a time and paying attention to your breath. When the inevitable thoughts arise, practice just letting them go. If you can't make yourself sit still, you can try listening to calming music (Pandora is a great option, and free), also shown to lower cortisol.

3. **Progressive muscle relaxation.** A similar technique to the relaxation response, progressive muscle relaxation is when you focus on a single body part and try to relax it. This is a common practice at the end of yoga class, which may be why we feel like we're floating out the door when we get up from the mat to leave. One study of undergraduates showed that an hour of instruction in progressive muscle relaxation reduced cortisol levels and raised secretory immunoglobin A (SIgA), one of the biomarkers of long-standing stress.[66] Stress lowers your SIgA (as described earlier in this chapter).

4. **Yoga: "OM," not "Ah."** I had a practical reason for beginning a regular yoga practice when I was in med school: I loved surgery. Although the many hours of surgical training meant I couldn't take very good care of myself, I wanted to stay healthy so I could learn as much as possible. And I wanted to stay focused during long cancer surgeries, when I held retractors inside women's bodies for hours on end, often in an awkward position. Yoga at four a.m.—it worked! My immune system improved; I didn't get sick; and I experienced minimal strain despite extended hours in the operating room. Recent evidence, from a group of medical students practicing yoga, supports this experience.[67] Data

suggest that the benefit of yoga arises from not just the physical poses but also from yoga as an integrated philosophical package. One recent study of college students doing yoga found that only the integrated-yoga students showed a decrease in cortisol.[68] Yoga lowers cortisol in women with breast cancer and lowers blood sugar in healthy people.[69] Other studies confirm that yoga lowers blood pressure in healthy college kids and people with heart disease, as well as women with cancer.[70]

5. **Mindfulness-based stress reduction (MBSR).** More than twenty-five years ago, Dr. Jon Kabat-Zinn promoted MBSR, based on ancient Buddhist concepts, as a form of natural medicine for addressing stress. MBSR is extremely helpful if you have trouble quieting your mind during meditation: when a thought floats into your consciousness, you simply observe it, label it, and gently let it go, without getting caught up in it or feeling guilty about it. For instance, while meditating, if you start thinking about your lunch, or what you'll say at tomorrow's meeting, you tell yourself something like "planning for the future," and let it go. As you become more proficient at this, you become less attached to your thoughts, and thus less reactive. In short, MBSR promotes awareness of the present moment with a compassionate, nonjudgmental stance, which over time leads to a shift in perception and response.[71] MBSR increases activity in the part of the brain that governs learning and memory, while decreasing activity in the area responsible for worry and fear.[72] Not surprisingly, MBSR lowers cortisol, improves sleep, decreases worry, and reduces depression, anxiety, and distress in people with various stress-related health problems.[73] Additionally, mindfulness was shown to reduce stress and abdominal fat in overweight and obese women.[74]

————————A STUNNINGLY SIMPLE————————
MEDITATION TECHNIQUE

Alternate-nostril breathing does four lovely things: lowers your pulse, reduces your blood pressure, raises the efficiency of your breathing, and, astonishingly, raises your ability to solve problems.[75] In Sanskrit, it's called Nadi Shodhana, and yogis have been performing it for thousands of years. It's only recently that we Westerners have learned that breathing unilaterally through the right nostril activates the sympathetic nervous system and left hemisphere of the brain, and that unilaterally breathing through the left nostril activates the parasympathetic nervous system (the relaxation response) and right hemisphere of the brain.[76]

The technique involves sitting on the floor and covering one nostril while breathing through the other. Cover your right nostril with your right thumb, and inhale through your left nostril while counting slowly to ten. Then hold your breath for a count of ten. Notice the sensations in your lower lungs and soft belly, particularly as you reach the higher numbers. Sit up straight, but keep your core soft. Move your right ring finger to cover your left nostril, release your thumb to uncover your right nostril, and exhale through your right nostril for a slow count to ten. Then inhale through your right nostril, and hold for a count to ten. Is the movement of air through the right nostril as smooth as it was through the left? Move your thumb back to cover your right nostril and exhale through your left. Repeat for three more rounds. Do this in traffic, on line at the grocery store, whenever you need a serenity boost.

Step 2: Herbal Therapies

Ancient traditions regularly used herbs known as *adaptogens* to reduce the effects of ingrained stress. Through correcting imbalances in the neuroendocrine and immune systems, these types of herbs normalize physiology that's been disturbed by prolonged stress. Despite thousands of years of use, we still lack studies proving their effectiveness. Yes, there is anecdotal evidence, but buyer beware, even though it appears that the potential for doing good is greater than the possibility of doing harm.

Navigating between modern scientific evidence and ancient wisdom is tricky. One of my clients tried ginseng because she heard that it helps memory, and it amped up her anxiety and gave her heart palpitations. Be careful with herbal therapies, as you may be sensitive to them. The herbal adaptogens I recommend below have been supported by randomized trials in humans.

Meet the Ginsengs

Ginsengs are a family of adaptogens characterized biochemically by the presence of ginsenosides or their cousins, eleutherosides. There are many different species, and they typically grow in cooler climates. Nearly every traditional culture has a ginseng to call its own. In China and Korea, it's *Panax ginseng*. In Ayurveda, the traditional medicine of India (the word means "scripture for longevity"), it's ashwagandha. In Russia, it's Siberian ginseng, or *Eleutherococcus senticosus*. In Peru, it's maca. Other ginsengs include neem, licorice, and rhodiola. Please note that ginsengs are calming for most people, but stimulating in others.

Asian ginseng (*Panax ginseng*). Several randomized trials support using *Panax ginseng* for hypercortisolism. In one trial, participants who took a multivitamin that included ginseng showed improvement in every quality-of-life measure on a validated questionnaire.[77] The group that took the plain multivitamin had no improved quality of life; in fact, some of the controls gained weight, and their diastolic blood pressure increased. The extract has also been shown to reduce fatigue and stress and, in seventy-five Italian patients with bronchitis, to improve immune function by reducing bacterial counts.[78] Data from a randomized trial from England's Northumbria University showed that a single dose helped lower blood sugar and improved cognition, working memory, and calmness.[79] Despite thousands of years of use, one review states that well-conducted, randomized clinical trials do not support using ginseng to treat any condition, although this review predated the 2010 trial from England.[80] I recommend 200 to 400 mg per day if you tolerate it.

Korean red ginseng (heated *Panax ginseng*). Red ginseng is *Panax ginseng* that has been steamed, which changes the chemical composition. Women who suffer from symptoms of menopause such as fatigue, insomnia, and depression tend to have higher stress and anxiety scores, as well as lower levels of DHEAS (the hormone is referred to as DHEA, but 90 percent is stored with a sulfate molecule attached called DHEAS, and this is the level we measure).[81] Korean red ginseng was given to a group of menopausal women for four weeks at a dose of 6,000 mg (6 grams) per day. It decreased menopausal symptoms and significantly lowered the ratio of cortisol to DHEAS. (According to seven randomized trials, Korean red ginseng also helps erectile dysfunction, but let's not get distracted.) Dosage in trials varies significantly from 250 mg to 6,000 mg, which relates to whether standardized extract or crude root is used, or the equivalent amount in tincture form is used. I recommend dosage of standardized extract of 250 to 500 mg per day, and limit use to 3 months or less.

Ashwagandha (*Withania somnifera*). Ashwagandha is the most commonly used herb in Ayurvedic medicine. In Sanskrit, ashwagandha means "odor of the horse," because the roots bring to mind (to some minds, anyway) the scent of a sweaty horse. For more than six thousand years, it has been used to induce sleep and as a sexual tonic; some herbalists call it Indian ginseng, because of its purported stress-relieving properties.

Despite all those years of use, remarkably scant data exists on ashwagandha in humans. One randomized trial of ashwagandha (300 mg twice a day, prepared from the root) combined with other naturopathic treatments showed a significant benefit in reducing anxiety, compared with the results of standard psychotherapy care.[82]

However, the naturopathic care included dietary counseling, deep-breathing relaxation techniques, and a standard multivitamin, so it's not clear that the ashwagandha is what made the difference. Even so, many expert herbalists such as Tieraona Low Dog, MD, of the University of Arizona Center for Integrative Medicine, believe that ashwagandha is an excellent tonic to buffer the effects of high stress. She prescribes it to people in her practice who feel overwhelmed, tense, or anxious, yet don't meet the rigorous criteria that clinicians use to diagnose major depressive disorder or generalized anxiety disorder. I favor ashwagandha, because it is less sedating than other ginsengs, for women with anxiety and/or sleep issues. Fortunately, ashwagandha may be used safely with antidepressants if you are already taking one, which is not true for other herbal therapies such as St. John's wort. I caution you that if you are on an antidepressant or other medication for mental health, you should consult your doctor before adding an herbal supplement. I recommend the amount used in the randomized trial: 300 mg twice per day.

Relora (*Magnolia officinalis, Phellodendron amurense*). Relora is an herbal combination that has been shown to reduce evening cortisol and stress-related eating, but only in overweight and obese women. Relora also reduces anxiety in premenopausal women. Dosage is 250 mg three times daily.

Rhodiola (*Rhodiola rosea*). Rhodiola is a plant used in Asian and eastern European traditional medicine to enhance physical and mental performance, stimulate the nervous system, fight depression, and improve sleep. It seems to alter levels of dopamine, norepinephrine, and serotonin in the brain. In one study that included both sexes, rhodiola was shown to have an effect on stress-related fatigue, including improved mental performance and concentration, and decreased cortisol levels.[83] Taken with gingko, rhodiola has been shown to lower cortisol and improve exercise endurance in men by increasing oxygen consumption and preventing fatigue.[84] Rhodiola has been shown to be an effective treatment for depression.[85] Personally, because I tend toward high cortisol, particularly in the morning, I take rhodiola at a dose of 200 mg once or twice per day.

FROM THE FILES OF SARA GOTTFRIED, MD

Patient: Lily

Age: Forty-eight

Plea for help: "*I'm in good health but am feeling off recently, anxious. My mom is dying. She lives in Florida, and I'm flying back and forth from California to see her at least once a month. I want to be there, but it's incredibly sad and a burden to be so far away, with unhelpful siblings. I wake up at four a.m. with a long list of stuff to do and feel like I'm a perfunctory taskmaster marching through the list.*"

Lily is a professional singer who has great self-care in place but often plays gigs that run late into the night. Her menstrual cycle is regular. She's an avid exerciser; she likes to run in the hills near her home for four miles at a stretch and attends a weekly yoga class. Lily also notes increasing hot flashes and night sweats.

When I tested her cortisol, it was high in the morning: normal is 10 to 15 mcg/dL, and Lily's was 27 mcg/dL.

Treatment protocol: Lily had a history of a blood clot in her leg, so I didn't want to prescribe estrogen for the hot flashes and night sweats. She started taking 500 mg per day of Korean red ginseng from her local health food store. She added a calming yoga sequence to her day (Yin Yoga), which she could practice at home, twice a week.

Results: Within two weeks of starting the protocol, Lily's mother died of metastatic cancer. Lily mentioned a favorite quote from William Faulkner: "Given a choice between grief and nothing, I'd choose grief." As she moved through the painful process of grieving her mother, Lily stayed on her protocol, and found her short Yin Yoga practice to be a great refuge for staying present with her feelings. After six weeks, we remeasured her cortisol. At 14.3 mcg/dL, her serum cortisol was in the normal range, and she no longer suffered with hot flashes or night sweats.

Step 3: Bioidentical Hormones

For high cortisol, I recommend only Step 1 and 2, except for one situation: high cortisol combined with low DHEA. You must have a blood or saliva test of both cortisol and DHEA to assess if you are a candidate. Small doses of DHEA, the precursor to testosterone, help to lower cortisol levels for women witlh adrenal dysregulation. Many randomized trials show benefits to women taking DHEA orally, particularly at midlife, although in aggregate, the data are mixed. DHEA improves mood.[86] One recent trial showed that taking 50 mg of DHEA a day (a higher dose than I recommend) increases cognitive performance (visual-spatial testing) after menopause and raised serum testosterone (the hormone of vitality and confidence), which tends to fall in women after menopause and in adrenal dysregulation.[87]

Other studies show that DHEA has a profound antidepressant effect, and even works in treatment-resistant depression.[88]

Many folks who suffer with autoimmune and rheumatological conditions, asthma, or even a bad case of poison oak, for which there is no cure, are given prescriptions for synthetic cortisol, or corticosteroids, in the form of prednisone or one of its cousins. Short-term treatment with prednisone (50 mg/day for a week) decreases production of both cortisol and DHEAS. It takes about three days for your hormones to return to baseline after treatment. This suggests that by taking a small dose of cortisol, you may be able to actually calm down your adrenals, perhaps by overriding the pattern of overactivity, and reset the balance. However, I don't believe the risks outweigh the benefits when there are so many less risky and proven approaches (Step 1 and Step 2 of The Gottfried Protocol).

When it comes to DHEA, I like to prescribe the minimum effective dose. For many women, it may be as low as 2 to 5 mg per day of DHEA. Higher doses may cause hair loss, greasy skin and hair, and possibly breakouts with cystic acne.

Some chiropractors and naturopathic physicians hand out glandular supplements like candy, claiming that dried pulverized adrenal and pituitary glands of animals can adjust cortisol levels. But searching the medical literature going back to the 1950s, and reviewing the findings of Hans Selye, who popularized modern stress research, I could find no rigorous data in humans to support this practice. Although many of my clients swear by their glandulars, I do not feel we have sufficient evidence or safety data to prescribe glandulars for high cortisol.

FROM THE FILES OF SARA GOTTFRIED, MD

Patient: Me

Age: Thirty-five

Plea for help: Stressed out, gaining weight, and overwhelmed by my life as a working mom, I had persistently high cortisol, particularly in the morning, on my diurnal cortisol. My afternoon cortisol was sometimes normal and sometimes low. In summary, I was in amygdala hijack almost daily.

Treatment protocol: I self-prescribed a softgel of fish oil (4,000 mg/day), phosphatidylserine (400 mg/day), and rhodiola. I started meditating twenty minutes per day five days a week. Although my salivary cortisol started to come closer to the normal range, it remained high in the morning, especially with consumption of caffeine. So I gave up caffeine and joined a meditation group to provide more structure and accountability.

Results: Within six months, I had normal cortisol levels. One of the greatest rewards of meditation is insight. As I became more comfortable with meditation, I noticed that a key feature of stress-crazed overwhelm is that it robs me of discernment. In other words, when I was overwhelmed, my external circumstances did not change, but it felt like they did. It felt to me as if my husband was more critical and annoying, my kids, more demanding. That's called Mirroring 101. My family was reflecting back to me my own internal state. I learned that I find the correct dose of meditation to get to insight; twenty minutes is my sweet spot. I also learned that stress is an inside job. *Even though it often feels as though the stressors are external, with time and wisdom I've determined that the locus of control is internal when it comes to stress response.* I try to choose how I respond to stressors rather than going into amygdala hijack. I've learned that contemplative practice is a nonnegotiable aspect to my day: it has improved my attention, made me more mindful of what I eat—which helped lead to a 25-pound weight loss— and given me a deeper sense of real choice during my day. I am more patient with my kids, better organized, happy in my work, and more joyful overall. Yes, I still lose my cool, but I've become far more skillful at what was clearly my Achilles' heel: high cortisol and the roller-coaster ride it can take you on.

Ultimately, I got it. I understood what William James meant by "The greatest discovery of any generation is that a human can alter his life by altering his attitude." Now, I'm good as long as I remind myself to breathe deeply and cultivate insight throughout my day. I imposed a laptop curfew at seven p.m. I taught myself how to *uplevel and downlevel my nervous system* more consciously and expertly.

Part B: The Gottfried Protocol for Low Cortisol

As mentioned in The Gottfried Protocol for High Cortisol, the following solutions are for informational and educational purposes only. Start first with the lifestyle resets, and consult a physician about the advisability of applying further approaches to your symptoms or medical condition, particularly herbal therapies such as licorice, which may cause blood pressure to rise excessively.

Step 1: Targeted Lifestyle Changes and Nutraceuticals

Get some exercise, perhaps African dance. A fascinating study of college students compared mood and cortisol levels before and after they attended one of three ninety-minute classes: yoga, African dance, or a biology lecture. African dance raised cortisol and mood, yoga lowered cortisol and raised mood, and the lecture changed neither mood nor cortisol.[89]

Develop a modular mind-set. Before I began medical school, I was a bioengineer, and my best friend, who happened to be a rocket scientist, was a remarkably calm woman who never seemed to get stressed out like me. She had a great way of approaching problems, which I call the modular approach: she would take a problem and, rather than trying to solve the whole gigantic hairy thing at once, break it down into component parts, or modules. When I try this, I find it remarkably helpful.

Nutrients. The interesting backstory to adrenal healing is that much of the research on antistress effects of nutrients and herbs was conducted by Soviet researchers in the 1970s (and are published in Russian). One study showed that a combination of vitamin C (200mg three times per day) plus an intravenous combination of vitamins B_1 and B_6 restored cortisol production and diurnal rhythm.[90] You don't need an IV. I suggest vitamin C at 600 to 1,000 mg per day, plus a good vitamin B complex.

Step 2: Herbal Therapy

Botanical therapies that are proven to raise cortisol include the following:

Licorice (*Glycyrrhiza*). Licorice raises urinary cortisol.[91] Planning a pregnancy? Be careful with licorice consumption because it can alter your baby's HPA function. One study of children of women who consumed varying amounts of licorice found that the more licorice the moms consumed, the higher the children's cortisol levels.[92] *Warning:* Take licorice with caution because excess cortisol raises blood pressure, so high doses can cause high blood pressure. About 20 percent of the population is at risk for high blood pressure. With licorice this may occur at doses as low as 1 to 2 grams. Consider deglycyrrhizinated licorice, a capsule or chewable tablet with the chemical bits removed that raise blood pressure. I generally recommend that people with low cortisol try a small dose of root extract: 600 mg, standardized to 25 percent (150 mg) glycyrrhizic acid— and check their blood pressure with a home device and at their local doctor's office.

Grapefruit juice. In patients with Addison's disease, licorice and grapefruit juice have been shown to raise cortisol levels. In one study, licorice raised median cortisol serum levels and urinary cortisol, whereas grapefruit juice significantly raised serum cortisol.[93]

Step 3: Bioidentical Hormones

Visit an antiaging physician and chances are high that you'll leave with a prescription for hydrocortisone or some other prescription for cortisol augmentation with a promise that it will renew your vitality. This makes me nervous because any adrenal support should be given extremely cautiously and with an entire whole-foods and lifestyle adjustment for sustained results. In other words, you need the foundation of nutrient-dense whole foods (not processed foods, and especially not refined carbohydrates, which worsen adrenal problems), restorative sleep, and supplements to fill nutritional gaps before resorting to a quick-fix prescription pill. Furthermore, if you take external cortisol for more than a few months, you could develop secondary adrenal insufficiency.

Here's what I suggest instead. If you still suffer with the symptoms listed in the questionnaire despite trying Step 1 and Step 2 of The Gottfried Protocol (pages 116–118), I strongly encourage you to ask your doctor to test your cortisol. If your serum, salivary, or urinary cortisol is low, then consider the bioidentical cortisol in Isocort, an adrenal-support pill from Bezwecken in which the cortisol is derived from fermented plants. The recommended dose is one or two pills up to three times a day—not to exceed six pills a day— taken with a meal.

As with high cortisol, I do not recommend supplements derived from animal glands for similar reasons.

Signs of Cortisol Balance

When your level of cortisol is appropriate and not turning your brain into Swiss cheese, you feel calm, cool, and collected most of the time. You bounce out of bed in the morning. Because you slept well, there are no bags under your eyes, you eat normally with no blood sugar swings, you feel like your body has a good rhythm, and your total load—the amount of physical and psychological stress you've got on your plate—is manageable and engaging. You eat nutrient-dense food. You strike a balance in your life between input and output. Sugar: you could take it or leave it.

- You feel buoyant, positive, and upbeat.
- You eat every four to six hours, without feeling shaky, irritable, or low in blood sugar.
- When faced with stress, you don't recoil in horror. Everything feels "figure-out-able."
- You sleep well at night and wake up refreshed.
- You focus on problems you can modify, not the problems you can do nothing about (the latter happens to be a hallmark of anxiety, and sometimes mild insanity).
- Your blood pressure and fasting glucose (blood sugar) are normal, which means that you don't crave coffee and all things chocolate.
- You have the time to accomplish your tasks, usually with pleasure and not future-tripping on what's next.
- You recall where you put your keys and your children (most of the time).
- When your kids bug you, your partner acts out, or something goes wrong, you take a deep breath and let your belly expand. You are more proactive, less reactive.
- You know how to calm yourself swiftly and effectively. You are skillful at coping with stress through breath, exercise, time with girlfriends, massage, and mindfulness.

- At night, it takes about twenty minutes to fall asleep. You awaken eight hours later (or after however many hours is the perfect number for you and to urinate twice or less), feeling fully restored and ready to embrace what the day will bring.

CHAPTER 5

LOW-PROGESTERONE BLUES AND PROGESTERONE RESISTANCE: HEAVY PERIODS, PMS, INSOMNIA, AND INFERTILITY?

From puberty and throughout your fertile years (fertility ends at menopause, which occurs, on average in the United States, at age fifty-one), your ovaries produce estrogen, progesterone, and testosterone. Estrogen is the diva—it's responsible for your breasts, hips, smooth skin, and a brain with a particular female orientation (plus tending to about three hundred other jobs and nine thousand genetic tweaks).

Don't Underestimate Progesterone

When I went to med school, I was taught that declining estrogen was responsible for the hormonal havoc of women in perimenopause, which starts sometime around age thirty-five to fifty, occasionally earlier or later. But it turns out that progesterone is far more crucial than scientists once believed. In fact, most of the havoc—from PMS to heinous sleep—stems from problems with progesterone.

You can't consider progesterone without discussing estrogen. In proper proportion, they are like the two sides of a seesaw, shifting rhythmically back and forth over the course of the menstrual cycle. It's essential to maintain the delicate balance between these two hormones to feel your most vital.

As you get older, the amount you make of each can fluctuate

from month to month and year to year. When your progesterone is low, the result is estrogen dominance, and it's as if the progesterone side of the seesaw slammed into the ground. The consequences can be rage, headaches, cysts, miserable periods, and sleep disorders. (Or as my husband summarizes, *"Run for the hills!"*) Keep in mind that progesterone that's either too high or too low can cause a range of problems. You can become fat and moody, and you're more likely to develop endometriosis and problems with uterine bleeding, possibly even cancer. When you have too much estrogen, you have a greater risk of infertility and endometrial cancer, a malignancy arising in the lining of your uterus. Proportionate balance is the goal.

In addition to balancing estrogen, progesterone is important for your overall sense of equilibrium or well-being. It raises body temperature (making it "thermogenic" and a boost to metabolism) and helps your thyroid perform efficiently. It is a natural diuretic, which means it helps you release excess fluid in your body. Psychiatrist Dr. Louann Brizendine, author of *The Female Brain,* considers allopregnanolone, a derivative or metabolite of progesterone (a metabolite is one of the natural substances made in a biochemical reaction in the body; for example, the metabolite glucose is the downstream metabolic consequence of eating an apple), "the luxurious, soothing, mellowing daughter of progesterone; without her, we are crabby; she is sedating, calming, easing, neutralizes any stress, but as soon as she leaves, all is irritable withdrawal; her sudden departure is the central story of PMS."[1] I can even say that progesterone provides contentment. That's why women report feeling a Valium-like effect in the second half of pregnancy: progesterone stimulates something called GABA receptors, and GABA (gamma-aminobutyric acid) has sedative qualities. Progesterone literally soothes you when you get enraged. It helps you sleep. When you produce the right amount, you feel more levelheaded and relaxed.

The Science of Low Progesterone

Remember, if you want to streamline your reading, skip this section, and go next to "The Solution: The Gottfried Protocol for Low Progesterone" (page 134).

Estrogen and progesterone have everything to do with menstruation and reproduction. During each menstrual cycle, they work together to build up and release your uterine lining. For women from about twelve to forty-five, it's like building a brick wall each month. During the first fourteen days of the cycle, estrogen creates the bricks, the tissue in the wall of your uterus. In the last two weeks of the cycle, progesterone makes sure you don't pile up too many bricks and, like mortar, it stabilizes the wall.

Progesterone is released primarily in your ovaries, when a follicle—a small cyst in the ovary containing a ripe egg—bursts at ovulation. When that happens, progesterone levels spike, shutting down estrogen production and stabilizing the uterine lining so that the menstrual period doesn't start too early or produce irregular spotting. Progesterone protects your uterus from developing too much of an inner lining from the exposure to estrogen. It does this by making sure the cells of the uterine lining shift from "grow, grow, grow" to "mature and prepare for the next stage," which is either menses or pregnancy.

If conception does not occur, the whole wall of bricks and mortar falls, released as your period approximately every twenty-eight days, when progesterone levels start to drop. If conception does occur, progesterone levels rise.

In pregnancy, progesterone—now produced by the placenta—is the main hormone that stabilizes the implantation of the fertilized egg. Combined with estrogen, progesterone is responsible for making your uterine lining into a superthick shag carpet for the fertilized egg to nestle in and grow. Progesterone is also released to support the developing fetus and promote breast-feeding.

Pregnant or not, hormones such as estrogen and progesterone

swim through your blood toward particular cells seeking to bind with receptors, which are like locks on the doors of those cells. Cells with progesterone receptors are in the uterus, brain, breast, and pituitary, among other places. When estrogen binds with its receptors on cells often enough, it switches "on" a new progesterone receptor on that cell; when progesterone binds with *its* receptor, estrogen activity slows down. In other words, estrogen and progesterone continually engage in a tango-like dance.

We call it a negative-feedback loop. When estrogen peaks, as on Day 12 of the menstrual cycle, that switches the progesterone receptors on. As part of this lovely dance, the progesterone receptors get to work regulating estrogen by removing the estrogen receptors so your body can get ready for the next menstrual cycle (through *apoptosis,* or programmed cell death). Apoptosis is how progesterone regulates estrogen and is absolutely necessary in regulating cell growth and differentiation, plus getting the body ready for the following month's cycle.

Progesterone Diaries: Hormone, Brain Chemical, and Progesterone Resistance

Problems with progesterone—the trigger for that dreaded PMS— usually develop at ovulation or shortly after. At that time, a mass of cells (*corpus luteum*) forms to protect the ripe egg. Then the ovary, believing it's "time to get pregnant," jumps in to produce progesterone to prepare a hospitable environment for a fertilized egg. In some women, there's a problem in the communication between the estrogen and the progesterone. The ovary doesn't get the signal to produce enough progesterone. This window between ovulation, or release of the ripe egg, and menstruation is called the luteal phase (after the corpus luteum). We'll expand on how this is related to fertility in a bit.

The most common problem with progesterone and its derivatives is PMS, but other signs of imbalanced progesterone include anxiety and disrupted sleep, which are far more common problems in women than men.[2] In women with PMS, the best evidence points to a problem between progesterone, GABA, and serotonin interaction.[3] In another dance, with even more complicated steps, progesterone (and its derivative, allopregnenolone) are produced in the ovaries, the adrenal glands, and the brain, and they affect both the uterus and the brain. These, along with pregnenolone (described in chapter 4, "High and Low Cortisol"), are *neurosteroids,* meaning they have two jobs. They are both hormones and neurotransmitters, and they alter both neural and hormonal pathways. No wonder your body, brain, and loved ones suffer when the partners aren't dancing to the same rhythm.

Here's the short version: In certain women with PMS, progesterone after ovulation changes the GABA receptor so that it is no longer able to respond to progesterone and other neurosteroids. This creates a form of "progesterone resistance" because the neurosteroid receptor is unresponsive. It's like a complicated key that fits snugly into a lock and opens a door. Progesterone is the key to the lock (in this analogy, the receptor for GABA). Since the progesterone is supposed to unlock the door, and the lock is jammed, there's *no calm for you* in the luteal phase. Enter PMS. All bets are off—and more progesterone doesn't open the door, although a more nuanced approach (see "The Solution: The Gottfried Protocol . . ." later in this chapter) just might unlock the door.

Unfortunately, we don't understand fully why some women have more progesterone resistance (jammed locks) than others. We do understand that part of the story involves progesterone, allopregnanolone, and GABA, but there are many other unknowns at the time of writing this book, including the interaction between GABA and serotonin. Some women note that a few days of a selective serotonin reuptake inhibitor (SSRI) in midcycle immediately brings relief (whereas in depression, most people need six or more weeks of taking a daily pill). This is likely because some SSRIs increase the formation of the progesterone derivative, allopregnenolone.[4] Although I caution against using such medication when the symptoms are caused by underlying hormonal problems, you might consider asking your doctor if taking an SSRI for a few days would alleviate PMS symptoms.

Do You Have Luteal Phase Defect?

Conventional doctors sometimes label low progesterone with the dismal-sounding phrase *luteal phase defect* (LPD), although the term was more popular a decade or two ago. As noted above, the second half of the menstrual cycle is known as the luteal phase, so LPD simply means that your ovaries aren't producing enough progesterone in the second half of your cycle. Accordingly, doctors may just offer you progesterone, especially if you're in early pregnancy and have a history of miscarriage.

Gynecologists look to several features to determine if you have luteal phase defect: the second half of your menstrual cycle is ten days or less, or you have low progesterone on Day 21 of the menstrual cycle, or both. (In other words, your menstrual cycle is considered shortened if it lasts twenty-four days or fewer.) Some clinicians argue there is no rationale to ordering serum levels of progesterone as a way of diagnosing LPD in recurrent miscarriage, but you'll find that most specialists in infertility order progesterone tests routinely.[5] However, in addressing miscarriage, it's not all about progesterone—you may need to look at other factors, such as anatomical problems in the uterus, genetic problems, and abnormal thyroid function. LPD is found in up to 10 percent of women with infertility, and in 35 percent of women who experience recurrent miscarriage.

Interestingly, recreational athletes have an even higher rate of luteal phase defect. As many as 48 percent of women considered to be recreational athletes were affected by low progesterone.[6] From the way this study defines *recreational athlete*—a woman who exercises for at least one hour four times per week—the term applies to me and my entire group of yoga- and Pilates-attending girlfriends.

Although questions remain, there is strong evidence that low progesterone associated with luteal phase defect is a factor in infertility and miscarriage for many women. See The Gottfried Protocol later in this chapter for ways of dealing with your low progesterone.

Perimenopause and Aging Ovaries

Tick tock. You'd think we have enough to worry about without fretting over the biological clock. But real changes do occur starting around age thirty-five, roughly the beginning of perimenopause. The first of these early changes is lower progesterone.

At about thirty-five, most women begin to have anovulatory cycles, which means no ripe egg is released from the ovaries during the menstrual cycle. Your levels of estradiol—the main form of estrogen produced from age twelve until the end of perimenopause—start to fluctuate wildly, while progesterone levels drop. Higher estrogen levels that aren't held in check by progesterone are the result of fewer ripe eggs: as the supply diminishes, you have some months in which you don't release a ripe egg, and some months when you release an egg but your progesterone level is below normal. The control center (your hypothalamus and pituitary in the brain) keeps screaming louder and louder for the ovaries to get the progesterone levels higher. Estrogen rises but the aging ovaries just can't make enough progesterone. This means the tango couple can't figure out who's leading and who's following—and you get caught up in the confusion.

Temporarily left unchecked by low progesterone levels, estrogen continues its stimulating business, which results in increased endometrial thickness, heavy bleeding, and lots of breast tenderness.[7]

Wild fluctuations in estrogen combined with low progesterone may lead to migraines and irritability and, in some cases, overt rage. Your periods may come early, be heavier, or both. You might not shed the entire uterine lining, which would mean a light period during one cycle and a heavier one the following month. These symptoms can be periodic, but in some women they're more frequent. Given the higher estrogen levels and lower progesterone levels, the potential for breast cysts and endometrial problems increases. Research shows that women who have the highest endogenous levels of estradiol (meaning the estradiol their body creates) have the greatest risk of breast cancer.[8]

GENETICS MATTER WHEN IT COMES TO MENOPAUSE

We used to think that a woman's age at menopause was determined simply by when she exhausted the supply of eggs in her ovaries. But the latest thinking is that genetics and environment play major roles.

Your age at menopause is highly correlated with your mother's age at menopause. It stands to reason that low progesterone, the first step toward menopause, is also genetically determined. It's good to find out if you have a genetic predisposition to that problem, because then you can look into boosting your progesterone using The Gottfried Protocol. Start the inquiry by asking your mother about her age at menopause, and when her menstrual cycles started to change.

A recent Harvard study identified ten places in DNA where your age of natural menopause is determined.[9] Of course, exposure to environmental factors, such as endocrine disruptors and birth control pills, can affect when you have your final period.

Stop, Thief: Stress and Pregnenolone Steal

Although progesterone is mostly made in the ovaries, a small amount is produced in the adrenal glands, where it can be converted into other hormones, such as cortisol. Your adrenal glands have a crucial job: to respond to stress by producing cortisol and the neurotransmitters epinephrine and norepinephrine, which help you focus, and tend and befriend as needed in a dangerous situation.

Progesterone is made from *pregnenolone,* the main "prehormone," or biochemical precursor, from which all sex hormones are derived. It may not surprise you to learn that there's a link between progesterone and cortisol: just as pregnenolone is the prehormone of progesterone, progesterone is the prehormone of cortisol. It's another step in the delicate dance of balancing your body's hormones.

Cortisol from your adrenal glands is the main stress hormone. Your body will make cortisol no matter what. Still, when you are chronically stressed, your body uses cortisol faster than it can be produced, so you need to get more. Where do you get it? You take it from cortisol's prehormones: pregnenolone and progesterone, fittingly called Pregnenolone Steal. If you have a lifestyle that keeps you in high demand for cortisol (see chapter 4 for assessment), your body will steal from your supply of progesterone by shunting pregnenolone so that it can make more cortisol.

As if that weren't bad enough, when chronic stress causes cortisol levels to rise, the cortisol also will block your progesterone receptors. Progesterone and cortisol compete for the progesterone receptors. If progesterone can't bind with a receptor because cortisol is having molecular sex with it, you will feel low in progesterone even if your serum level is normal, *because progesterone cannot get inside of your cell's nucleus.* Your mood worsens, particularly before your period. Your stress resilience drops, you feel anxious, and you can't calm yourself down. Since progesterone is a diuretic, you'll notice fluid retention, and perhaps breast tenderness as well.

Clearly, stress relief is essential for more than regulating high or low cortisol. That's why I put a big focus on ways for harried women to manage stress.

Other Hormones That Take Down Progesterone

From chapter 2, "A Hormonal Primer," you are well aware of the cross talk between the ovaries, adrenals, and thyroid, which I liken to Charlie's Angels. When it comes to low progesterone, a slow thyroid can lower progesterone too, and vice versa.

Finally, one other minor hormone worth mentioning is prolactin, the hormone that originates in the pituitary of the brain and controls breast milk production (or lactation); women with high prolactin usually have a milky discharge from both breasts. If you have this, see your doctor immediately. Prolactin has many other jobs, related to water and salt balance, growth and development, ovulation, behavior, and immune regulation. Making too much prolactin can lower your progesterone level and stress raises prolactin.

Low progesterone is one of the top three hormone imbalances, and it's also one of the easiest to mend. Rather than jumping to the solution for your low-progesterone symptoms, I encourage you to perform root-cause analysis. When you understand why your progesterone is low, you'll get better results because you can customize your solution.

Low Progesterone: Do You Have It?

When I say a patient needs to balance her estrogen and progesterone, I have something quite specific in mind, a clear solution based on solid numbers. Here it is: You want your serum progesterone on Day 21 or 22 of your menstrual cycle to be 10 to 25 ng/mL. Additionally, you want the *ratio* of your salivary progesterone to your estradiol to be *1 to 300*. To put it another way, during the luteal phase, the amount of progesterone in a normal woman who is fertile and ovulating is three hundred times the concentration of estradiol, ideally measured five to six days before your period starts.

I find that 300 is ideal for most women. That's what helped me prevent the symptoms I had related to low progesterone, such as

PMS, fibroids, painful periods, and mood problems, including a proclivity toward depression (now resolved!).

Progesterone is your security guard, standing sentinel at the uterine gate. If you've been low in progesterone for a while, see your clinician. You may need to have a pelvic ultrasound or a biopsy to make sure you don't have an excessively thick uterine lining. (If you do have a thickened lining, your doctor may want to perform a biopsy to exclude abnormal growth of cells in your uterus.) If your menstrual cycle is shorter than twenty-one days, you must see a medical professional to investigate for precancer or cancer of the uterine lining.

Four other, more serious conditions related to low progesterone include the following:

1. **Endometriosis.** The most common cause of pelvic pain, endometriosis affects up to 10 percent of the women in the United States.[10] That's five million suffering women. It occurs when cells of the endometrium, or uterine lining, migrate and implant outside the uterus, usually on the ovaries or other pelvic organs, causing inflammation and sometimes extreme pain. In one study, nearly half of the women with endometriosis had either low blood progesterone or a short luteal phase.[11] Progesterone resistance seems to contribute to the development of endometriosis.[12] Women with endometriosis don't make enough progesterone receptors, particularly in the endometriosis growths. That makes it difficult to shut down estrogen activity, so estrogen levels rise, especially around the aberrant growths.[13] Endometriosis treatment involves prescribing progesterone (usually as synthetic progesterone pills, or progestins).

2. **Endometrial precancer and cancer.** As we've seen, low progesterone allows estrogen to build up too much tissue in the endometrium, or uterine lining. That puts you

at a greater risk for both precancer or cancer of the endometrium.[14]

3. **Anxiety**. Since progesterone helps keep us calm, it follows that some women with low progesterone feel anxious. Even when given to nonanxious volunteers, progesterone and its downstream daughters such as allopregnanolone have shown antianxiety effects.[15] Paradoxically, for some women who take progesterone, the result is the opposite: restlessness and malaise. It turns out that while high doses of progesterone can lead to calm, low doses seem to create anxiety.[16] The dose response is based on how progesterone interacts with the GABA receptor. I find for my clients that it's best to try several doses of progesterone to determine the ideal amount.

4. **Disordered sleep.** One of the most distressing symptoms of perimenopause is poor sleep. It's not life-threatening, but lack of proper sleep can affect every part of our mental and physical being. In 2011, pharmacists filled 60 million prescriptions for sleeping pills, up from 47 million in 2006.[17] Unfortunately, sleeping pills are not a real solution. The most popular prescription pills add a mere forty minutes or less of sleep to your night. They are approved only for short-term use. In fact, new data links prescription sleeping pills with a greater risk of cancer and death.[18] There's an alternative for women with sleep issues at middle age: taking oral progesterone at a dose of 100 to 300 mg has been shown to restore normal sleep in postmenopausal women (note that this is a higher dose than normal, and I reserve it only for women with sleep issues). In normal women with undisturbed sleep, progesterone had no effect on their sleep, which is good news.[19] However, other studies show that women have mood problems at higher doses of progesterone, so I recommend caution in finding your ideal dose.

────RECAP: DR. SARA'S TOP 5 REASONS──── FOR LOW PROGESTERONE

1. Aging. Especially relevant from thirty-five onward as you march toward menopause, age is associated with fewer ripe eggs, less ovulation, and low progesterone.

2. Stress. If your problem is unmanaged and chronic emotional stress, cortisol blocks your progesterone receptors, and your body will make cortisol at the expense of pregnenolone and progesterone, causing Pregnenolone Steal.

3. Little or no ovulation. Ovulation is key to the regular, monthly production of progesterone during your fertile years. If you don't ovulate, either because you've run out of eggs or you have another hormonal problem such as excess testosterone, you will have progesterone deficiency.

4. Low thyroid. Thyroid hormone is essential to the smooth operation of the hormone pathways I've described. You need adequate thyroid hormone to make pregnenolone from cholesterol, and then to make progesterone. If you are low in thyroid hormone, you will not make as much progesterone. Additionally, there's a vicious cycle that occurs: when you have low progesterone, it raises thyroid requirements. Your thyroid gland has to work harder. If your thyroid gland is already borderline, it will worsen your low progesterone.

5. High prolactin. Some women make too much prolactin, a hormone in the pituitary of the brain that controls lactation in women. High blood prolactin interferes with the function of the ovaries in premenopausal and perimenopausal women, and as a result, secretion of ovarian hormones such as progesterone, and eventually estrogen, decreases.

The Solution: The Gottfried Protocol for Low Progesterone

Addressing progesterone deficiency is sometimes more complicated than simply adding more hormone to the equation. The problem of progesterone resistance means that some women don't respond to the addition of progesterone cream or pills.

You can increase your body's progesterone level in several ways: vitamin C and chasteberry for women who are premenopausal, and over-the-counter progesterone cream or progesterone pills for women who've reached menopause. When you're premenopausal, your ovaries still may be able to produce progesterone, but they need a nudge. Once you've had your final period and a year has passed (the official definition of menopause), topical or oral progesterone is the best choice. I suggest tweaking your protocol to adjust to the realities of your life stage, so use these steps as a starting point.

Step 1: Targeted Lifestyle Changes and Nutraceuticals

Vitamin C is the lone but mighty solution in this arena. It's the only over-the-counter nutraceutical treatment for low progesterone proven to be effective. At doses of 750 mg/day, vitamin C has been shown to raise progesterone in women with both low progesterone and luteal phase defect.[20] In a randomized trial, women were randomly assigned to receive either vitamin C or a placebo. Within three menstrual cycles, the group receiving vitamin C saw progesterone levels increase on average from 8 to 13 ng/mL. (Remember, your goal is 10 to 25 ng/mL.)

If you have garden-variety low progesterone—that is, not associated with luteal phase defect—we don't know if vitamin C will raise your progesterone level. But we're not talking massive doses here. Taking 750 mg/day is completely safe, even though the recommended daily allowance is an abysmally low 75 to 90 mg/day. Incidentally, a daily dose of 500 to 1,000 mg of vitamin C also helps prevent cancer and stroke, keeps your eyes working well, boosts immunity, and increases longevity. Because it's water soluble, any excess vitamin C is excreted in your urine. It's a win/win situation.

Hang out with others. Progesterone is another stress-related hormone, and affiliation helps women to calm down. "Closeness" exercises with a partner were shown to raise progesterone in the saliva.[21]

Hold the joe. Has your doctor asked you about caffeine? I'm guessing the answer is no, because many American physicians are addicted to caffeine themselves. Sorry to be the bearer of bad news, but one of the first steps I recommend in treating low progesterone is weaning yourself from caffeine. Caffeine boosts energy temporarily by raising cortisol, but as we've seen, high cortisol can block progesterone receptors: your daily jolt may be decreasing the ability of your progesterone to bind to its receptor and do its job. While caffeine has not been shown to lower progesterone levels in women who are still having monthly cycles, two studies have linked caffeine with PMS symptoms.[22]

I won't sentence you to the interim irritability and headaches, though. I have a systematic approach: switching from regular coffee to yerba mate or green tea, and from yerba mate or green tea to decaffeinated green tea, and then to flavorful herbal teas, such as rooibos and fruit teas.

Skip the zin. While you are abstaining from coffee and nonherbal tea, consider ditching other drinks that can adversely affect your hormonal balance. Alcohol intake is associated with premenstrual anxiety, mood problems, and headache.[23] Drinking more than three to six alcoholic servings per week increases risk of breast cancer.[24] If that's not enough to convince you, consider that alcohol increases belly fat.[25] This makes sense to me because when you drink a glass of wine, your liver shifts to burning alcohol for fuel instead of burning fat in your body. This sidetracks your fat-burning mechanism and may slow down your rate of fat burning by more than half.

Step 2: Herbal Therapy

There are several herbs worth mentioning, but *chasteberry* is the most effective and safe. Other botanical therapies that raise progesterone include *bladderwrack* and *saffron*.

Chasteberry (*Vitex agnus-castus*). Also known by several other terms, including chaste tree, chaste tree berry, and vitex, this herb is available as capsules or liquid tincture, and the average dose is 500 to 1,000 mg/day. It is proven to reduce PMS and infertility, presumably by raising progesterone.

Chasteberry, used by the ancient Greeks more than two thousand years ago, restores normal progesterone levels in the body. Most researchers believe that chasteberry increases the release of luteinizing hormone from the pituitary, which raises progesterone and normalizes the second half of the menstrual cycle. The progesterone boost stimulated by chasteberry has been demonstrated in blood-hormone levels, in endometrial biopsies documenting progesterone effect on the uterine lining, and in analysis of vaginal secretions.[26] Some postulate that chasteberry works by lowering prolactin, another hormone that affects menstrual cycles, while others believe that chasteberry affects dopamine (the brain chemical or neurotransmitter of reward-driven learning, pleasure, and satisfaction), acetylcholine (the neurotransmitter that governs communication between the nerves and muscles), and/or opioid receptors (located in the brain and organs—these receptors bind to morphine, endorphins, and other similar chemicals).[27] Bottom line? We don't yet know how it works. In Germany, where integrative medicine is practiced as the standard of care, chasteberry is approved for menstrual irregularity, PMS, and breast pain.[28]

A Stanford University School of Medicine study shows that in women with low progesterone, fertility rates are higher among those taking chasteberry. After six months of treatment, 32 percent of the women taking chasteberry became pregnant, compared with

10 percent of the group taking a placebo.[29] Unlike with most pharmaceuticals, fewer than 2 percent of the women taking chasteberry have adverse effects. Among this small percentage, the most common complaints are malaise and gastrointestinal complaints, including nausea and diarrhea.

Chasteberry has been proven to help low progesterone in more than sixty years of clinical research, including five randomized trials.[30] As I wrote in the Introduction, randomized trials are my gold standard of best evidence. When performed properly, they allow the least amount of bias and demonstrate causation—unlike lesser-quality study approaches, such as observational studies or case-control studies. As we try to find what truly, effectively helps women with hormone imbalances, any kind of bias is the enemy.

CHOOSE YOUR CHASTEBERRY

Have you decided to go the chasteberry route? The number of products out there can seem dizzying; it's hard to know what to look for and where to find it. I've spent twenty years testing products, following the studies, and experimenting for the benefit of my patients. For my patients, I recommend two formulations: Fertility Blend and Agnolyt.

Fertility Blend. This is a capsule of chasteberry at a dose that is proprietary (i.e., top secret, but it's been proven to raise progesterone). I recommend it even if you don't have an issue with fertility but have symptoms of low progesterone. Why? Studies show that it raises serum progesterone levels and increases fertility. One nonrandomized but large study found that chasteberry increases fertility, which led to a well-designed randomized trial that documented increased fertility in women taking chasteberry.[31]

Agnolyt. Agnolyt is considered one of the best-known extracts of chasteberry. A company in Cologne, Germany, makes this proprietary blend of chasteberry fruit tincture, which contains

9 grams of 1:5 tincture for each 100 grams of aqueous alcoholic solution. Most herbalists are able to create a tincture with this formula, or you can purchase the proprietary blend from Europe.

Bladderwrack (*Fucus vesiculosus*). Bladderwrack, an edible brown seaweed, has been used for thousands of years in Ayurveda, the traditional medicine of India. If your low progesterone symptom is a shortened menstrual cycle, consider bladderwrack, which has been shown in one study to raise progesterone levels and lengthen a shortened menstrual cycle.[32] I do not recommend bladderwrack if you have a thyroid condition (described in chapter 9), as it contains iodine and may worsen your symptoms.

Saffron (*Crocus sativus*). While less proven than chasteberry in women with symptoms of low progesterone, saffron is a safe option for depression, painful periods, and PMS.[33] Yes, the same saffron that you add to your paella. This is not as wacky as you might think— saffron has been used medicinally for more than 3,600 years, and it is effective for treating depression, according to six randomized trials, including two that show it's as effective as Prozac (for both depression and PMS, dosage was 15 mg twice a day).[34]

FROM THE FILES OF SARA GOTTFRIED, MD
Patient: Lucinda
Age: Thirty-four
Plea for help: "I'm anxious, and it's a problem. It peaks a few days before my period and I can go from zero to sixty in a nanosecond if, for instance, my fiancé picks a fight or does anything annoying. And I have bloating. Ridiculous bloating."

Until a few years ago, Lucinda's menstrual cycle was regular. Now she cycles consecutively for a few months, then skips one or more periods. When her period comes, it's heavy and painful. Along with premenstrual anxiety, Lucinda can routinely gain five or more pounds in her luteal phase, the time from ovulation until the start of her period. She calls the premenstrual bloat her "belly goiter" but, joking aside, feels the amount of bloating is rather freakish. Lucinda and her fiancé are planning their wedding, and once the ring is on her finger, she is eager to get pregnant. She and her fiancé are currently using condoms, which I favor—when used correctly and consistently, they provide reasonable contraception and, unlike birth control pills, do not delay fertility.

Treatment protocol: Lucinda came to me not long after she'd purchased progesterone cream. I recommended she try chasteberry for three months, because progesterone cream can sometimes prevent ovulation, which is not helpful if you want to proceed rapidly to babymaking.

Results: Within six weeks, Lucinda had reverted to a regular cycle, every thirty days. Her anxiety resolved, which was particularly useful as she made plans for her wedding. It took a while longer to reduce her bloating. But we worked on her food plan and tried a modified elimination diet of cutting out dairy, refined carbohydrates, alcohol, and gluten. Together with the boosted progesterone, the modified elimination diet resolved Lucinda's bloating completely. She felt confident and healthy, and ready to start a family. "I finally feel like myself again," Lucinda explained at a subsequent appointment, "and no one is happier about this than my fiancé!"

——BIRTH CONTROL PILLS: THE BALANCE SHEET——

Millions of women agree to take the birth control pill (BCP) for contraception, to treat an underlying hormone imbalance, or both. BCPs block ovulation and thicken your cervical mucus so that sperm have a reduced chance of meeting up with a fertilized egg. Here is the balance sheet of the advantages and disadvantages of taking a BCP.

ADVANTAGES

- **Effective contraception** of 99 percent if used properly and taken daily.
- **Lowers androgens,** so birth control pills reduce acne, but the pill may lower sex drive by the same mechanism and may cause pain with intercourse.
- **Cancer reduction:** Taken longer than one year, you reduce risk of ovarian cancer. Five years of birth control pill use is associated with a 90 percent reduction in future ovarian cancer. BCPs also cut in half your risk of thyroid cancer.

DISADVANTAGES

- **Doesn't help PMS,** and may make it worse (exceptions are for the BCPs containing drosperinone, a synthetic progestin, but these are also linked to greater risk of blood clots of six- to sevenfold).
- **More blood clots;** increased risk up to triple (greater if drosperinone used).
- **Lowers free thyroid hormones and testosterone.** BCPs increase thyroglobulin, a protein that binds thyroid hormone. If you are on thyroid medication, you may need to adjust your dose. Additionally, BCPs raise sex hormone binding globulin (SHBG), a protein that binds free testosterone and may make it biologically inert.
- **Depletes B vitamins.** You need B vitamins, especially vitamins B_1, B_2, and B_6, to keep your neuroendocrine system working as an ally.
- **Delayed conception.** For women who stop the BCP to become pregnant, return to normal ovulation may be delayed. Other contraceptives, such as the copper IUD, have no delay in fertility. Stress also seems to interfere with return to fertility in women who stop the BCP.
- **May cause weight gain.**

- **Possible risk of breast cancer.** Data are mixed, although if there's any increased risk, it's modest. We know that synthetic progestins in menopausal hormone replacement increase the risk of breast cancer, and the same may be true of the synthetic progestins in BCPs.

BOTTOM LINE

If you take BCPs, add a vitamin B complex. If you have PMS and want a birth control pill, choose one containing drosperinone as long as you do not have an increased risk of blood clots. While BCPs may reduce your risk of ovarian cancer and thyroid cancer, they may modestly increase your risk of breast cancer, so take care to adjust based on family history and individual risk.

Note: For a full list of citations, see http://thehormonecure book.com.

———DR. SARA'S LOW PROGESTERONE:——— CHASTEBERRY WORKED FOR ME

In the Introduction to this book, I detailed the hormonal mess I was in my midthirties, when I tested my hormone levels. It turned out my progesterone on Day 21 was 6 ng/mL, which is low. I remembered reading literature by Katharina Dalton, MD, the physician who popularized treatment of PMS with natural progesterone cream. In *Menstrual Syndrome and Progesterone Therapy*, she claimed that 83 percent of her treated patients experienced total relief. One anecdote had stayed with me: Dalton aided in the defense of a woman who had killed her boyfriend; the defense strategy was that she'd been temporarily insane due to PMS. I could relate.

The problem with Dalton's data was that it wasn't tested in a randomized trial. After searching the scientific literature, I found two randomized trials. In both, progesterone was taken in whopping doses: 400 mg twice per day in one study, and 300 mg four times per day in the other. Each *failed* to show any benefit. I found five randomized trials extolling the virtues of the chasteberry tree and decided to give it a try. I took it in a capsule form, 1,000 mg/day. Within one month, my period returned to arriving every twenty-eight days, and I was feeling calmer. Within two months, my PMS had resolved. And when I checked my progesterone, it was 17 ng/mL, which is optimal. Success!

The lesson learned: use chasteberry first. Since women lose ovarian response to chasteberry as they age, if you don't respond to this herb within six weeks, I recommend starting progesterone as a cream, gel, or pill, under the direction of your doctor.

WILD YAM DOES NOT WORK

Wild yam (*Dioscorea villosa*) is often touted as a natural way to augment your progesterone levels and help reduce hot flashes. However, the active component of wild yam, *diosgenin*, can be converted into progesterone in a lab, but not in the human body. Not surprisingly, a randomized trial of wild yam cream versus placebo for menopausal symptoms showed no difference in symptoms or progesterone levels.[35]

Step 3: Bioidentical Progesterone

Some women are at the point in their ovarian lives where chasteberry isn't an option: because they are in late perimenopause or menopause, their ovaries can no longer respond. Time for Plan B.

Why would you care about low progesterone when you're in menopause? I'll tell you: many menopausal women have symptoms of low progesterone and are reluctant to use the official "hormone replacement therapy," as they should be. Since chasteberry will not work for them, I recommend trying a small dose of progesterone cream. Bioidentical progesterone is biochemically the same as the progesterone you make in your ovaries. In most over-the-counter creams, 20 mg equals about ¼ teaspoon. Rubbing ¼ teaspoon (about the size of a dime) into your arms where they're hairless and the skin is thin, for fourteen to twenty-five nights per month, is often enough to relieve the symptoms of low progesterone.

There are three randomized trials demonstrating the efficacy of progesterone cream for women with symptoms of low progesterone, such as hot flashes. One examined a dose of 20 mg a day, and when it came to hot flashes, 83 percent in the cream group experienced fewer flashes (versus 19 percent in the placebo group), but several of the women experienced vaginal bleeding.[36] If you have bleeding, this must be investigated immediately. Another trial looked at a dosage of 32 mg per day, and found that the progesterone cream raised serum levels but did not change hot flashes, mood, or sexual drive.[37] Lastly, one trial of progesterone cream at various doses showed no change in hot flashes—this time using Progestelle progesterone cream at doses of 60, 40, 20, and 5 mg or placebo.[38] It's possible that the different formulations of progesterone cream are responsible for the inconsistent results; anecdotally, many of my patients find progesterone cream to be extremely helpful.

FROM THE FILES OF SARA GOTTFRIED, MD
Patient: Donna
Age: Forty-seven
Plea for help: "I'm in blended-family hell," Donna says her first visit with me, "with adolescent daughters who are serotonin stealers. I just feel drained and angry most of the time. No sex drive. Needless to say, this isn't helping my marriage, and things are slowly falling apart."

Donna is a therapist in private practice. She has two daughters, ages fifteen and thirteen, and a stepdaughter, age ten. Donna describes fluid retention and lousy sleep before her period, no libido, and no energy to run or practice yoga. She also experiences a heavier period.

Treatment protocol: Donna has classic symptoms of low progesterone, including retained fluid, heavier periods, insomnia, poor self-soothing and decreased stress resilience. We started her on progesterone cream, 20 mg per night rubbed into the inner surface of her upper arms.

Results: Within four weeks, the progesterone cream had decreased her insomnia, menstrual flow, and bloating. After eight weeks, Donna reported dramatic changes that not only improved her life but also positively impacted everyone around her. For the first time in years, she told me that she felt home again in her body, embodied and in control. She felt motivated to get back into yoga and running and possessed the mettle to cope with her daughters again. When little things happened, she didn't fly off the handle, but managed them with grace and ease. I often find that small doses of progesterone are the small hinges that swing big doors for perimenopausal women.

BIOIDENTICAL PILLS

You might need to augment your progesterone with a bioidentical pill, cream, troche, or vaginal suppository. Pills work remarkably well if insomnia is your main symptom. The FDA has approved Prometrium, which is bioidentical, micronized progesterone: natural progesterone that has been broken down—micronized—to enable your body to metabolize it more easily. Taken orally, it is identical to the progesterone you've always made while cycling. It is a *somnolent,* which means DO NOT OPERATE HEAVY MACHINERY. More to the point, it helps you sleep restoratively.

A word of caution: use Prometrium, not Provera (medroxyprogesterone acetate), the most common progestin, or synthetic form, of progesterone. Many physicians prescribe progestins to patients suffering from irregular periods, fibroids, and/or heavy bleeding. But progestins cause terrible mood problems. In my opinion, it should not be used. Though the words frequently are used interchangeably by physicians and the media, progesterone and progestins are different biochemically, which means they have very different effects on the body. In study after study, Provera has been shown to increase the risk for breast cancer, depression, weight gain, blood clots, and cardiovascular disease (stroke and heart attacks). In the best evidence of progestins and heart disease, women aged forty-five to sixty-four were randomly assigned to receive Provera, Prometrium, or a placebo. Provera was shown to reduce HDL, your good cholesterol (and we need all the HDL we can get). Prometrium did less harm to HDL.[39]

Prometrium has been shown to be safe. One study, of more than eighty thousand women followed for eight years, showed no increased risk of breast cancer when using Prometrium.[40] An important point about progesterone is that one of its main security jobs is to protect the endometrial lining from overgrowth, precancer (hyperplasia), and cancer. The only bioidentical progesterone shown to prevent buildup in the uterine lining is Prometrium.

Prometrium, taken in 100 mg or 200 mg tablets, can do anything progestins can do, but better and more safely. (Occasionally, women need higher doses to correct estrogen dominance, or for improved sleep.) The only contraindication is a peanut allergy, because Prometrium is suspended in peanut oil in a soft-gel sphere. Women with peanut allergies might consider compounding natural progesterone in another base oil, which would have to be ordered by a physician who's comfortable working with a compounding pharmacy.

Bottom line: make sure your doctor prescribes biodentical progesterone, NOT progestins, for you. The only situation in which progestins might be appropriate is for incarcerated sex offenders, because progestins removes sex drive in both men and women. *Seriously!*

FROM THE FILES OF SARA GOTTFRIED, MD

Patient: Joan

Age: Forty-four

Plea for help: "*My sleep became horrendous this past year. It has totally wiped me out. My husband and I have sex once a week, but really, I can't be bothered. Emotionally, I'm like a taut wire, ready to snap. I'm completely wiped out.*"

Joan is an executive coach who works part-time and bears the bulk of the caretaking for her three-year-old son. A bulimic in recovery, she had difficulty with infertility in her thirties. Her periods are heavy, and as a result, she has low ferritin, which is the most sensitive indicator of iron levels.

Treatment protocol: Joan's heavy periods bordered on hemorrhage. Because of that and her disrupted sleep, I wrote a prescription for Prometrium, which acts as a somnolent. From Day 12 through Day 26 of her cycle, she takes 100 mg each night.

Results: Joan began sleeping through the night immediately. Her periods became lighter, and her ferritin climbed back to normal levels. With improved sleep, she felt more patient and energetic. She noted that her sex drive peaks around Day 12. She and her husband have learned to take advantage of every morsel of increased interest.

————THE GOTTFRIED PROTOCOL FOR PMS————

Some statistics thrill me, like the one that says 70 percent of women with PMS turn first to integrative strategies to help themselves.[41] While low progesterone may manifest as PMS, not all women with PMS have low progesterone. It's more complicated, as I described earlier, and relates to progesterone "resistance." Given that 60 to 80 percent of women overall experience PMS, here are the integrative strategies, supported by at least one randomized trial, that improve PMS.

STEP 1: TARGETED LIFESTYLE CHANGES AND NUTRACEUTICALS
TAKE YOUR CALCIUM, MAGNESIUM, AND VITAMIN B.

Calcium, as calcium carbonate or citrate—600 mg taken orally twice a day—reduces PMS by 50 percent.[42] Magnesium, 200 mg/day, helps with bloating, as does vitamin B_6, 50 to 100 mg/day.[43] Taken with magnesium, B_6 reduces PMS-related anxiety.[44] B_6 is involved in the production of many neurotransmitters, including serotonin, which controls mood, sleep, and appetite, and dopamine, which controls pleasure and satisfaction. Be cautious: higher-than-recommended doses can cause nerve toxicity. Recently, vitamins B_1 and B_2 were shown to be lower during PMS, and low vitamin D was also associated with PMS, but we do not yet have randomized trials supporting their use for treatment.[45]

Lay off the cupcakes. Here's a shocking statistic for you. Women with PMS consume *275 percent* more refined sugar than women who don't have PMS.[46] Consumption of excess refined carbohydrates causes loss of magnesium through the urine. Together with the data showing an association between caffeine and PMS, I advise women *to eliminate sugar and caffeine* from their diets for ninety days when they have PMS.

Get acupuncture. In a recent review of ten randomized trials, acupuncture was shown to improve PMS symptoms by 55 percent with no risk of harm.[47]

Exercise moderately and frequently. Exercising at moderate intensity for thirty minutes four times/week decreases PMS. For all you marathoners, frequency is more important than intensity.[48]

Guided visualization, a technique that uses imagery to induce feelings of calm, has been shown to increase vaginal temperature, a proxy for a rise in progesterone, and to improve PMS.[49] I'm not sure why this works, but it may reduce cortisol—less stress, more progesterone.

Homeopathy is a form of complementary medicine in which clinicians treat clients with diluted preparations called *remedies*. Homeopathy in PMS has been shown to reduce symptoms in a small group by 90 percent.[50] You would need to see a homeopath for this individualized therapy, which might be worthwhile and confers little risk.

Light therapy was shown to lower PMS symptoms in one randomized trial. For two cycles, fourteen women sat in front of a bright light (10,000 1x cool-white fluorescent light), compared with dim red light, for two weeks before their period. Reductions in both depression and PMS symptoms were seen in the group treated with bright light.[51]

STEP 2: HERBAL THERAPIES

Chasteberry. Chasteberry at doses of 500 to 1,000 mg/day raises progesterone levels.

St. John's wort. This herb has been shown effective at relieving both behavioral and physical symptoms of PMS.[52] One trial looked at a combination of chasteberry and St. John's wort (*Hypericum perforatum*) for the PMS-like symptoms in perimenopausal women. They found that the combination of herbs was more effective than placebo for PMS symptoms, particularly anxiety.[53] We already know that St. John's wort is superior to placebo for depression, based on a review of twenty-three randomized trials of 1,757 patients.[54] But consult with your doctor if you already are taking an antidepressant or antipsychotic medication.

STEP 3: BIOIDENTICAL HORMONES

Because of conflicting evidence, I do not recommend progesterone for PMS.[55] However, bioidentical hormone replacement can be useful for irregular menstrual cycles once you've been thoroughly evaluated by your local physician, and it improves sleep in perimenopause.

Progesterone in Balance

When you've got your progesterone at its proper level—not too little and not too much—you feel like Goldilocks in the just-right bed: sleepy at the right times, triumphant, and content.

- You hardly notice your period until (surprise!) there's a spot of blood on your underwear.
- You have regular periods, at least every twenty-five days, with no spotting or flooding.
- Your weight remains stable throughout your menstrual cycle.
- Every night, eight hours of sleep is a regular, delightful experience, from age thirty-five well into menopause.
- You graduate from couples therapy. *Yes!*
- After menopause, estrogen and progesterone are in a perfect tango, with no breast tenderness or scary need for a biopsy after a mammogram.

CHAPTER 6

EXCESS ESTROGEN: DEPRESSED AND CHUNKY?

When I hit puberty, I was already reading about hormones (remember, I'm a geek). I blamed estrogen for many of my new physical quirks: painful periods that interrupted my childhood at age ten; breasts and hips that grew too fast and caused stretch marks; and breakouts that perplexed even my dermatologist. Hormones in general, and estrogen in particular, felt inscrutable, volatile, and beyond my comprehension. Little did I know that hormones would become the canvas of my life's work.

I mentioned this in the last chapter, but it's worth repeating: estrogen is the hormone that most defines you as a woman. In fact, estrogen is the primary female sex hormone, made by all animals with a spine ("Mom, duh! Those are called *vertebrates!*" as my daughter reminds me), as well as some insects, which qualifies estrogen as the most ancient of hormones. In humans, the female brain becomes exquisitely sensitive to estrogen at puberty, and this continues until about your mid-forties, when the brain becomes less sensitive again—that is, the ovary is increasingly numb to the admonitions of the ovaries, and vice versa.

At puberty, release of estrogen increases the feel-good chemicals of oxytocin, the arbiter of love and affiliation, and dopamine, the neurotransmitter of pleasure, satisfaction, and reward-based learning. With its biochemical girlfriends, oxytocin and dopamine, estrogen kick-starts your period at around age ten to fifteen.

Estrogen: Archetype of Femininity

Here's the short version of what estrogen does:

- Externally, estrogen gives you hips and breasts. More estrogen makes you *zaftig,* the Yiddish term for voluptuousness.
- Internally, estrogen buffers mood and keeps you on task. Estrogen is nature's Prozac, adjusting the level of available serotonin—another important neurotransmitter—so that it's in more ready supply. Serotonin regulates your mood, sleep, and appetite, and acts as a general gatekeeper of other neurotransmitters in your brain.
- Estrogen is responsible for the first half of your menstrual cycle, building up the cells lining your uterus to protect a developing fetus. If conception does not occur, the lining is released about every twenty-eight days as your period. If conception does occur, estrogen, combined with progesterone, thickens and deepens that lining for the fertilized egg to settle into and grow.
- Estrogen lights a libidinous fire and gets you obsessing about babies until about age forty-five, when you start thinking that sleep sounds a lot better.

Estrogen balance is directly related to progesterone. Ideally, you have a rhythm between these two hormones, which should function like well-matched dance partners. Estrogen is the flirtatious, curvy member of the team; progesterone plays a less dramatic, supportive role.

Balance is crucial because estrogen and progesterone have opposing yet interdependent effects, similar to the Chinese concept of yin and yang. Estrogen stimulates the lining of the uterus to grow; progesterone stops the growth, stabilizes it, and then releases it in a coordinated fashion called menstruation. Estrogen stimulates breast cells to grow; progesterone prevents cysts from developing in painful breasts. Estrogen causes you to retain salt and water; progesterone is a natural diuretic. Estrogen creates progesterone receptors, the locks on a cell's nucleus into which a hormone inserts like a key; progesterone makes estrogen receptors jam and shut down.

It takes two to tango. When they work in tandem, maintaining the body's delicate equilibrium, you dance to a passionate rhythm. When your estrogen and progesterone are synchronized, your bones are strong, dense, and pliable. Your skin is hydrated, smooth, and well girded by collagen. Your metabolism is forgiving. Your cardiovascular system stays clear of meddlesome debris, like clots and plaque. You know that you have reached this balanced state when you measure your levels of estradiol (the main estrogen of the reproductive years) and progesterone in saliva on Day 21 of the menstrual cycle, and the ratio of progesterone to estrogen is 100 to 500, and optimally 300.

Estrogen as Dominatrix: Background on Estrogen Dominance

Just like couples on a dance floor, problems can arise when one partner dominates . . . and the other doesn't follow. Estrogen is the hormone that dominates, not progesterone. Excess estrogen can lead to a host of annoying ailments: water retention and its first cousin, breast tenderness; painful periods, perhaps endometriosis; mood swings, or your garden-variety free-floating irritability—take this a step further, and you have full-fledged anxiety or depression. You might feel foggy, sleepless, and weepy. Maybe you've noticed that you have more headaches, or that your face is redder than you want it to be. These, my friends, are signs of excess estrogen.

When estrogen levels are high in relation to progesterone, women often experience a wild ride of emotions before their periods. During perimenopause, the emotional roller coaster can be in play all month long. Beyond mood swings, symptoms can include hair loss, headaches, breast tenderness, bloating, difficulty losing weight, depression, fatigue, insomnia, decreased libido, foggy brain, and/or memory loss. Studies on rats show that high estrogen can interfere with the ability to learn and pay attention.[1] Basically, you feel like crap. And that's on a good day.

The Highs and Lows of Estrogen Dominance

Because estrogen and progesterone levels are so entwined, let's look at the different combinations that relate to high estrogen:

1. High estrogen relative to *normal* progesterone. This combination is common in overweight women, and in women who have been exposed to xenoestrogens, which are synthetic chemicals that mimic estrogens. Ovaries are the main source of estrogen, but fat cells make estrogen too. More fat cells mean higher estrogen levels.

2. High estrogen relative to *low* progesterone. This combination, called estrogen dominance, is more common. Beginning around age thirty-five, as a natural consequence of aging, you begin to run out of ripe eggs. More than half the women over thirty-five have this combination. Estrogen dominance—the medical term is *dysestrogenism*—isn't a problem in every woman. But many women with estrogen dominance show myriad symptoms of hormonal unrest. After taking the quiz in chapter 1, "Getting Started," you might have decided you're one of them.

Today, it is common to have too much estrogen before you reach age fifty. This is an epochal shift in our estrogen hormones over the past century. I believe the reason is twofold: women are more emotionally stressed, and they're more exposed to artificial estrogens than ever before.

The Science of Excess Estrogen

Caution: Proceed with reading the science section if you're curious about the scientific underpinnings of excess estrogen. Otherwise, skip ahead to "The Solution: The Gottfried Protocol for Excess Estrogen" (page 171).

What happens in your body that causes estrogen levels to rise? Simply put, you need to properly metabolize your estrogen—to break it down and eliminate it—or it will build up in your blood and cause estrogen dominance. In other words, *you need to use it, then lose it.*

Your body makes several kinds of estrogens. During your re-productive years, 80 percent of the estrogen is made in the ovaries as estradiol; 10 percent is estriol; 10 percent is estrone. When you go through menopause, this ratio changes, and you primarily make estrone.

Estrogen starts as estradiol, but it can be broken down into estrone and metabolites. It's crucial for your body to break down the estrogen in order to maintain balance. You must inactivate es-trogen to maintain normal levels, and inactivation occurs mostly in the liver via phases: hydroxylation and conjugation. Hang with me while we briefly visit each of them—I promise it won't be painful.

Phase I: Hydroxylation. To understand the ways that foods and supplements affect your estrogen levels, you've got to know the basics of how we process estrogen in the body. The first phase of healthy estrogen metabolism is a chemical process, performed by the liver, *hydroxylation.* In this phase, the estradiol and estrone are con-verted into one of four other forms of estrogen: 2-hydroxy-estradiol, 2-hydroxy-estrone, 16-alpha-hydroxy-estrone, or 4-hydroxy-estrone (see Figure 3, page 156). You can think of estradiol and estrone as parent estrogens, and the metabolites as their offspring, some well behaved and some unruly.

Healthy, well-balanced bodies metabolize estrogen by the forms that begin with 2: 2-hydroxy-estradiol or 2-hydroxy-estrone. Women who have or are at high risk of developing breast and endometrial cancer have been found to make too much 16-alpha-hydroxy-estrone.[2]

Phase II: Conjugation. In the second phase of estrogen metabolism, a chemical process, *conjugation,* binds the estradiol and estrone hormones to glucuronic acid, which occurs naturally in our bodies. This binding process enables the estrogens to be excreted more easily in the bile, stool, and urine. Good-bye, used-up estrogen.

If Phase I is impaired, too much estrogen accumulates in your blood and may become carcinogenic.[3] Over time, accumulated estrogen may trigger breast, endometrial, or cervical cancer in women, and prostate cancer in men. It's like a library where no one checks out any books, but the librarian keeps buying more. If Phase II is impaired, some estrogen will be excreted, but not enough. Either way, the library shelves and aisles are overflowing. The excess estrogen keeps recirculating in the body, and the result is *dysestrogenism,* which means you've got a problem regulating your estrogen levels.

Let me give you a brief example to illustrate this point. When your diet is based on a food plan with too much fat, such as the Standard American Diet, you may raise your estrogen levels excessively. Here's why: dietary fat encourages your gut to reabsorb estrogens by slowing down the conjugation process that causes you to excrete excess estrogens. On the other hand, more dietary fiber increases conjugation—that is, more fiber lowers estrogen levels in the body—and you poop and pee more estrogen out of your system.

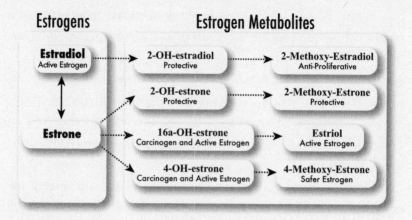

Figure 3. Estrogen and Metabolites. Estrogen metabolism occurs primarily via four pathways, starting either with estradiol or estriol. Some studies have found that a relatively high ratio of 2:16 (2-OHE to 16-alpha-OHE) is associated with a low breast cancer risk, which reflects dominance of one pathway over the other.

What Causes Excess Estrogen: Dr. Sara's Top 7 Root Causes

Several factors can interfere with normal estrogen metabolism, causing you to produce or accumulate too much of the "less good" estrogens, or too much estrogen relative to progesterone. These factors include the aging ovaries, wayward cortisol levels, exposure to xenoestrogens, and nutritional factors such as fat, fiber, and alcohol consumption.

1. Perimenopause Revisited and Diminished Ovarian Reserve

We can blame perimenopause for so many things! In the two to ten years before your final period, your estrogen levels fluctuate madly. Overall, women experiencing perimenopause show higher estrogen relative to progesterone, compared with women in their twenties and thirties.[4] In the years preceding menopause, typically from age thirty-five to fifty, your ovaries produce *more* estrogen, in some cases double the level of estrogen found in the normal menstrual cycles of a woman in her early twenties. I know this becomes confusing: initially, estrogen levels drop slightly starting in your late twenties, and then estrogen levels *increase* when your ovaries are running out of ripe eggs, usually after age thirty-five. Ob-gyns have a fancy name for it: diminished ovarian reserve (DOR).

Women are born with one to two million eggs in their ovaries, but by the time you reach perimenopause, you are down to one to three thousand. As your control system (once again, your hypothalamus and pituitary) senses that you are running out of eggs, you make more hormones to stimulate the eggs to hatch so you can become pregnant before it's too late—that is, you make more follicle-stimulating hormone (FSH) and luteinizing hormone (LH), and FSH rises faster than LH.

As *your ovaries age based on the decreasing number of ripe eggs,* the production of estradiol climbs. Once estradiol rises above 50, this blocks FSH production in the pituitary. These are examples of basic feedback loops in your body, and they mean that your control hormones keep rising in order to try to get the ovaries to do what they did when you were twenty-four. When FSH climbs above 10, you're less fertile.

Why does estradiol production rise as women age, until one to two years prior to the final period? We don't completely understand the process, but it's a bit like sprinters who jump the gun at the start of a race. Your eggs are in a follicle that is supposed to follow a particular script of responding to FSH and producing estrogen, and after the egg hatches from the follicle, producing progesterone. On Day 3, all should be quiet in the follicle but poised and ready for the hormonal cue to sprint out of the starter blocks when the gun (FSH and LH) goes off (are released from the pituitary). Instead of waiting for the gun—which is what your follicles do superbly in your twenties if you are normal—your follicle at around age forty-something will "jump the gun" and start growing and producing estradiol. This is bad for fertility and can be associated with excess estrogen.

Ultimately, estrogen plummets at the end of perimenopause—when you are closer to your final menstrual period.

2. Cortisol-Linked Estrogen Dominance

Premenopausal women treated with hormone therapy—specifically, estrogen plus progesterone—have been shown to develop a high level of cortisol at night.[5] Taking exogenous estrogen raises cortisol levels. Similarly, high levels of cortisol can block your progesterone receptors. Over time, that will lead to lower levels of progesterone, and the result is estrogen dominance.

3. Xenoestrogens

Xenoestrogens are chemicals that can mimic estrogen. (*Xeno* means "foreign.") These are synthetic chemicals that have an estrogenlike reaction in the body. They come from artificial chemicals that you get exposed to in your daily life, such as plastics in the environment. Think of them as uninvited guests at a costume party. They act like all the other guests, drinking and chatting convivially, but they are really party crashers who will disrupt the whole affair when they take off their masks.

Yet the problem is not only that they are crashing your endocrine party. Xenoestrogens are stored in fat tissue for decades, and your greatest concentration of fat is usually in your breasts. When xeno-estrogens bind to your estrogen receptors, they can activate some of them, such as those in the breast, and block others, such as those in the bone. Recall that receptors are like the locks on a cell's nucleus. When estrogen passes from the blood into the cells, it attaches to one of two types of estrogen receptors to trigger a particular task, such as stimulating breast-cell growth or slowing bone loss.

Lengthened exposure to estrogen creates a significant risk factor for breast cancer. Recently, flame retardants such as polybrominated biphenyls have been linked to estrogen disruption and a higher rate of abnormal Pap smears.[6]

Xenoestrogens are known endocrine disruptors. They interrupt the action of natural, endogenous hormones, with reproductive and developmental consequences. Just living our normal lives, we are exposed to more than seven hundred of these dangerous chemicals; they can be found in toothpaste, deodorant, sunscreen, food preservatives, the lining of cans that hold food, and many kinds of plastic.

Be wary of your cosmetics: one report describes a woman who developed both breast and endometrial cancer after using the same estrogen-containing cosmetic cream for seventy-five years.[7] The same researchers tested sixteen other commercially available facial moisturizers and found that six of them contained estrogens. Your quest for youthful looks may have the opposite effect, causing excess estrogen to enter your body through your moisturizer.

Since the 1990s, menarche (onset of menstruation) has been occurring in the United States at younger and younger ages. Researchers have spent many years and many dollars trying to figure out why. You guessed it: xenoestrogens have been clearly implicated in the early onset of menstruation and puberty.[8]

Xenoestrogens are not just disrupting women's hormonal balance, they are also wreaking havoc on men's sperm count and prostate cancer rates. Moobs (man boobs)? They are a sign of estrogen dominance in men—estrogen out of balance with testosterone—which leads to less muscularity and more fat deposits, including at the breasts and love handles. This is not some conspiracy theory. Study after study shows that xenoestrogens can cause high estrogen.

Estrogen pollution doesn't affect only humans; animals exposed to estrogens also suffer the consequences. Scientists have noted profound changes from the rising load of xenoestrogens in our oceans from man-made waste.[9] There are documented cases of polar bears with hermaphrodite offspring; seals with increased uterine fibroids, or benign growths of the uterine muscle; male fish and turtles with female characteristics and genital confusion.

Just to maintain perspective, normally in the United States, slightly more baby boys than girls are born, and we are not yet seeing an impact on gender beyond the Arctic. However, we are facing an environmental crisis with our biochemistry and neuroendocrine balance.

If you discovered from the questionnaire that you have high estrogen, don't panic. You can learn what the most common xenoestrogens are and find ways to avoid them. Among the hundreds of xenoestrogens lurking in the environment, two of the most common—and the most damaging—are bisphenol-A and phthalates.

Bisphenol-A (BPA). You might have seen someone in your yoga class carrying a water bottle with a sticker claiming that it is "BPA free." She isn't being holier than thou. BPA is a synthetic molecule used to make hard, polycarbonate plastics and some epoxy resins. It has been known to disrupt estrogen receptors since the 1930s. Among the many places BPA occurs are water bottles and some medical devices. Although U.S. manufacturers have stopped using it in baby bottles, the FDA didn't outlaw BPA in baby bottles and children's drinking cups until July 2012.

Perhaps most insidiously, it is used to coat the inside of food cans. A few years ago, the Environmental Working Group (www .ewg.org) published a pivotal study demonstrating that BPA leaked from canned-food linings into *more than half* the canned foods and drinks randomly purchased at supermarkets in the United States. For some reason, the worst offenders were chicken soup and canned ravioli.[10] Not a very comforting fact about perhaps your favorite comfort foods.

BPA exposure is ubiquitous. In one study, BPA was documented in 93 percent of Americans older than six years of age.[11] Despite the mounting and convincing evidence, some people still argue that there's no connection between environmental toxins and our health, and that it's all environmentalist hysteria. Extensive research has shown that high BPA levels in the blood have been associated with cardiovascular disease and diabetes, as well as with abnormal elevation of liver enzymes.[12] Elevated BPA has been linked to higher cytomegalovirus antibody levels, meaning that the immune system is less able to battle chronic infections.[13]

Furthermore, BPA disrupts your natural hormones, including production of estradiol in the ovaries.[14] By interfering with estradiol's protective effect against colon-cancer growth—the estradiol-induced activation of the apoptotic cascade, or programmed cell death—BPA exposure has been linked to an increased risk of colon cancer.[15]

Phthalates. Like BPA, phthalates are industrial chemicals. Used in soft, flexible plastics and in polyvinyl chloride (PVC) products, they are everywhere in modern life. They're found in nail polish, shampoos, shower curtains, baby toys, vinyl flooring, car interiors, and medical devices such as IV bags.

Studies on phthalates show a detrimental effect on men, women, and children, including an increased risk of diabetes.[16] In children, the chemicals influence thyroid-hormone signaling in the developing brain.[17] Phthalates can affect male reproductive development and thyroid function.[18] In women, they can affect the level of reproductive hormones, such as free testosterone, and sex-hormone-binding globulin. One type of phthalate, called DEHP, blocks estradiol production in the ovaries. This causes anovulation, or lack of egg production in the ovaries, which in turn leads to estrogen dominance.[19] This can lead to other problems, such as buildup of the uterine lining, with subsequent excessive bleeding and infertility.

————PRECAUTIONARY PRINCIPLES————

Enough of the doom and gloom. What can we do to reduce our exposure to these frightening chemicals? Here are my top recommendations:

• **Reduce your canned food.** Prepare your own fresh beans and soups. It's easier than you think! I use my Crock-Pot almost exclusively for beans and soups. Do your homework. Some companies are introducing BPA-free cans.

• **Eat from glass, stainless steel, and ceramic containers.** Don't drink or eat from plastic containers containing PVC. Find containers labeled "BPA free" and use them only when glass or other, safer options aren't available.

• **If you must use food from a plastic container or covered in plastic wrap, don't microwave.** Use glass or microwave-safe ceramic for microwaving.

• **Look for natural alternatives to the cosmetics, nail products, hair products, deodorants, and lotions rife with endocrine disruptors and estrogens.** Consult the Environmental Working Group database, called Skin Deep (www.ewg.org/skindeep), for safe cosmetics. Avoid sodium lauryl sulfates, parabens, formaldehyde, fragrance, and hydroquinone.

• **When you walk into your home, remove your shoes.** This is not some generic Zen advice. After walking on lawns and public gardens, you will carry pesticides and other endocrine disruptors into your home.

• **Buy shoes made from natural materials.** When you wear plastic shoes, such as flip-flops and clogs, the chemicals can be absorbed into sweaty feet.

• **Wear organic-cotton clothing to prevent exposure to the pesticides and insecticides used in growing cotton.** Dichlorodiphenyltrichloroethane (DDT), a xenoestrogen banned in the United States in 1972, has been detected in cotton imported from other countries. Unlike the European Union, the United States does not regulate the quality and safety of imported fabrics. *Buyer beware.*

• **Swap your pesticide-ridden sheets and mattresses for organic.** As Alejandro Junger, MD, has said about sleeping on conventional mattresses covered with conventional sheets, "Sleep in a cloud of formaldehyde, and insomnia, not to mention headaches, asthma, and skin rashes, can likely result."[20]

4. Obesity and weight gain

We know the health risks to women with obesity: sleep apnea and asthma; diabetes; heart disease; cancer of the breast, uterus, colon, and gallbladder; and premature death. According to the U.S. Surgeon General, women who gain more than 20 pounds from age eighteen to midlife double their risk of postmenopausal breast cancer. That's only a few pounds a year! Indeed, estrogen is fifty to one hundred times greater in overweight menopausal women than in lean women, because fat cells also produce estrogen, and that probably accounts for the greater risk in breast cancer associated with being overweight and female. Recall that 66 percent of adults in the United States are overweight or obese; for an average woman of forty, at 5 feet 4 inches in height, she is overweight if she weighs more than 145 pounds.

In the United States, obesity has been increasing steadily over the past twenty-five years. In 2010, more than one-quarter (26.4 percent) of the women in this country were considered obese—the highest percentage in our history.

You may also have heard reports that cases of type 2, or adult-onset, diabetes have been steadily rising in this country. Diabetes involves insulin and its ability to regulate blood sugar. Excess weight and lack of exercise can lead to high levels of insulin. Cells that get too much insulin can become resistant to it. Chronically high insulin increases estrogen; estrone, specifically, increases the cells' resistance to insulin. Ultimately, you get into a vicious cycle: higher insulin creates higher estrogen, which can lead to higher insulin and insulin resistance, which tends to make you gain weight, which leads to making more estrogen. This is a downward spiral with seemingly no end in sight. Enough to get you out there walking, and to just say no when the waitress offers the dessert menu?

There is a difference in estrogen levels, however, depending on menopausal status. Before menopause, women make estrogen *mostly in the ovaries,* though remember that fat cells still do produce estrogen. After menopause, women make estrogen *mostly in the fat tissues.* Overweight or obese women have more fat cells than lean women, so they produce more estrogen.

Before menopause, overweight women have lower estrogen than women of normal weight.[21] Why? Because premenopausal women with a high body mass index are more inclined to ovulate irregularly, which results in lower levels of circulating estrogens.

After menopause, the opposite is true—overweight women consistently have higher estrogen levels.[22] Also, excess fat after menopause is more likely to produce estrogen out of testosterone, a process called aromatization.[23] Obesity lowers sex hormone-binding globulin, which raises free estrogen in the blood.[24] Weight gain also correlates with endometrial cancer, another downstream consequence of estrogen overload. In one study from the National Cancer Institute of more than one hundred thousand women, those who gained more than 44 pounds since age eighteen had a fivefold increased risk of endometrial cancer.[25] Overall, 40 percent of women with endometrial cancer are obese.

In summary, higher estrogen in postmenopause is a risk factor for breast cancer, and you can modify your estrogen level. Reduce your excess estrogen by getting your weight down to normal and changing your food plan.

5. Diet

Many women have found that a diet high in conventionally raised red meat and refined carbohydrates is likely to cause estrogen overload. That could be because of hormones in the meat, or perhaps from the type of bacteria cultivated in the gut by people who eat a lot of meat.[26] When estrogen is metabolized, it leaves the body in your urine and feces. If you don't have a certain type of bacteria in your gut to process it, the estrogen will stay in your system. When this happens, you don't follow the Golden Rule of Estrogen—"use it and lose it." Instead, you keep recycling estrogen and the process may lead to overload. The "wrong" bacteria are predominant in people who consume large amounts of meats and refined carbs.[27] That's why the modified hunter-gatherer (or Paleo) diet that I often recommend for my patients works well for women with high estrogen, because of the emphasis on pastured meats and dairy that lack synthetic hormones and antibiotics as well as the avoidance of refined carbohydrates. I call this approach the Paleolista Food Plan, which also emphasizes nuts and fresh, low-glycemic fruits and vegetables. I abhor white bread, white sugar, and white rice for many reasons, but one important reason is that they reduce progesterone and worsen estrogen dominance. My recommendation: reduce your intake of refined carbohydrates as a key step to rebalancing your neuroendocrine system. For more on the food plan I recommend, please see the Appendix.

Alcohol. Consumption of alcohol raises estrogen levels and slows down fat burning. In postmenopausal women, drinking one or two servings of alcohol a day raises estrone and DHEAS, another hormone that can be converted into estrogen.[28] In one study, estrone was elevated by 7 percent with one serving (15 grams) of alcohol per day, and by 22 percent with two servings (30 grams) per day, within four weeks. In the same study, DHEAS increased by 8 percent with one portion and 9 percent with two portions of alcohol per day.

How about wine, you ask? Yes, the French famously drink wine at lunch and dinner. Wine lowers your risk of heart disease and stroke, but excess estrogen can increase your risk of breast cancer. So what's a sophisticated girl to do? Here's what: calculate your risk of breast cancer, heart disease, and stroke, and then decide. Here are your online tools to figure risk:

For stroke: http://stroke.ucla.edu/#calculaterisk
For heart disease: www.mayoclinic.com/health/heart
    -disease-risk/HB00047
For breast cancer: www.cancer.gov/bcrisktool

The proven safe threshold for women in general is two or fewer servings of alcohol per week. If you are at low risk for stroke and breast cancer, I would say it's OK to have a glass of wine with dinner a few days per week. If you are at high risk for breast cancer, I suggest drinking minimally, if at all. And remember that alcohol interferes with your fat-burning mechanism, if you're concerned about those extra pounds.

6. Nutritional deficiencies

Specific nutritional deficiencies can also lead to excess estrogen. Low magnesium, for example, is associated with high estrogen levels in both premenopausal and postmenopausal women.[29]

Vitamin B_{12}, folate, and an amino acid called methionine are other supplements that can help produce "good" estrogens and decrease formation of "less good" estrogens. How can you find out if you are deficient in any of these nutrients? If you have five or more of the symptoms in the questionnaire corresponding to this chapter, ask your doctor for a blood test to measure your magnesium, zinc, copper, vitamin B_{12}, and folate levels.

7. Mercury

Jane M. Hightower, MD, is an internist who cares for patients in the Bay Area. She has built a thriving practice around mercury toxicity, although that was never her intended path. Her interest began when she saw a series of patients with vague symptoms, such as fatigue, nausea, and brain fog, and found that a common link was a robust appetite for fish consumption.

She began a yearlong study of mercury levels in her patients, and the results thrust her into the limelight as an advocate for a poorly recognized public-health threat: mercury toxicity. In her book *Diagnosis: Mercury,* she describes the reasons for mercury toxicity in our fish supply and the problems her patients have experienced. Particularly poignant are the stories of female patients with high mercury levels and children with learning disabilities. These women thought they were doing everything right while they were pregnant: they avoided caffeine, they didn't drink alcohol, they ate fish once a week . . . and now they feel tremendous guilt about the harm that fish may have caused their offspring.[30]

The shocking part is that Dr. Hightower found her female patients had *ten times* more mercury in their blood than the Centers for Disease Control's national average.[31] Some of the children had forty times the national average, which likely relates to contaminated oceans and mercury-laden fish from local grocery stores and restaurants in the Bay Area. For fish with less mercury, check out websites that list fish according to mercury content (for example, www.montereybayaquarium.org's Seafood Watch site).

Dr. Hightower has raised awareness of mercury toxicity from our food supply. Mercury can also be found in high-fructose corn syrup, fungicides and herbicides, dental fillings, thermometers, some drugs, and some vaccinations.

Mercury also acts like the aforementioned xenoestrogens by binding your estrogen receptors.[32] If you have five or more symptoms of excess estrogen, I encourage you to talk to your doctor about testing for mercury levels in your blood or urine.

High Estrogen, Breast Cancer, and Genes

Science bears out the link between high estrogen and cancer.[33] We know that early onset of menstruation is a risk factor for breast cancer.[34] Excess estrogen levels in the first half of the menstrual cycle significantly predict breast cancer for women who have not yet reached menopause.[35] However, during premenopause the risks appear less powerfully associated with estrogen, perhaps because our estrogen levels fluctuate more.[36]

We also know that high estrogens are linked with greater breast density.[37] In fact, women with the highest breast density have quadruple the risk of breast cancer, when compared with the least-dense group.

Higher estradiol levels put you at a higher risk for the type of breast cancer that involves estrogen receptors. It does not seem to put you at risk for the type of breast cancer that lacks estrogen receptors.[38] High estrogen has been linked strongly enough with breast and ovarian cancer that high-risk women are routinely advised to consider prophylactic removal of the ovaries through the laparoscope. I performed many of these preventive surgeries while undergoing my residency training at the University of California at San Francisco, where genetic counseling for breast cancer is robust and data driven. If you wonder if that type of surgery is for you, please consult your doctor.

Does this mean that every woman with excess estrogen is destined for cancer? Of course not. That's where triggers and the exciting and emerging world of epigenomics come into play.

Imagine that two women have the same levels of estrogen. One develops cancer; the other doesn't. What gives? Each inherited twenty-three pairs of chromosomes from her parents. But these aren't fixed in stone; it's more like sand. Many of the genes you inherit can be expressed in one way or another, depending on triggers. The triggers can be internal (how you react to stress) and external (xenoestrogen exposure, radiation, what you eat, whether you are sedentary or active). They can have what's called an epigenetic effect, which refers to the changes in gene expression caused by mechanisms other than the DNA sequence. Certain triggers may override your gene expression, silencing a bad gene or promoting a good gene.

I consider epigenomics to be good news. It means that you can get your body to work for you instead of against you. By making lifestyle changes, such as reducing your alcohol consumption, exercising more, and losing weight, you can potentially encourage a gene that tells your body to make more of the "good" estrogens instead of the "less good" estrogens.[39] Overall, there's no change in your DNA sequence, but nongenetic triggers can cause your genes to behave, or express themselves, differently. This is where being proactive establishes your hormone cure.

Look no further than the Amish for a good example of a trigger determining gene expression. This hardworking group of people has a high incidence of a particular obesity gene known as FTO—yet very few Amish are obese. Why? Because each day, they labor on their farms for three hours or more. The hard physical work keeps the obesity gene from expressing obesity.

The Bottom Line on Mammograms

After being told for years that women should have annual mammograms starting at age forty, you may have read about the dramatic turnaround in recommendations for mammogram screenings that occurred in 2009.[40] The respected epidemiology group U.S. Preventive Services Task Force (USPSTF) now recommends that after age fifty, women should have a mammogram every two years. This is a congressionally mandated panel of independent experts who systematically review our best evidence in the area of primary care and prevention.[41] I trust these people. Turns out that having more mammograms over the years may lead to more unnecessary biopsies (because of false positives) and perhaps increased damage to breast tissue from radiation.

Exceptions to the two-year rule are women with an increased risk of developing breast cancer, including women who have a strong family history of breast cancer, bear the genes BRCA 1 or 2, or take antidepressants.

Another exception is women with dense breasts, in which case you may want to have your mammograms more frequently and the first mammogram done earlier.[42] Make sure your mammographer is checking for "percent of fibroglandular volume," an objective measure of how much white is on your mammogram (density on an X-ray) as opposed to black space (tissue that is not dense, such as fluid). This has been shown to predict breast cancer risk better than other measures of density or risk factors alone.[43]

Antiestrogen Prescriptions, Friend or Foe?

Wouldn't it be great if a magic pill existed to prevent breast cancer? Recently, the *New York Times* reported on a new drug often prescribed to prevent breast cancer in women. The drug, exemestane (the brand name is Aromasin), joins the class of drugs including tamoxifen and raloxifene, which are FDA-approved for prevention of breast cancer.

Although tamoxifen and raloxifene have been shown to help prevent this kind of cancer, they are rarely used for this purpose. That's because they can cause serious side effects, such as blood clots, uterine polyps, and even endometrial cancer. You may wonder why in the world a doctor would prescribe a pill to prevent breast cancer that actually causes another type of cancer, and I completely agree with the illogic of that practice. That's why there's such controversy about the prescription medications now available to help prevent the downstream effects of excess estrogen and another situation where discussing risks and benefits with your clinician is the best option.

Paul Gross, the lead author of a study showing the benefit of exemestane, considers it "a very safe therapy that looks highly effective in preventing breast cancer." While it may be safe, exemestane drops your estrogen to almost nothing. As a result, my patients report that while taking the drug, their skin sags, they can't focus, their libido drops, and their memory is shot. They say it makes them feel "neutered." The million-dollar question here is, at what cost are women willing to endure the risks associated with these types of drugs?

I have found that answers rarely lie in a bottle of pills, and I follow instead my great-grandmother's bidding to find the internal solution rather than resorting to external prescriptions. Prescription pills are often more complicated and dangerous than the drugmakers and some physicians want you to believe. And there's more: once a prescription drug is approved for a particular purpose, such as breast-cancer prevention, it often takes five to ten years before we have a full grasp of the side effects and adverse reactions.

My opinion is that when it comes to lowering excess estrogens and reducing risk of breast, endometrial, and cervical cancer, effective lifestyle and nutritional strategies are infinitely less risky than lesser-known prescription medications. Like everything in life, positive results often require a little work.

The Solution: The Gottfried Protocol for Excess Estrogen

Step 1: Targeted Lifestyle Changes and Nutraceuticals

Reduce alcohol. We know that alcohol raises your level of estrogen and can disrupt the function of the liver. Even one glass of wine a day increases breast cancer risk by 11 percent. Yikes! If you have five or more symptoms of excess estrogen from the questionnaire in chapter 1, I recommend fewer than four servings a week. Better yet, stick to a glass of wine only on a special occasion, and you'll be good to go.

Cut caffeine. In premenopausal American women, diet sodas and green tea raise estradiol levels. Yet Japanese women lower their estradiol levels with green tea, suggesting that race modifies your estrogen metabolism, perhaps explaining why Japanese women have a lower risk of breast cancer.[44] I am a fan of eliminating caffeine, both to balance your estrogen levels and to calm your cortisol.

Avoid xenoestrogens. As I hope I've shown you, endocrine disruptors such as bisphenol-A and phthalates can cause havoc. Do what you can to minimize your exposure to environmental toxins. Avoid canned food, plastic food containers, and fish with a high mercury content. Take off your shoes when you go inside. Buy organic when you can, especially fruits and vegetables that don't have skin you have to peel. All of these steps can add up.

Eat less meat and dairy from conventionally raised animals. After menopause, consumption of red meat can increase your breast cancer risk by 22 percent.[45] Dairy consumption after menopause correlates with higher estradiol levels.[46] When you eat red meat, choose organic, grass-fed beef, and I recommend eating it the way author Michael Pollan suggests: as a condiment (reduce quantity).

Consume more prunes. Perhaps the advice of your grand-mother was spot on: consumption of prunes has been shown to reduce 16-alpha-hydroxy-estrone, the "less-good" estrogen associated with breast and endometrial cancer.[47]

Close the fiber gap. We know that increased fiber will lower your estrogen levels and likely reduce your risk of breast cancer.[48] However, premenopausal women respond differently from post-menopausal women.[49] Regardless of age, I recommend that you consume 35 to 45 grams of fiber per day as part of a healthy food plan; most women only consume about 13 grams per day. Even with seven or more servings of fresh fruits and vegetables per day, most women need medicinal fiber, taken as a supplement.

Lose weight. If you are obese or overweight, weight loss will reduce your excess estrogen levels and lower your risk of breast cancer and other conditions.[50] It also will protect your body from a number of ailments associated with carrying around extra weight. Aim for a body mass index of 21 to 25.

Exercise regularly. I know you know this. Exercise decreases estrogen levels, lowers risk of breast cancer, and helps you make more of the good estrogens.[51] It also makes you feel good and lowers stress.

Go to sleep by ten p.m. We know that going to sleep by ten p.m. provides optimal production of melatonin, a hormone that lowers estradiol. Blind women have a much higher production of melatonin than women with normal eyesight do, and their risk of breast cancer is 50 percent lower.

Take DIM. Di-indolemethane (DIM) is the most potent promoter of 2-hydroxylase, the enzyme that helps to correct dysestrogenism by making more 2-hydroxy-estrone and 2-hydroxy-estradiol. In other words, DIM has been shown to favor the production of protective estrogens and reduce bad estrogens. Overall, DIM lowers your excess estrogen. This is not nutraceutical mumbo jumbo. One randomized trial showed a significant improvement in abnormal Pap smears among women given DIM versus a placebo.[52]

DIM occurs naturally in the Brassica, or cruciferous, vegetables, such as cabbage, broccoli, Brussels sprouts, and cauliflower. My patients often ask, "Can't I just eat more broccoli?" One study showed that eating 500 grams a day of broccoli does improve your 2:16 ratio, or good to bad estrogen ratio, by 30 percent.[53] In postmenopausal women, however, every 10-gram increase in consumption of Brassica vegetables is associated with an 8 percent increase in the 2:16 ratio—a positive outcome.[54]

Unfortunately, you have to eat bushels of Brussels sprouts to benefit your estrogen balance. You can ingest DIM in a capsule or tablet. The dosage is approximately 200 mg/day. Higher doses do not result in higher blood levels.[55] The patented version, made by BioResponse Nutrients, and also available from Integrative Therapeutics, has been shown to be the most stable, bioavailable (available to your cells when you consume it), and effective.[56] If you have five or more symptoms of estrogen overload, I recommend taking DIM at the dose recommended on the bottle, which is usually 200 mg per day.

FROM THE FILES OF SARA GOTTFRIED, MD

Patient: Tania

Age: Forty-two

Plea for help: "I want to rock my forties, but constantly fall short. I'm more agitated, more frustrated; little things get to me. My attention and productivity suck. I'm too young to feel so old. What's the problem?"

Tania is the HR director for a start-up tech company in the Bay Area. She overworks, overeats, overdrinks, overdiets, and overprovides to her two young kids and husband. Her blood pressure crept up since her first child, and she never lost the baby weight. She's gaining weight, in fact, and feels burned out. Other symptoms of excess estrogen include mood swings, headaches, rosacea, heavy periods, and bloating. I suspected the excess estrogen was related to the high stress of grueling work combined with the demands of motherhood.

Treatment protocol: I started Tania on DIM, the extract of cruciferous vegetables that helps lower estrogens. She took a six-week mental
health leave from her job and began an exercise regimen of Pilates and
the elliptical trainer four days a week. She adopted the Paleolista Food
Plan—more lean protein, no refined carbs, and vegetables, vegetables,
vegetables—with clear guidelines as to types and quantities of food.

Results: After six weeks, Tania had lost 15 pounds and felt terrific.
Her family-practice doctor was delighted with her lower blood pressure
and began weaning her off diuretics. No more headaches. Periods were
lighter. Energy level? Dramatically better.

Step 2: Herbal/Botanical Therapies

Eat seaweed. In Japan, where women have a sixfold lower risk
of breast cancer, people eat seaweed regularly. A randomized trial
looked at Alaria, a type of brown alga. After consuming 5 grams per
day for seven weeks, the group that took Alaria had significantly
lowered estrogen levels.[57] However, Alaria contains iodine, and
most people in the United States are not iodine-deficient. Iodine
consumption may trigger problems in people with Hashimoto's or
autoimmune thyroiditis, so consult your doctor if you have this condition. If you know that you do not have antibodies to the thyroid,
you can probably consume small amounts of Alaria, but keep in
mind that the recommended daily allowance of iodine is just 150
micrograms per day (less in children).

Supplement resveratrol. Resveratrol is a potent botanical—
derived from grapes, berries, and other plants—that helps direct
estrogen metabolism away from the less-good estrogen, 4-hydroxy-
estrone, and toward the more protective pathways. Another antioxidant, N-acetylcysteine, does this to a lesser extent. Although the
combination is synergistic, this has been shown only in in vitro
studies of cells.[58] In another study, resveratrol was shown to block
the estrogen receptor.[59] I recommend resveratrol as an antioxidant,
but only from food sources, such as grapes and blueberries, not
from wine.

Take turmeric (*Curcuma longa*). Turmeric is best known as the ingredient in curry that adds the yellow color. Turmeric has been shown to counter the proliferative effect of estrogen on cancer cells.[60] Turmeric is one of the most potent anti-inflammatory agents we know. So I believe it's a good idea to take it. Sprinkle a teaspoon of organic turmeric on whatever you're eating for lunch or dinner. If a tablespoon per day of turmeric on your food is not your idea of haute cuisine, then consider a supplement. Here's a favorite: Meriva, a patented delivery form of turmeric phytosome, which contains *Curcuma longa* root and phospholipid extract, available as Curcumax Pro from Integrative Therapeutics or Curcuma-Sorb from Pure Encapsulations. Follow directions on the bottle (for Curcumax, it's one tablet twice per day following meals; for CurcumaSorb, it's one 250 mg capsule, up to six times per day in between meals).

Hop to it (*Humulus lupulus*). You've probably heard of hops. It's the aromatic herb that flavors beer. Turns out that one of its components, xanthohumol, is active against breast, colon, and ovarian cancer cells. Hops have been shown to reduce estrogen levels via aromatase, an enzyme that converts testosterone into estrogen.[61] This doesn't mean you should run out and buy a six-pack. Integrative Therapeutics has hops in its Revitalizing Sleep Formula, a supplement I sometimes take to help get some shut-eye. This supplement contains 30 mg of hops as Humulus Lupulus Flower Extract 66:1. Another option is the same company's AM/PM Perimenopausal Formula, which contains 100 mg of hops in the bedtime formulation. Other hops-containing sleep formulas include Tori Hudson's Sleepblend and Julian Whitaker's Restful Night Essentials.

Step 3: Bioidentical hormones

Melatonin. Melatonin lowers estrogen and may prevent breast cancer.[62] Low melatonin has also been linked to a greater risk of endometrial cancer, another estrogen-dependent cancer.[63] I recommend 0.5 to 1 mg at night if you have sleep problems.

FROM THE FILES OF SARA GOTTFRIED, MD

Patient: Maggie

Age: Fifty-four

Plea for help: "*My fibroids are growing, and I'm bleeding all the time. Help!*"

Maggie is a philanthropist and an activist. With her many board positions and activities, she wants her mind to stay alert and work quickly, and she believes estrogen contributes to her executive functioning. After going through menopause and reading Suzanne Somers's books, she became interested in the Wiley Protocol.

A pelvic ultrasound showed that since her previous ultrasound, Maggie's fibroids had increased in size—a sign of excess estrogen. Even after menopause, most women menstruate while on the Wiley Protocol.

Treatment protocol: Dropping her estradiol fourfold from the Wiley dosing, I recommended a standard dose of 0.05 mg estradiol patch (also bioidentical but a much smaller dose, and approved by the FDA for women with menopausal symptoms), which she changed twice a week. Maggie also started taking DIM (see page 172).

Results: Maggie experienced a few days of estrogen withdrawal, after which she adjusted to the estradiol patch. After three months, another ultrasound showed that her fibroids had shrunk by more than 50 percent, back to the previous year's dimensions. I recommended getting off the estradiol patch at that point, but Maggie prefers her quality of life on estrogen, so we plan to monitor her every six to twelve months for fibroid growth and to discuss the risks, benefits, and alternatives to hormone therapy. That's how frequently I like to meet with my patients to discuss the latest findings with hormone therapy and to examine the body for changes.

Estrogen in Balance

When you have your estrogen in the sweet spot, you feel feminine and content. Your moods are steadier, your face is clear, and your body feels well rested.

- With lubrication and sufficient blood flow to the genitals for youthful arousal, you respond sexually, and your orgasms feel as robust as when you started enjoying them regularly.
- Your breasts feel normal in size, neither too big (excess estrogen) nor droopy or pancakelike (low estrogen).
- If you're cycling, you maneuver through your menstrual cycle noticing ovulation, but not burdened by ovarian or breast cysts or painful, heavy periods.
- If you have fibroids or endometriosis, you enter "remission." Your symptoms resolve. Your fibroids or endometriosis starts shrinking.

CHAPTER 7

LOW ESTROGEN: ARE YOU DRY AND CRANKY?

Estrogen is the hormone that makes and keeps you feminine. With more than three hundred jobs, estrogen is the ultimate multi-tasker. Among hundreds of other duties, it builds and maintains the structure and function of the vaginal, urethral, and vulvar tissues; it stimulates and develops the female reproductive organs, preparing and maintaining the uterus for pregnancy; and along with its partner, progesterone, it regulates the menstrual cycle.

As I described estrogen's intricate tango dance with progesterone in the previous chapter, I pointed out that it is much more common to have too much estrogen than too little, at least until your last year of perimenopause. I think of estrogen as a woman's life force, which means having too little can feel like a slow death. One patient with low estrogen told me she was "dry, cranky, and barely holding it together."

> Before I came to see you, my doctor heard my litany of symptoms, patted my hand, and told me I needed to get used to the idea of aging. He said, "You're just not going to look as good as you used to." I wanted to punch him, but I'm so unsure of what's happening that I no longer trust my instincts. I'm weary from the vigilance. (Patricia, age forty-six)

While most women don't notice the subtle dips in estrogen as they age, some women are exquisitely sensitive. If you've had a child and remember going through an emotional roller coaster postpartum, that was just a preview of coming attractions in perimenopause, which typically begins sometime between age thirty-five and age fifty. I find that women who struggle with mood swings after giving birth are particularly at risk. Some women are extremely sensitive to their estrogen levels, which can be measured with the same accuracy as thyroid or progesterone. Sensitivity to estrogen makes you more vulnerable to emotional swings in response to estrogen upheaval, which occurs most commonly at puberty, at postpartum, and during perimenopause. And if you're simultaneously postpartum and in perimenopause . . . well, consider the estrogen patch your new tattoo and put your gynecologist on speed dial. This is a situation where the benefits may outweigh the risks.

The Science of Low Estrogen

Caution: If you can't focus because of lack of estrogen in your brain, skip the following section and move directly to "The Solution: The Gottfried Protocol for Low Estrogen" (page 188).

When I use the term *estrogen,* most of the time I'm referring to *estradiol,* the estrogen in highest concentration during the reproductive years. From puberty until perimenopause, 80 percent of the estrogen you make is estradiol. Ten percent is *estriol,* the main estrogen of pregnancy. The other 10 percent is *estrone,* the main estrogen of menopause. Low estrogen can affect some of the areas most near and dear to a woman's heart: appetite and weight, sleep, sex, and fertility.

Weight and appetite. Low estrogen stimulates appetite. Researchers from Yale found that estradiol uses the same biochemical pathways in the body as leptin, a hormone released by fat that, when activated, pushes your "hunger button" and tells you that you need food.[1] When your estrogen levels are in the normal range, leptin is kept from triggering your appetite. Conversely, the lower your estrogen, the hungrier you become. Here's what happened to Catherine, age forty-two: "I noticed an increased amount of hunger starting about three years ago, at age thirty-nine. I would wake up in the middle of the night needing to eat to go back to sleep. Now that I'm on estradiol cream, I smear a bit on after waking up at night, and the hunger goes away."

Sex. Estradiol makes the genital skin sensitive, full of innervation and blood supply. When a woman's estradiol is low, the hormonal-control centers in her brain assume that she's in danger, and the last thing she needs is to become pregnant. So the vagina becomes dry, and the nerves that densely populate the clitoris, G-spot, and labia minora (the inner lips of the vulva) start to disappear. Sometimes the elastic, compliant, blood-supplied tissues dry up like a desert. Getting wet feels like a distant memory, and orgasms may be so subtle that you barely notice them. One patient wryly remarked, "It's as if there's a pile of blankets between my husband's attempts to get me going and my clitoris. It takes so much more effort. Why bother?"

Mood. Estradiol fills your tank with serotonin, the feel-good neurotransmitter. When estradiol starts to fade in perimenopause, serotonin levels drop. This can sometimes lead to depression.[2] In fact, many of my perimenopausal patients tell me they feel that they're going crazy, meaning that their moods have suddenly become unpredictable and stormy.

Bones. Bone loss, whether mild (osteopenia) or more serious (osteoporosis), is a problem for women with low estrogen, especially after menopause. Many doctors will monitor your estradiol levels to assess if you've got enough estrogen in your bloodstream to keep your bones healthy, dense, and flexible.

Hot flashes. Night sweats. Insomnia. We don't completely understand the mechanism behind hot flashes and night sweats. But as many premenopausal women know, the thermoregulatory control in the body gets wiggy and unpredictable as estradiol levels start to decline.

―――――DR. SARA'S 5 COOL TIPS FOR HOT FLASHES―――――

Hot flashes and night sweats are a common recipe for disrupted sleep and unhappy women in perimenopause and menopause. Eighty-five percent of Western women experience them. Here are my suggestions:

1. Paced breathing—this cuts flashes by 44 percent! Not too shabby. Breathe deeply twenty minutes twice per day with a five-second inhale, a ten-second hold, and a five-second exhale.[3] I do this while driving, which is not how the researchers intended you to apply their methodology, but I'm a working mom who multitasks.

2. Acupuncture—I'm a fan of outsourcing your neuroendocrine repair, at least in part. Acupuncture has been shown to reduce hot flashes and night sweats.

3. Vitamin E—proven to reduce hot flashes in several trials.

4. Pollen extract—an herbal remedy called Femal was shown to reduce flashes and improve quality of life.[4]

5. Rhubarb—who knew? Proven to reduce hot flashes in two trials.

Subfertility. Infertility. Diminished ovarian reserve. If you've been trying to get pregnant for less than a year, you're considered subfertile, rather than infertile. However, if you are aged thirty-five or older, infertility is diagnosed after trying to conceive in earnest for six months. Once you reach menopause, of course, you are infertile. Many of my patients come to me with diagnoses of premature menopause (diminished ovarian reserve).

Low Estrogen and the Connection to Your Ovaries and Eggs

Fertility and estrogen are inextricably linked. Indeed, the female estrogen factory is located in the ovaries. The factory reaches peak production when we're in our midtwenties, then output starts to decline slowly. After age twenty-five, it takes a few years before fertility starts to wane, usually around ages thirty-two to thirty-nine. The first phase of perimenopause—the two to ten years of symptoms leading to the final menstrual period—is heralded by low progesterone. The most dramatic decline in estrogen occurs immediately before your final menstrual period.[5]

It's important to note, though, that low estrogen is common in women in their twenties, thirties, and forties. Subtle changes in the earlier years, such as night sweats before your period or dryness in the vagina, could be a tipoff that your estrogen levels are declining.

Women are born with a finite number of eggs, generally one to two million. By puberty, we're down to 300,000 to 500,000 eggs. That's because of apoptosis, or programmed cell death. The rate of apoptosis varies with each woman, which accounts for the difference in age at menopause. By age thirty-five, 60 percent of a woman's eggs are ripe: ready and able to be fertilized. By forty-five, that number drops to 15 percent. In the United States, on average, menopause occurs at age fifty-one. As you run low on ripe eggs, the communication system between your brain and ovaries figures this out and raises the hormone called follicle-stimulating hormone (FSH).

Most Western women ovulate four hundred times over the course of their lives, far more than ever before in our history. Most women have plenty of ripe eggs for their reproductive plans, but some women run out of ripe, fertilizable eggs before they turn forty, hence the term *premature menopause*. By contrast, women in other cultures may ovulate just seventy times, because of multiple births beginning at an early age, plus long periods of breast-feeding, during which ovulation is suppressed.

Low Estrogen: Test Yourself?

The standard test for egg supply used to be measuring your follicle-stimulating hormone (FSH) and estradiol on Day 3 of your menstrual cycle, and/or your antral-follicle count, which tells you how many ripe eggs you have in each ovary. FSH can vary from cycle to cycle, so I recommend taking multiple tests over three to six months.

FSH is predictive of diminished ovarian reserve or menopause only if it's high. Mounting evidence suggests that the most accurate way to measure ovarian reserve is a relatively newer test based on your levels of anti-mullerian hormone (AMH). AMH is a protein, made in the follicles of the ovaries, which recruits and coordinates the formation of egg follicles. As a woman runs out of ripe eggs, her AMH falls. It seems that AMH is more reliable for detecting diminished ovarian reserve than its predecessors; your AMH can also predict your age at menopause.[6]

Here's why it's important to know your hormone levels. If you really are prematurely menopausal—that is, menopausal prior to age forty—and want to have a child, knowing your hormone levels will help you to figure out what to do next. (Egg donors become the best bet.) If you are subfertile, trying and failing to get pregnant over the course of less than a year, estradiol and FSH levels may help determine an important root cause, and again, help you determine how to proceed.

If pregnancy isn't an issue but you have other symptoms of low estrogen, wouldn't you want the knowledge that could prevent you from feeling lousy and experiencing adverse symptoms such as thinning hair and painful sex?

Many women ask their gynecologists for a hormone test and receive a variation on the same reply: "Hormone tests haven't been shown to be helpful." Or "Hormone levels are erratic, so the tests are of little value." I beg to differ. Most gynecologists wouldn't think twice about ordering hormone tests for women who are infertile. Why withhold testing from women who have precursors to these conditions, such as night sweats before menses, or who are simply curious about their egg quality? The data show that it's as easy to compare your current and previous levels of estrogen as it is to compare your cholesterol levels.[7] What doctor would hesitate to check your cholesterol?

If you are still menstruating, I recommend asking your doctor for a blood test on Day 3 of your cycle. If he or she argues, stand firm. It's your body, your health, and your future at stake.

The Estrogen-Food Connection

Here's a secret that I didn't learn at Harvard Medical School: food impacts estradiol levels. Studies bear this out. For instance, vegetarians have lower estrogen levels than omnivores and lifelong vegetarians have a lower risk of breast cancer.[8] Japanese women, who suffer from hot flashes far less than American women and have lower rates of breast cancer—and lower estradiol levels—eat more whole soy and less meat.[9] Overall, women in the United States have a five-fold increased risk of breast cancer compared with Japanese women who eat a traditional diet, which has less fat and more fiber. Sadly, the risk of breast cancer among Japanese women has been rising over the past three decades as their traditional diet has eroded.[10]

How much you eat can also affect your estrogen. Lower body fat can cause lower estradiol levels, which can lead to amenorrhea, or cessation of menses for three months or longer. When a woman's body fat is lower than 21 percent of total body mass (normal range depends on age, but for women aged twenty to thirty-nine, I recommend 21 to 33 percent; for women over forty and older, I recommend 23 to 34 percent), the hormonal-control centers in her brain keep her from making enough estrogen to ovulate or to build up her uterine wall. You see this in women suffering from anorexia nervosa, bulimia, and other eating disorders. Extreme exercise or training is another cause of decreased body fat, and is the reason many competitive athletes don't get their periods.

While this may sound appealing to some women, such as young athletes, it can have long-term consequences, among them weak bones and perhaps cognitive deficits. Additionally, exercise-associated amenorrhea may be linked to problems in blood vessels that may counter the exercise-induced benefits to the heart and accelerate the risk of atherosclerosis, the disease behind heart attacks and strokes.[11] If you are younger than forty and experience three months without a period, you should see a physician for a complete evaluation.

The Gluten Iceberg: Is Pizza Causing Your Problems?

Not all estrogen/eating issues are as dramatic as anorexia, bulimia, or overexercising. Lurking below the radar, despite causing a host of symptoms, is gluten intolerance, possibly as full-blown celiac disease or as a milder form. Gluten is a protein found in most pastas, bread, crackers, pizza crust, and the like. More than 1 percent of the American and European populations—that means at least three million Americans—have celiac disease, a genetically based intestinal intolerance to gluten that is permanent. Most of these folks don't know they have this condition. In fact, 97 percent are undiagnosed and untreated. An additional 18 million Americans have gluten intolerance, meaning they don't have an immune response to gluten, but suffer various problems depending on their sensitivity and how much gluten they consume.

Typically, problems with gluten cause diarrhea, abdominal pain, and bloating. In women, however, sometimes the only tipoff is bone loss, irregular cycles, or difficulty getting pregnant. Gluten intolerance has been linked to altered estrogen levels and consequences such as amenorrhea (no periods for several months), infertility, and diminished ovarian reserve.[12] According to one study, in more than 19 percent of women with celiac disease, the main symptom was amenorrhea or another menstrual disorder.[13]

Short version: imbalanced estrogen is a common side effect of gluten intolerance.

Celiacs also have a greater risk of premature menopause and infertility, which can be reversed by eating a gluten-free diet. Several reports in the medical literature show that for women who are sensitive to gluten and suffering from either amenorrhea or diminished ovarian reserve, going gluten-free can reverse these conditions.[14]

The best blood-test screening for gluten intolerance appears to be measuring your level of antitransglutaminase antibodies. Tissue transglutaminase (tTg) is a mouthful, but it's important. It's an enzyme that modifies gliadin, a protein found in gluten. Essentially, it measures how hard your immune system is fighting off this particular protein associated with wheat. If your level of antitransglutaminase antibodies is elevated, you can get a definitive diagnosis of celiac disease by having a gastroenterologist snake a tube down to your stomach to get a small biopsy of your intestine and test it for signs of gluten problems.[15]

————WHY ESTROGEN LEVELS DROP————

Here's the complete, Harvard Medical School–certified list of reasons that estrogen levels fall:

- **Perimenopause and menopause.**
- **Hypogonadism.** Your gonads (ovaries in women, testicles in men) aren't making the hormones as they used to. Medically put, the gonads have "decreased functional activity." This may be genetic, such as Turner's syndrome, in which a woman is missing one X chromosome.
- **Hypopituitarism.** Decreased production of one of the eight hormones that modulate your endocrine glands, such as follicle-

stimulating hormone (FSH). Your pituitary is a neighbor to your hypothalamus and it produces the eight hormones mentioned in chapter 2.

• **Hypothalamic defects.** Decreased production of estrogen due to a problem with the hypothalamus, which is part of the control system for your ovaries. An example of this is Kallman's syndrome, a genetic disorder associated with loss of smell and lack of gonadotropin-releasing hormone, which results in low estrogen.

• **Pregnancy failure.** When a baby is not carried to term— which occurs in 15 to 20 percent of pregnancies—the mother's hormone levels drop, and her estrogen levels may plummet temporarily as a result.

• **Delivery of placenta after childbirth.** This temporarily causes you to enter a menopausal state because of your low levels of estrogen and progesterone—and lasts until your period returns.

• **Breast-feeding.** Depending on frequency, volume, and duration, breast-feeding lowers your estrogen levels and may prevent ovulation.

• **Anorexia nervosa, bulimia, and other eating disorders.** Lower body fat can cause lower estradiol levels, which can lead to amenorrhea, or a cessation of menses, for three months or longer.

• **Extreme exercise or training.** This also causes lower body-fat levels.

• **Gluten intolerance.** This is an increasingly common reason for estrogen-related problems such as amenorrhea, infertility, and diminished ovarian reserve.

The Solution: The Gottfried Protocol for Low Estrogen

Step 1: Targeted Lifestyle Changes and Nutraceuticals

Avoid coffee and other caffeine-loaded treats. Both caffeine and coffee have been shown to lower estradiol levels in premenopausal women.[16] I recommend decaffeinated coffee and herbal teas, which also may help reduce hot flashes or improve sleep if you choose an herb such as rhubarb or valerian. Another coffee alternative I enjoy is Dandy Blend, derived from dandelion greens, which is detoxifying.

Cut out gluten. Because of the link between gluten sensitivity and diminished ovarian reserve, I encourage women with low estradiol before the age of forty to stop eating gluten. There are many palatable alternatives, but the idea is to shift to whole, unprocessed foods, such as fruits and vegetables with lean protein at each meal, and gluten-free carbohydrates, such as brown rice or quinoa. Ideally, you'll eat five to seven servings of fresh fruit and vegetables per day.

Eat more whole soy. Soy is controversial—if you get a hundred nutritionists in a room, at least half would say it's evil, particularly soy derived from or contaminated by genetically modified organisms. Nevertheless, studies in Asia of women who eat whole and fermented soy show *reduced symptoms of low estrogen,* such as fewer hot flashes, and lower rates of breast cancer and osteoporosis.[17] Remember, Asian women eat less fat and more fiber than American women. Perhaps, like me, you're wondering why the paradox: why do Japanese women, whose diets compared with American women seem to favor lower estradiol levels, demonstrate *fewer symptoms* of low estrogen? Scientists hypothesize that the paradox relates to the higher consumption of whole soy. Soy is structurally similar to estrogen, so it makes sense that it acts like a weak estrogen in the body. One large meta-analysis, in which several studies are combined to address a particular question, showed that consuming soy brought no change in estradiol levels in premenopause and a small increase in estradiol after menopause.[18] However, studies of soy intake in Western women have shown conflicting results. At present there's insufficient support that dietary soy and extracts improve hot flashes or night sweats.[19] My opinion is that the paradoxical data mean that we're missing some important variable or factor (genetic? cultural?). Perhaps there are significant differences in how the various soy products and extracts show up in the body, or perhaps different ethnic groups are genetically programmed to handle soy differently, or perhaps *all of the above*.

Soy lowers FSH level in premenopause and can lengthen your menstrual cycle by up to one day.[20] Japanese women get soy in the miso soup traditionally eaten with breakfast, lunch, and dinner; they also eat far more tofu than American women. Try adding fresh organic tofu to your salad or stir-fry; sauté it in olive oil with fresh herbs and garlic for a light side dish. My recommendation: eat whole soy in moderation, less than twice per week.

Add flaxseeds to your meals. Flaxseeds contain lignans, one of the major classes of phytoestrogens, which are estrogenlike chemicals that also serve as antioxidants. One study showed that eating 2 tablespoons of flaxseeds twice per day (approximately 30 grams total) for six weeks reduced hot flashes—a key symptom of low estrogen—by half, and diminished the intensity by 57 percent.[21] Other studies have been inconclusive. Because flax also offers a good dose of fiber (at about 8 grams of fiber in 4 tablespoons), I believe, despite the need for more data, that flaxseeds are a healthful addition to your diet if you're low in estradiol. Flaxseeds have a nutty texture; they're available in most grocery stores. I add them to my cereal in the morning and to anti-inflammatory green smoothies.

Orgasm more. Female orgasm and sexual stimulation raise estradiol levels in women who are premenopausal.[22] This illustrates the "use it or lose it" concept: regular sexual connection and orgasm stimulate the blood flow that helps massage, soften, and thicken the tissue of the outer (vulva) and inner (vagina) pleasure equipment. Orgasm raises oxytocin, which works with estrogen in the female body to buffer stress and lower cortisol, and help women feel more connected and loving. One practice that I prescribe is Orgasmic Meditation, a combination of Buddhist practice and orgasm. Anecdotally, women who practice Orgasmic Meditation have fewer symptoms of low estrogen after menopause than women who do not.[23]

Don't exercise too much! Exercise helps low-estrogen symptoms only if you are lean. Women who are overweight can actually increase their vasomotor symptoms—such as hot flashes and night sweats—if they do too hard a workout. If you are overweight or prone to injury, it's better to walk briskly than to run; to jog one mile three times a week instead of six miles four times a week; to spin or bicycle at a moderate speed.

Get needled. Acupuncture has been shown to raise estradiol levels, although not sufficiently to help with vaginal dryness or bladder infections. It does reduce hot flashes, and it may be as effective as hormone therapy when acupuncture is combined with the Chinese herbal medicine Kun Boa Wan.[24] Although results are mixed, newer data suggest that acupuncture is worth a try.[25] Since there's no significant risk associated with acupuncture—not to mention a two-thousand-plus-year track record of safety—you might want to see if it works for you. I recommend weekly sessions for at least eight to ten weeks.

Pry open a pomegranate. Some women in menopause swear by pomegranate in one form or another for the treatment of symptoms of low estrogen. One trial showed that pomegranate seed oil at a dose of 30 mg twice per day for twelve weeks reduced hot flashes significantly, although the placebo treatment did as well. However, twelve weeks after treatment was completed, hot flashes were significantly improved in the pomegranate group but not the placebo group, suggesting a real effect.[26]

Take vitamin E. The oldest remedy in the book for certain symptoms of low estrogen, including hot flashes, vaginal dryness, and mood swings, is vitamin E. Reaching way back to the 1940s, studies found vitamin E at doses of 50–400 IU per day effectively decreased hot flashes and other low-estrogen problems compared to placebo. According to one study, supplementing with vitamin E was shown to increase blood supply to the vaginal wall and improve menopausal symptoms. You need four weeks of vitamin E to experience the effect.

Be magnanimous with magnesium. Among breast cancer patients, magnesium was shown to reduce hot flashes, fatigue, and distress, all common symptoms of low estrogen.[27] In this study, women took 400 mg of magnesium oxide every day for four weeks, escalating to 800 mg if they needed more because their hot flashes persisted. Higher doses can cause loose bowels, though, so check with your doctor before going beyond 400 mg per day.

Step 2: Herbal Therapies

Add maca to your smoothie. The magical herb maca (*Lepidum meyenii*) has consistently been shown to increase estradiol in menopausal women, and helps with insomnia, depression, memory, concentration, energy, hot flashes, and vaginal dryness, as well as improved body mass index and bone density.[28] Additionally, maca has been shown to improve libido and to lower anxiety and depression, all of which are symptoms of low estrogen.[29] It has been shown to help with the sexual side effects of a type of antidepressant called selective serotonin reuptake inhibitor (SSRI).[30] You can buy maca extract at your local health food store, in both a capsule and a liquid tincture. The common dose is 2,000 mg/day. Maca has a malty taste that I prefer to mask with 1 to 2 tablespoons of raw cocoa powder in my smoothies for breakfast.

Brew *Pueraria lobata* or *Pueraria minifica*. *Pueraria lobata* (PL) is a traditional Chinese herbal remedy for menopausal symptoms as well as an ingredient in traditional preparations for conditions affecting menopausal women, such as osteoporosis, coronary heart disease, and some hormone-dependent cancers. The scientific basis may be its phytoestrogen action on receptors for estrogen. In randomized trials, PL has been shown to reduce bone loss and, after two months, to improve cholesterol levels by lowering the bad cholesterol (LDL) and raising the good cholesterol (HDL).[31]

Say "right on" to rhubarb. I grew rhubarb in my medicinal garden until it took up too much square footage, similar to how cortisol dominated my hormonal garden. Siberian rhubarb (*Rheum rhaponticum*) contains active ingredients that lock in to estrogen receptors. One formulation of rhubarb, available in Germany for twenty years, is now available in the United States as rhaponticin (brand name Phytoestrol). Randomized trials show benefits for women with hot flashes.[32]

Take the herbal combo. St. John's wort, a perennial herb, had been recorded for its medicinal uses since as far back as ancient Greece. The yellow flowering tops are used to prepare teas, tablets, capsules, liquid extract, and topical preparations for mild depression, anxiety, and sleep disorders. In a randomized trial of premenopausal, perimenopausal, and menopausal women, hot flashes were seen to diminish after four weeks of treatment with this herb.[33] It has also been shown to improve sexual satisfaction in women in menopause.[34] St. John's wort is recommended at 300 mg three times a day. Note: you should consult your doctor first if you are taking an antidepressant.

Black cohosh, a member of the buttercup family, was used by Native Americans for a host of problems, including gynecological disorders. It appears most effective in improving symptoms of low estradiol when combined with St. John's wort.[35] The recommended dose of black cohosh is 40 to 80 mg/day. Higher doses may be associated with liver damage, so you should take the lowest dose that helps your symptoms. (Signs of liver damage include nausea, vomiting, dark urine, and jaundice.)

Breast cancer patients undergoing treatment with tamoxifen tend to have worsening of hot flashes and night sweats. In one study of such patients, black cohosh alone was shown to reduce hot flashes, sweating, sleep problems, and anxiety, although urogenital and musculoskeletal complaints remained.[36]

Butter yourself up? There's anecdotal evidence that, for women whose symptoms of low estradiol include vaginal dryness, an herbal balm called Shatavari Ghee, from Ayurveda, made from clarified butter and medicinal herbs, can help when applied externally. Shatavari is made from *Asparagus racemosus,* which contains phytoestrogenic activity. The ghee mixture is a popular remedy that you might hear about, but I do not recommend it because the evidence is too inconclusive.

Drink your ginseng. Recently, red ginseng was found to decrease hot flashes on the Kupperman Index and the Menopause Rating Scale, two research tools used to assess menopausal symptoms related to low estrogen.[37] Additionally, red ginseng at a dose of 3 grams per day, versus placebo for twelve weeks, was associated with lowering total cholesterol and low-density lipoprotein, both of which climb as estrogen drops after menopause. A previous study showed that 6 grams per day of red ginseng for thirty days improved cortisol-to-DHEA ratio and quality of life in postmenopausal women with symptoms of fatigue, insomnia, and depression.[38] *Panax ginseng* is known to improve mood and add to a general sense of well-being in postmenopausal women.[39] German health authorities recommend ginseng as a "tonic for invigoration and fortification in times of fatigue and declining capacity for work and concentration."[40] A common dose as an oral pill is 200 mg/day.

Hop to your hops. Hops (*Humulus lupulus*) are used in brewing beer, to balance the sweetness of the malt with a bitter, tangy flavor. They are also used in other beverages as well as in herbal medicines. Hops are approved by the German Commission mentioned above for sleep difficulty, anxiety, and restlessness. (The Germans love their beer, but the commission recommends getting your hops in pill or tablet form.) Hops appear to help with symptoms of both high and low estrogen, as you might recall from chapter 6. Higher doses are usually more effective than lower doses, but with hops, studies show that 100 mg is superior to 250 mg—a good example of the importance of always taking the lowest effective dose possible.

Because of the drop-off in effectiveness, hops may be best as an in-between treatment, while you are waiting for other, more lasting measures to kick in. I often give my patients hops while we're trying other treatments, such as flaxseeds and bioidentical hormones, since those may take six or more weeks to become effective.

Value your valerian. Low-estrogen symptoms such as sleeplessness and anxiety have been treated for centuries with valerian, a medicinal herb with therapeutic uses described by Hippocrates. A new randomized trial in menopausal women showed that valerian at 530 mg of extract improved sleep in 30 percent of treated insomniacs, versus only 4 percent of the placebo-treated group.[41]

Here's more good news: when valerian is taken to help with sleep, there is no documented change in reaction time, concentration, or alertness the next morning.[42] It's recommended that you not combine it with alcohol, because of a theoretical concern that it may make alcohol more toxic. In any event, side effects, which include migraines, dizziness, and gastrointestinal disorders, are very rare.

The skinny on valerian? Take it if your difficulty sleeping is one of your symptoms of low estrogen. Based on the best data, the dosage should be 300 to 600 mg of valerian root extract, usually as a pill, or 2 to 3 grams of dried herbal valerian soaked in a cup of hot water for ten to fifteen minutes, taken thirty minutes to two hours before bedtime. Personally, I take the amount shown to help menopausal women at a dose of 530 mg of root extract.[43]

FROM THE FILES OF SARA GOTTFRIED, MD
Patient: Jennifer
Age: Forty-eight
Plea for help: "Night sweats are ruining my sleep! Hot flashes are ruining my business! I'm the together one in my family—my husband is an artist

and temperamental, and my kids are teenagers—and I cannot stay sane for long without good sleep."

Jennifer is a hairdresser, so neither she nor her clients can tolerate her sweating like she's in spinning class while she's trying to cut and color hair. She has what I would call "an intrusive case" of vasomotor symptoms. Since her mother developed breast cancer while taking Prempro, a drug combination of Premarin, a synthetic estrogen, and Provera, a synthetic form of progesterone (see details in the Introduction), she wanted to avoid hormone therapy.

Treatment protocol: The best herbal therapy to start with is either Remifemin (black cohosh) or AM/PM Perimenopause, which contains black cohosh, valerian, hops, and chasteberry. She chose AM/PM Perimenopause, which contains a different pill for the morning versus the evening, and that appealed to her. The morning dose (conveniently labeled AM) contains black cohosh, green tea, chasteberry, and rhodiola, which I describe in chapter 4 and can sometimes be activating. The evening dose (conveniently labeled PM) contains black cohosh (again), L-theanine, hops, and valerian.

Results: In an e-mail just a month later, Jennifer let me know she was sleeping deeply once again. She was thrilled to be able to do so without taking a hormone, which she feels raised her mother's breast cancer risk.

HERBS THAT DON'T WORK (YET)

Some remedies rumored to help with low estrogen are just that: rumors. Here are the facts. It's possible that these herbs just haven't been studied properly. I'd wait for better evidence.

Dong quai. Used more than twenty centuries ago as a female tonic, dong quai was studied in a three-month randomized, placebo-controlled study of seventy-one women.[44] It showed no benefit for hot flashes or in blood-hormone levels, and no effect on endometrial thickness. Other studies also have shown no estrogenic effects.[45]

Red clover. While most of the data on red clover are mixed, the three largest randomized trials showed no change in or relief of low-estrogen symptoms or in estradiol levels associated with the use of red clover.[46]

Step 3: Bioidentical Hormones

If your symptoms don't resolve with Steps 1 and 2, I urge you to review the risks and benefits of taking estrogen with a trusted clinician who is willing to prescribe hormones.

For women who already have shown a sensitivity to diminishing hormones, the loss of estradiol at menopause may be linked to depression. I believe these women should first be treated with estrogen, not an antidepresssant. In one study, antidepressants were associated with an 11 percent increased risk of breast and ovarian cancer.[47] Another study shows that women respond better to stress after menopause when they have estrogen augmented via an estradiol patch (see below).[48]

Perimenopause and menopause, of course, are much more common reasons to augment the meager amounts of estrogen women produce as they approach their final menstrual period. Why shouldn't these women consider replacing the estrogen their bodies are missing? One of my Mission Ignition (the online teleseries) members framed it this way:

> I have all the classic perimenopause symptoms, and yet even with all I do with nutrition, exercise, and meditation, the impact on my everyday life is significant—muscle fatigue, anxiety, memory, insomnia, libido. Tweaking my chemistry may be my next step, but it's so complex and nuanced, it's hard to know where to start. And, even with updated research, I am still concerned about the long-term health impact of hormone therapy, bioidentical or otherwise. But I also think hormonal imbalance could breed disease. Really, what's worse? Being a ditzy, pudgy, anxious, dull wife or tweaking my internal chemistry a bit for balance and peace of mind? (Melinda, age forty-seven)

Reasons NOT to take estrogen. Estrogen must be prescribed by a clinician, and there are a few important reasons not to take it, as well as some serious risks, which you need to discuss with your doctor. These include pregnancy, heart disease, a history of fibroids or of blood clots in your legs or lungs, undiagnosed vaginal bleeding, active gallbladder disease, severe liver disease (because the liver processes estrogen and sends it to the gut via bile), some types of estrogen-sensitive ovarian cancer, breast cancer, atypical hyperplasia of the breast, and endometrial cancer before the cancer treatment is complete. In some cases, taking estrogen can worsen these conditions.

I am confident recommending estradiol patches to appropriate patients, provided they do not have issues that make them unsafe, such as a history of blood clots or if they are ten years past menopause (beyond ten years from menopause, risk of heart disease rises). Because these patches are approved by the FDA, there is excellent regulatory oversight. Examples are Vivelle Dot and Climara, taken at the lowest doses that relieve symptoms. I've found that, for most of my patients, doses of 0.25 mg or 0.0375 mg work effectively.

Estrogen's neurohormonal benefits. Estrogen's ability to raise serotonin, which is associated with improved mood, sleep, and appetite, is well proven.[49] At the latter half of perimenopause, which normally begins around age forty-three to forty-seven, estrogen withdraws from the daily hormonal menu. Many women find that estrogen withdrawal causes serious mood changes, which we've recently learned is related not just to estrogen levels but also to whether you have the short or long gene for serotonin transportation in the brain. Data from a randomized trial that examined perimenopausal women aged forty to fifty-five who had either major or minor depression showed that the estrogen patch caused remission of symptoms in 68 percent of women assigned to the patch, and 20 percent in the placebo group.[50] In short, estrogen has an antidepressant role, particularly in mood disorders affecting women over forty.

Media distortion. That said, I believe the media coverage of hormone replacement has been widely distorted and even fear-mongering. The controversy probably began with the Women's Health Initiative (WHI) study, published in 2002, which looked at women treated with the *synthetic* estrogen Premarin, a potent concoction derived from the urine of pregnant horses. Premarin contains many forms of estrogen that are not known to human females, such as equilin. The WHI study of women on Premarin found increased risks of colon cancer, blood clots, stroke, dementia, and gallbladder removal.[51]

Fortunately, estrogen continues to be avidly studied. As one veteran journalist, Cynthia Gorney, who sports an estrogen patch, put it: "The problem with the estrogen question . . . is that you set out one day to ask in what sounds like a straightforward way—Yes or no? Do I or do I not go on sticking these patches on my back? Is hormone replacement as dangerous in the long term as people say it is?—and before long, warring medical articles are piling up."

Writing in *The New York Times Magazine,* Gorney, who is also a professor at the UC Berkeley Graduate School of Journalism, reported on a multidisciplinary meeting of hormone experts from around the world, where she heard the latest opinions on estrogen and depression, dementia, and what happens when you ratchet back up a woman's estrogen levels:

> *One after another, their notes and empty coffee cups piling up around them, heart experts and brain experts and mood experts got up to talk about estrogen—experiments, clashing data, suppositions, mysteries. . . . I typed notes into my laptop for hours . . . and the whole time I was typing . . . I had one small but persistent estrogen-replacement thought of my own: If I make the wrong decision about this, I am so screwed.*[52]

So what are we to do? Any woman with a uterus who takes *systemic* estrogen of any type, such as a cream, patch, or pill, *must coun-*

terbalance the estrogen with progesterone, preferably delivered orally as a pill, to prevent buildup of excess tissue in the uterine lining, which may turn into precancer or cancer. Most prohormone folks would have you believe that bioidentical creams compounded specifically for you are the best bet, and favor either estradiol cream applied to the skin of the arms or bi-est cream, a combination of estradiol and estriol.[53] But I believe in the lowest possible doses of estrogen balanced with progesterone, if you have a uterus.

After her journalistic inquiry, Gorney settled on wearing a dime-size patch containing bioidentical estradiol. This is what I normally recommend. The estradiol patch is applied like a Band-Aid; you put it on yourself at home. Some patches stay on for 3.5 days (that is, you replace the patch twice a week, as with the Vivelle Dot). Others you replace once a week, such as Climara, the brand name for another bioidentical estrogen patch. Bottom line: weigh the pros and cons and risk factors for you, and consult with your doctor.

Local estrogen—in the vagina. Recall that your body makes both estradiol and estriol (see Figures 2 and 3 on pages 46 and 156). Short version: Estradiol is the main estrogen in your fertile years, and estriol is the main estrogen of pregnancy. Both can be prescribed as a cream for the pleasure equipment of your genitalia to make sex more fun if you suffer from vaginal dryness, bladder infections, or irritation. Additionally, a Cochrane Review showed that estrogen creams, tablets, and plastic rings containing estrogen are equally effective. I recommend that both types of creams, estriol and estradiol, be applied with a finger, not the nasty plunger that comes with the cream. (The plunger shoots the cream up to the top of the vagina, where there are no estrogen receptors, which are like locks on the door to a lubricated vagina; estrogen is the key.) I recommend applying 1 gram of the cream to the outside of the vagina (vulva), labia minora, clitoris, and opening to the vagina (introitus). Apply a second gram to the lower third of the vagina, where you do have estrogen receptors. That's a total of 2 grams.

I use a velvet vulva puppet in my office to demonstrate; there's a video showing the technique at http://thehormonecurebook.com/ videos. Within two weeks, estrogen cream applied locally to the vulva and vagina should encourage the crucial nerve endings to come back home. If your breasts become sore, or you don't feel right in some other way, you may be absorbing too much estrogen and should see your doctor. In that case, you should lower your dose until your body gets used to having estrogen again.

FROM THE FILES OF SARA GOTTFRIED, MD

Patient: Joanna

Age: Thirty-four

Plea for help: Hot flashes and weight gain

Joanna came to me after having been diagnosed four years earlier with diminished ovarian reserve, with a high FSH (75.5, about ten times higher than what it should be at age thirty-four) and an estradiol level < 10 (about ten times too low). During that time, she had found her way to a Tibetan physician, who put her on a strict dietary program, with no caffeine, sugar, yeast, or wheat. After six months, Joanna's FSH was normal (7.6), and so was her estradiol (62), and she was cycling regularly again.

"But the minute I default into my bad sugar and caffeine habits, my menstrual cycle disappears. I get weepy and overwhelmed. I have night sweats," she woefully described to me. Unfortunately, Joanna was unable to sustain the elimination diet, I suspect because of her addiction to flour and sugar. While several 12-step programs, such as www.foodaddicts.org and the HOW (honest, open-minded, and willing) Program of Overeaters Anonymous (www.oa.org), have helped many people with this problem, Joanna did not want to pursue that route.

Treatment protocol: I prescribed bioidentical hormones—specifically, an estradiol patch called Vivelle Dot, at 0.0375 mg, plus 100 mg of Prometrium, a bioidentical form of progesterone (proven in a randomized trial to help your cholesterol), twice a day from Days 12 through 26, to get her cycling again.

Results: After two months, Joanna came back, thrilled with the results. She told me that the estradiol had boosted her mood and that she could finally get a night of long, deep, uninterrupted sleep, which totally transformed her waking hours. She is now trying to get pregnant—and she's enjoying the sex.

————GOOD NEWS ABOUT LOW ESTROGEN————

It's not all doom and gloom if you are low in estrogen. Lower estradiol in premenopause is associated with a lower risk of breast cancer and less dense breast tissue on mammograms (another risk factor for breast cancer, and lower estradiol confers lower risk of breast cancer) in women aged forty to forty-five.[54]

There's even an upside to hot flashes. Women who have hot flashes have half the risk of developing breast cancer compared with women who have never had hot flashes. In fact, the worse the flashes, the lower the risk.[55] Additionally, a Harvard study by one of my mentors showed women with hot flashes early in perimenopause were 11 percent less likely to have a heart attack or a stroke.[56]

FROM THE FILES OF SARA GOTTFRIED, MD
Patient: Georgia
Age: Fifty-two
Plea for help: Waning sensuality, dry and painful sex, several bladder infections

Georgia is a charismatic artist who went through a divorce and now, back in the dating world, wanted a vaginal tune-up. "Just give me the big guns," she said. "I'm on a mission to have some really good orgasms ASAP. I tried an over-the-counter vaginal moisturizer from the drugstore, and that was messy and not effective."

When I examined Georgia's vulva and vagina, I found telltale signs of low estrogen. This included loss of rugae, which refers to the redundant folds of the vulvovaginal area. Rather than a medium rosy pink, the marker of robust blood flow, her vulvovaginal area was pale pink, almost white. In addition, her clitoris, instead of being plump and full, was rather shrunken.

Treatment protocol: We discussed trying Shatavari ghee, the medicated clarified butter thought to balance hormones (she had heard about it from a friend who is an Ayurvedic doctor). Because there is a lack of data showing benefit, we settled on a six-week trial of Estrace (estradiol) vaginal cream, which Georgia could buy at her local pharmacy with my prescription. She opted for Estrace cream in part because her insurance paid for it.

Results: Georgia returned to my office six weeks later with a big grin. When I examined her genitalia, her vagina looked hot pink, a sign of increased blood flow. "Sex is yummy again. Thank you! My new boyfriend calls you Dr. Hotfried."

——BIOIDENTICAL VERSUS SYNTHETIC ESTROGEN:—— SHOW ME THE DATA!

There's a popular movement to favor bioidentical hormones over synthetic hormones. Bioidentical hormones are exact replicas of the hormones your body makes during your fertile years, including estradiol and progesterone, which are the two hormones commonly referred to as "bioidenticals." Synthetic hormones have a different chemical structure, which allows them to be patented by pharmaceutical companies. It's important to recognize that bioidentical hormones include both U.S. Food and Drug Administration (FDA)–approved forms as well as non-FDA–approved forms made by compounding pharmacies, such as bi-est, which contains both estradiol and estriol.

Some alternative providers insist that bioidenticals solve every problem a menopausal woman has and are vastly superior to synthetic and animal-derived counterparts. Academic and mainstream thought leaders think you're being taken for a ride. Where's the truth? I suspect it's somewhere in the middle. When I counsel a woman about taking hormone therapy, I recommend bioidentical estrogen and progesterone, including transdermal estradiol and oral progesterone, but with an important caveat: *I assume that the risks of bioidentical hormone therapy are the same as synthetic until proven otherwise.*

Overall, compounded bioidentical hormones often lack the regulatory oversight and rigorous testing that I believe women deserve.[57] Based on current data, I prefer to prescribe FDA-approved forms of bioidentical hormones, particularly the estradiol skin patch and oral micronized progesterone (Prometrium) pills.

Estrogen in Balance

As I said at the beginning of this chapter, estrogen is the hormone that most defines you as a woman. Without it, you may feel, as one patient put it, "neutered." More estrogen means more testosterone, and that often boosts your sex drive too. You feel more generous, successful, and sensual. When you've got your estrogen levels in balance, life feels joyous and right again.

Signs of Estrogen Balance

- You have regular periods (estrogen and progesterone work together on this one). If you're postmenopausal, you'll notice the other signs.
- Your joints and vagina feel well lubricated.
- Orgasm regains its central role in your libidinous life, and that sense of dullness is a distant memory.
- You roll with the punches; you don't feel so stressed and overwhelmed.

- Sleep is a crucial part of your self-care regimen, and restores your energy, although you *don't* prefer it to sex with your partner.
- Your mood is stable throughout your menstrual cycle.
- You have improved brain function: the fog lifts, your memory and recall improve.

CHAPTER 8

EXCESS ANDROGENS: DO YOU HAVE PIMPLES, OVARIAN CYSTS, AND ROGUE HAIRS?

Listen up: the combination of excessively high androgens is the most common hormone problem of women in their fertile years, and perhaps even before puberty. After menopause, high androgens are associated with serious health problems, such as heart disease, stroke, mood problems, and cancer. High androgens wreak havoc hormonally for women from the embryo to maturity.

Androgens are a group of sex hormones that strongly affect your liveliness, libido, mood, and self-confidence. When an embryo is about six weeks old, these hormones kick-start gender identity.

Virilization: Normal in Males, Abnormal in Females

In males, androgens stimulate the embryo to increase the length and diameter of the penis and to develop the prostate and scrotum. The sex differentiation process that unfolds inside the uterus—and differentiates the boy from the girl fetus—is *virilization,* defined as the development of male physical characteristics such as the penis, and later, after puberty, muscle bulk, body hair on the chest and face, and a deep voice.

In females, lack of androgens causes the embryo's ambiguous genitalia to commit to a female pattern, as a default setting. In a young girl, mildly high androgens might range from nuisance symptoms, such as acne, to more severe and serious symptoms requiring an endocrinologist's evaluation, such as early signs of puberty (pubic hair growth before age eight), or equally worrisome, signs of female virilization. Virilization is normal in males, *but requires swift medical attention in females*. In adolescent and adult females, virilization—as evidenced in enlargement of the clitoris, increased muscle strength, deepening of the voice, and/or menstrual irregularity due to lack of ovulation—indicates a problem. Most worrisome is that it may be a result of tumors of the ovaries, adrenals, or pituitary glands.

Because they control the development of typically male characteristics, androgens are considered "masculinizing" hormones, but they also account for emotional well-being, assertiveness, and sense of *agency*—the capacity a person has to act powerfully in his social structure or an innate sense of belonging. Androgens are the biochemical underpinnings of dominance and desire, and even though males have more androgens than females do, having the right amount of androgens is just as essential to women's health and well-being.

High Androgens and Polycystic Ovary *What?*

High androgens are everywhere you turn. A good friend of mine has this problem. Two of my cousins have it. Eighty-two percent of women with excess androgens have what is known as *polycystic ovary syndrome* (PCOS), a condition where the sex hormones become unbalanced for reasons we don't quite understand. Women with PCOS—the top cause of infertility—start making more androgens, which causes the symptoms of high androgens such as acne and rogue hairs.

Here's what confuses most people: *not all women with excess androgens have PCOS, and not all women with PCOS have high androgens*. While they do overlap, the difference is that PCOS is characterized by insulin resistance and ovarian cysts. Sadly, PCOS goes widely undetected; among women eventually diagnosed with it, 70 percent had not been previously diagnosed.[1]

Regardless of whether you suffer from excess androgens, PCOS, or there's an overlap, it's important to treat the root causes. (See "The

Solution: The Gottfried Protocol for High Androgens" at the end of the chapter.) Excess androgens are thought by most doctors to affect women from teenage years to menopause, but new data shows women are affected far more seriously and much longer than previously believed, from in utero to menopause.

The Science of High Androgens

The best-known androgen is *testosterone,* the hormone that inspires motocross, wrestling, and bar fights. Although it is often thought of as the male hormone, women need to have some testosterone in their bodies as well. In fact, I believe women require *testosterone to feel confident and sexy.* The difference between men and women lies in the quantity of testosterone: women produce approximately 250 micrograms (0.25 milligrams) of testosterone a day, while men typically produce ten to forty times more than that. Of all the androgens circulating in your blood and tissues, testosterone is the superstar. It promotes muscles, bigger bones, and immune function, including the bone-marrow manufacture of red blood cells.

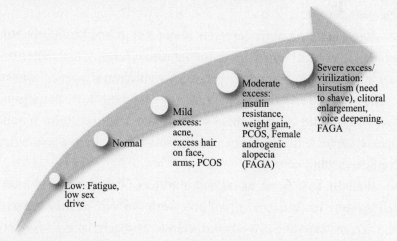

Figure 4. Spectrum of Androgen Levels in Women. Androgens normally decrease by 1 to 2 percent per year beginning in your twenties, so higher levels of androgens are less common after menopause. In reproductive-aged women, polycystic ovarian syndrome (PCOS) is common, affecting the majority of women with symptoms of androgen excess.

In men, testosterone is produced in the testes and adrenal glands; in women, it is produced in the ovaries and adrenal glands. Both sexes use testosterone to get the brain's sexual engine fired up. In general, testosterone is released throughout the body, sending word to your erogenous zones that you are ready for sex. When testosterone is functioning properly, it revs up the hypothalamus, boosting erotic feelings and sensations. Growing research supports the role of testosterone in female desire, with evidence of low desire associated with low testosterone and increased desire with replacement.

Women reach their peak testosterone levels in their midtwenties, after which comes a slow but steady decline, about 1 to 2 percent per year, of available testosterone. Fifty percent of the testosterone in a woman's body comes from conversion of two other types of androgens—DHEA and androstenedione—in the skin and fat tissues; 25 percent from the adrenal glands; and 25 percent from the ovaries. By menopause, testosterone levels are at half the peak level, mostly due to decline in adrenal production. (Even after your ovaries stop producing estradiol—the most common estrogen during a woman's reproductive years—the ovaries continue to make testosterone.)

We're learning more each day about the role of testosterone in women, particularly from studying females who have had their ovaries removed. Since ovaries produce testosterone, women whose ovaries have been excised are suddenly operating with 75 percent less testosterone. Most of these women feel the drop almost immediately, often with hot flashes and a substantial decline in libido, confidence, and verve.

If all this talk about mood and libido sounds familiar, it should: testosterone has an overlapping role with our old friend estrogen. You see, testosterone can be converted to estrogen; fat cells contain an enzyme, called aromatase, that converts testosterone to estradiol. The more fat you have, the more likely it is that you'll create an excess of both androgens and estrogens. We know that excess estrogen may make it extremely difficult to lose weight, which then reinforces the cycle of more fat, estrogen, and weight. We also know that too much testosterone is associated with mood problems such as depression and anxiety, weight gain, and what we call sexual issues (as in, *"Back off, Cowboy!"*).

Women with too much testosterone have deeper voices, more pubic and facial hair, and more muscular builds than women with normal amounts of this hormone (Figure 4, page 207). Occasionally, high testosterone is so significant that it causes balding, a full beard, or growth of the clitoris. We also know that criminal violence and aggressive dominance in women are linked to higher testosterone.[2] As if that weren't enough, recent data shows that women with higher testosterone levels have more depressive symptoms during the menopausal transition.[3]

Women with higher testosterone levels have been shown to have a greater appetite for risk.[4] A group of MBA students enrolled in a lab game in which they could choose to gamble or to take a certain amount of a guaranteed win, which increased each time. Measuring testosterone levels in the saliva on two occasions two years apart, the researchers found that the women with the highest testosterone levels were the most likely to gamble. Testosterone levels also predicted ultimate career choice: women with higher testosterone were more likely to have chosen riskier careers, such as investment banking and finance. These jobs tend to have fatter salaries, but also less security and a higher probability of turnover.

FROM THE FILES OF SARA GOTTFRIED, MD
Patient: Cheryl
Age: Fifty-five
Plea for help: "My clit is growing!"

Cheryl is a midlevel executive at a public relations firm who recently married for the second time. Her libido had been abysmal for the past ten years, yet she loves her new husband and wanted to feel more passionate toward him. Her woes led her to a doctor, who prescribed

2 percent testosterone cream, which she applied to her vagina. Within a few weeks, Cheryl had large, painful pimples on her cheeks and jawline and had to wash her hair more often.

When I performed an exam, her clitoris *indeed looked like a tiny penis.* The clitoris has a wide normal range and engorges with blood during sexual arousal; the nonaroused clitoris is normally 3 to 4 mm wide by 4 to 5 mm long. Cheryl's was 8 mm wide by 7 mm long. The testosterone in her blood was, not surprisingly, elevated: the normal range of free testosterone—I'll explain what that is in a minute—is 0.1 to 6.4 picograms/milliliter (pg/mL); Cheryl's was 10.6 pg/mL.

Sometimes high doses of testosterone can cause liver damage and lower the level of HDL (good cholesterol) in the blood. After checking Cheryl's liver enzymes and doing a cholesterol test, I was relieved to find normal levels.

Treatment protocol: Upon my recommendation, Cheryl stopped using the testosterone vaginal cream. After six weeks, both her clitoris and testosterone level were back in the normal range. I recommended instead a trial of maca, an herb proven to raise sex drive in menopausal women, to help her libido.

Results: Four weeks later, Cheryl reported that her hair and skin were less greasy, and lovemaking with her new husband was much steamier.

Meet the Extended Androgen Family

Besides testosterone, your body makes several other androgens, including the following:

Dehydroepiandrosterone (DHEA). Considered the prehormone to testosterone, DHEA can convert into testosterone when needed. High DHEA has been associated with depression in menopause and acne in women with PCOS.[5] DHEA has been used topically in the vagina to reverse atrophy and dryness.[6]

Androstenedione. A steroid sex hormone that is an intermediate in the production of testosterone and estrogen from cholesterol, androstenedione has both androgen and estrogen activity. In other words, it's promiscuous and likes more than one hormone receptor. Too much androstenedione can cause "minor" symptoms, such as acne and hair loss.

Dihydrotestosterone (DHT). Testosterone also can be converted to dihydrotestosterone (DHT). Three times more potent than testosterone, DHT is the main cause of male-pattern hair loss, which occurs in both men and women. High DHT can cause female androgenic alopecia, or FAGA.[7] Most women with FAGA have hair loss from the temples (the places where men commonly have bald spots).

Of all the circulating androgens, only testosterone and DHT can bind to androgen receptors. Translation: the other members of the family can't trigger the androgen sequence of events, whether good (building muscle and bone, boosting confidence and libido) or not good (hair loss, rogue hair growth). What the ancillary androgens offer is the intermediate prehormones needed for production of testosterone and estrogen.

Excess Androgens and Insulin Resistance

In my practice, I've seen many women who got the brushoff from their primary-care doctors when they expressed concern over thinning locks or raging acne. Yet the problems go far beyond losing or gaining hair or having a complexion like your teenage daughter's.

Most women with high androgens suffer from insulin resistance, and androgens and insulin have their own tango. Insulin resistance is when you need higher and higher levels of insulin for the same result—that is, to drive glucose into cells as fuel. It's the law of diminishing returns: over time, insulin becomes less effective at lowering blood glucose because the cell becomes numb. Eventually, you have high insulin and high glucose. This is bad because high insulin causes the ovaries to make excessive amounts of androgens, and insulin also gets the liver to make less sex-hormone-binding globulin (SHBG), the key protein that binds testosterone and keeps it from causing trouble. This combination results in more free testosterone charging around the bloodstream like a bull in a china shop. High glucose inches you toward prediabetes and diabetes.

Here's the lowdown: insulin is made in the pancreas, and under normal circumstances, its release is finely calibrated to produce just the right amount so that glucose is extracted from food in your gut, sent into your bloodstream, and then driven into cells, particularly the fat, muscle, and liver cells. In other words, the main job of insulin is to regulate your blood sugar. Think of insulin as the knock on the door of your muscle, liver, and fat cells. The cell hears the knock and opens the door to let in the glucose. Once insulin gets glucose inside the cell, the cell can get busy with crucial tasks such as growth, movement, and repair. With insulin resistance, insulin is banging on the door of the cell like an irate neighbor, yet the cell can't be bothered with opening the door anymore, so the pancreas gets the message to make more insulin. Then a vicious cycle is off and running, and the knock of the insulin just gets louder and louder—insulin levels rise and the cell is numb. Insulin is also a fat-storage hormone, so you deposit more fat, notably at your waist.

When you need higher and higher amounts of insulin to deliver glucose as fuel to your cells, you burn out the ability of the pancreas cells (islet cells, to be precise) to keep up with demand. *You lose pancreatic reserve.* When this happens, you cannot stabilize your blood sugar within the normal range anymore—defined as a fasting blood sugar of less than 87 mg/dL. Your blood sugar rises, initially to prediabetes levels, and possibly to the diabetes range.

Insulin Resistance Is a Bad Neighborhood for Your Cells

Insulin resistance heralds several serious problems, including excess weight, obesity, prediabetes, diabetes, dementia, Alzheimer's, stroke, and some cancers. Insulin is not something to mess with. Here's an analogy: insulin resistance fosters a *bad neighborhood* around the cells of your body, but instead of drive-by shootings, muggings, and other high crime influencing your vulnerable cells, you have too much sugar, inflammation, clogged arteries, and weight gain. These problems lead to accelerated aging, wayward hormones, and poor organ reserve.

It's the classic chicken or egg scenario: it's not clear whether high androgens cause insulin resistance or insulin resistance causes high androgens. Either way, we know that high insulin levels drive the ovaries to make more testosterone. Insulin resistance is also a major factor in the troubling condition called *metabolic syndrome,* a cluster of ominous signs that are linked to a greater risk of diabetes and heart disease; it affects one in four women in the United States.

Do you have a problem with insulin? Think back to Part F of the questionnaire in chapter 1. If you answered *yes* to the question about ovarian cysts, consider having an ultrasound to find out if you have multiple small cysts in a characteristic string-of-pearls pattern, the "Pearl Sign." If you do, your risk of type 2 or adult-onset diabetes is increased by a whopping 80 percent. Indeed, simply having menstrual irregularities or symptoms of high androgens increases your risk of diabetes by 50 percent. Or perform the *mirror test,* as described by Dr. Mark Hyman: Stand in front of a mirror without a shirt. Jump up and down. If your belly jiggles, you have a problem with insulin.

Of all of the problems I see in my practice, balancing insulin and glucose is the biggest challenge. This is because of the serious health consequences and the great difficulty most of us have eating less sugar and fewer carbohydrates. It's a common thread in my practice to see patients who struggle to limit pizza, pasta, and pie.

Experts estimate that between 25 and 50 percent of the U.S. population is insulin resistant, which can lead to a number of problems in women that relate to polycystic ovary syndrome (PCOS) and reinforces symptoms of excess testosterone.

Insulin resistance:

- raises the activity of aromatase, the enzyme chiefly responsible for estrogen production, which sets the stage for estrogen dominance and lack of ovulation.

- enhances the activity of 12/21 lyase, an enzyme that increases androgen levels.
- lowers sex-hormone-binding globulin (SHBG), allowing more free testosterone to roam the bloodstream and trigger rogue hairs and pimples.
- raises blood markers of inflammation (*biomarkers*) such as interleukins, cytokines, and adopokines, which initiate a perpetual cycle of inflammation.

How to Test for Insulin Resistance?

While scientists lack consensus on the best way to measure your sensitivity or resistance to insulin, here's my advice: ask your doctor to measure your levels of glucose and insulin after you've fasted for eight to twelve hours (check with your local lab). I believe the optimal range for blood glucose after fasting is 70 to 86 mg/dL; insulin should be less than 7 mcU/mL. Most gynecologists use a glucose-to-insulin ratio to determine if a patient is insulin resistant. Overall, a G:I ratio of less than 4.5 is abnormal.[8]

However, the Androgen Excess and PCOS Society (I kid you not) recommends that all women with PCOS get a two-hour oral glucose tolerance test to look for blood sugar problems every one to two years.[9] If you get this test, it's essential to add an insulin level to the fasting glucose prior to the test, and then check glucose and insulin one and two hours after drinking the "glucola," which is a standardized sugar drink laboratories provide.

Causes of Excess Androgens

While they vary according to the specific type of androgen, the main causes for high androgens are genetics, chronic stress, and excess body fat.

Genetics. It's often easy to blame our parents for everything, but sometimes that blame is appropriate. From looking at how symptoms cluster in families, we know that genetics plays an important role in androgen levels. Forty percent of women with PCOS have a sister with the same condition, and 35 percent have a mother with it. You can inherit the risk from either your mother or your father.

Chronic stress. Ah, our old friend *stress*. Seems connected to everything, doesn't it? Some women have high androgens simply because they are habitually stressed and their bodies are rebelling. Continual stress can throw your adrenal glands into overdrive, increasing the release of stress hormones, such as cortisol, and also increasing the level of androgens. When you produce too much DHEA, you get symptoms such as pimples and rogue hairs. Even mild anxiety raises your DHEA.[10]

Excess body fat. Extra body fat impacts androgen levels. In adults, body fat is necessary for normal gonadotropin levels. Gonadotropins are the control system for hormones: they determine how much estrogen, progesterone, and testosterone you make, depending on how much luteinizing hormone (LH) and follicle-stimulating hormone (FSH) your brain releases. Think of LH and FSH like mafioso who normally share the territory. They're the bosses of hormone underlings, estrogen and testosterone, who vary in brains and brawn. When you have excess body fat, the extra testosterone and estrogen you produce blocks the FSH. FSH gets demoted. This leads to LH dominating FSH, and from there, it's a short step to irregular menstrual cycles.[11] LH becomes the new mafia boss, and you no longer ovulate every month. Women with polycystic ovary syndrome (PCOS) almost always have an aberration in secretion of gonadotropins versus women with normal menstrual cycles.

Rare causes. Uncommonly, androgens rise because of an androgen-secreting tumor in the ovary. That's usually how the bearded lady got that way, although sometimes those women suffer instead from untreated PCOS. Another unusual cause is called congenital adrenal hyperplasia (CAH), a group of inherited disorders of the adrenal glands that affects both males and females. All people with CAH have in common a deficiency of an enzyme that is involved in the synthesis of cortisol, or aldosterone, another hormone made in the adrenals, or both. I recommend considering CAH before a diagnosis of PCOS is made, since the treatments are different.

PCOS: The Number One Reason Women Struggle to Get Pregnant

Most women with excess androgens have PCOS. It sounds like a scary syndrome, and it is. The most common hormone condition in women of reproductive age, PCOS affects 20 percent of women and can interfere with fertility by blocking regular monthly ovulation. If you are trying to conceive, I recommend asking—no, *demanding*—that your doctor do a blood test to check your fasting insulin, glucose, progesterone on Day 21, and leptin. This will clarify whether or not you have insulin resistance. Before you go the übermedical route, you may be able to improve your fertility with a few small lifestyle and food changes specifically targeted to women who want to get pregnant.

Women with PCOS typically develop many small cysts on their ovaries—often between *ten and one hundred small cysts*. We believe the cysts are a result of disturbed hormones and ovulation, so that eggs don't go through the normal maturation sequence of (1) a cyst forming around a ripening egg (the corpus luteum); (2) the release of luteinizing hormone (LH) from the brain to trigger the ripe egg to pop out of the cyst and head toward the fallopian tube for possible fertilization; and (3) the now-empty cyst getting reabsorbed into the ovary. Short version: the maturation sequence of the eggs is disturbed so that there is a breakdown and ovulation doesn't happen. And if you're not ovulating, you won't be getting pregnant.

The cysts in PCOS are not dangerous. It's more that the multiple cysts, along the periphery of the ovaries like a string of pearls, are along for the ride—they are a sign that ovulation is not happening. Over time, the cysts do not grow. They are not the type of cysts that require surgical removal and, unlike some other cysts, are not associated with an increased risk of ovarian cancer. Women are often treated for PCOS with a birth control pill, which suppresses LH and thereby lowers production of ovarian androgens. Not the sort of treatment you want if you're trying to get pregnant.

PCOS: Cause Unknown (But Several Associated Problems)

The exact cause of PCOS is obscure. However, we know that there are two main hormonal underpinnings: *high androgens* in 50 to 82 percent of women with PCOS, and *high insulin* in 50 to 80 percent.[12] Additionally, PCOS is often associated with obesity. Among women with obesity, 28 percent have PCOS, whereas only 5 percent of lean women have PCOS.

Symptoms of PCOS

Perhaps PCOS is often left out of many hormone books because the topic is so complex and hard to diagnose. Symptoms are varied and manifest differently over time, which makes it very difficult to determine a precise, uniform definition of the syndrome. Some women with all the other symptoms of PCOS do *not* have polycystic ovaries. Some, but not all, women with PCOS have hirsutism, or increased hair growth where it doesn't belong. Some women with PCOS are obese or overweight, but others are lean. Regardless, it's important to treat the root cause.

Nearly all women with PCOS share these symptoms:

- **Difficulty losing weight.** Up to 75 percent of women with PCOS are overweight. While losing weight is hard enough for most people, women with PCOS have an even harder time, probably because of their high insulin levels, which alert the body to store fat at all costs. High insulin also increases hunger and carbohydrate cravings. When women with PCOS have high insulin levels, it exacerbates all the features of PCOS.

- **Rogue hairs.** When you have too much androgen circulating in your bloodstream, it can stimulate your hair follicles to thicken and grow. The result can be increased hair growth on the upper lip, chin, breasts, between the breasts, back, belly, arms, and thighs. Hirsutism, or excess hair growth, in a male pattern, is present in 80 percent of women with excess androgens and is a diagnostic condition of PCOS.[13]

- **Inflammation.** Women with PCOS have chronic, low-grade inflammation, which may provide the molecular basis for PCOS.[14] I encourage you to reduce inflammation if you have PCOS by following the lifestyle reset, described in "The Solution: The Gottfried Protocol for High Androgens" (page 222).

PCOS Across the Life Span

How PCOS is manifested depends on age, genes, and environment, including lifestyle and body weight. Figure 5 provides the age-related ways that PCOS may appear, from tween years to middle age.

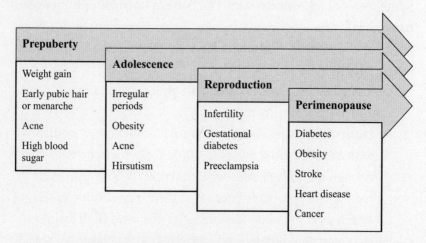

Figure 5. Signs of PCOS Across the Female Life Span. How a woman shows signs of PCOS varies according to her age and life stage, as well as her genetic and environmental influences.

Beyond Infertility: The Dangers of PCOS

PCOS is also linked to other significant health concerns:

Heart disease. PCOS puts you on the fast track to major diseases, like heart disease and stroke.[15] PCOS is associated with an undesirable cardiometabolic profile, as measured by belly fat, high blood pressure, inflammation, insulin resistance, and abnormal glucose metabolism—and a sevenfold increase in diabetes.

The risks can last a lifetime: insulin resistance, high ovarian output of androgens, and inflammation all persist after menopause.[16]

Cancer. PCOS may be associated with an increased risk of hormone-dependent cancer, such as breast cancer and perhaps endometrial cancer.[17] The underlying mechanism is that when women rarely ovulate, the ovaries continue to make estrogen but it's not balanced by progesterone, which is released by ovulation. Over time, this can lead to buildup of the uterine lining and precancerous changes.

Mood problems. Even among lean women with PCOS, there is an increased rate of body dissatisfaction and depression symptoms, as well as more anxiety, depression, withheld anger, diminished sexual satisfaction, and lower health-related quality of life.[18] Anxiety correlates with androgen levels and insulin resistance, but not with body mass index or age.[19]

Abnormal liver enzymes. Blood tests show that 30 percent of women with PCOS have high levels of liver enzymes, which indicates inflammation in the liver and probably scarring.[20] In other words, one in three women with PCOS has a liver that doesn't work normally. If you've been diagnosed with PCOS, you'll want to get your liver checked, and I recommend caution with alcohol and medications that overtax the liver and can harm it.

Diagnosing PCOS: Not as Easy as You Might Think

PCOS generally starts early in life, probably in utero, but it's very hard to diagnose until puberty, when a girl starts to have a menstrual cycle. Classic signs then appear, such as irregular periods, acne, increased hair growth (on the chin and chest), and sometimes acanthosis nigricans, a dark-colored, velvety discoloration on the underarms and back of the neck. I recommend diagnosing PCOS as early as possible, so that lifestyle changes can be instituted and, ideally, the unfortunate consequences of subfertility, obesity, diabetes, and heart disease can be prevented. If you think you may have PCOS, I recommend seeing your physician for hormone tests and a possible ultrasound.

Here's a recap of why awareness and diagnosis of PCOS are so important:

- PCOS is the top hormone imbalance in women up to age fifty.
- Overall, one in five U.S. women have PCOS, yet 70 percent don't know it.
- Of women with high androgens, most have PCOS, and the high androgens are associated with high insulin, obesity, and inflammation. It's a vicious cycle that is extremely difficult to break.
- High androgens (and by extension, PCOS) affect women across all stages of life, even though most people think about its role only in reproductive-aged women.
- Most of the treatments that doctors offer for PCOS (birth control pills or metformin) do not address the root cause of the problem, which is why I believe a systems-based approach such as The Gottfried Protocol is preferable to synthetic medication.

Highlights on Hair Loss

You've seen the infomercials. You've clipped the ads for your beloved. Rogaine (minoxidil) and Propecia (finasteride) are two treatments for hair loss. Before I tell you why I don't think you should be in a rush to slime your hair follicles every day or remove every molecule of testosterone in your body, let's first consider why we're doing so poorly with hair loss. Thirty percent of women report serious hair loss by age thirty. By age fifty, that statistic climbs to 50 percent. This is a major problem, of both vanity and sanity.

Sometimes hair loss is associated with high androgens, but more commonly, I find in women that the root cause is low iron, thyroid hormone imbalance, or insulin resistance. Before my patients start looking for a solution to their hair loss in a box from the drugstore or a pill bottle from a dermatologist, I encourage them to look inside their bodies. Remember that most symptoms women try to solve with a pill bottle are a message from the body that something is awry. To find a patient's particular reason for hair loss, I order the blood panel listed below.

Minoxidil, which you can buy without a prescription, is actually a drug for lowering blood pressure, but when applied topically, it slows hair loss and promotes regrowth. It dilates blood vessels, allowing more oxygen, blood, and nutrients to reach the hair follicles, resulting in new, thicker, and better hairs. If you are wigging out because of hair loss and need to do something while investigating root causes, I recommend parting your hair down the middle, snapping a few photos (your smartphone works nicely) to document the width of your part and your hairline, and applying the lower dose to your scalp (2 percent minoxidil, not the higher dose for men, which is 5 percent). Then wait patiently for four months and watch your hair grow. Unfortunately, there's no cure—when you stop using minoxidil, you will return to the rate of hair loss you had unless you've corrected the cause.

Taken orally, finasteride acts systemically to reduce androgens by inhibiting the enzyme that converts testosterone to DHT. While most people take these treatments to hang on to their hair, they are actually treating the downstream symptoms of high testosterone and DHT.

Both these treatments for hair loss have been studied primarily in men. Are they safe for women? Minoxidil has been used for more than thirty years, so it's got a longer track record.

There are a few other details you should know before taking these medications. Neither treatment addresses the root cause of hair loss. My advice is to try therapies aimed at the root cause of your hair loss first, and to ask your doctor for my top blood tests, including these:

- complete blood count (a measure of whether you are anemic and your immune system is functioning)
- ferritin (the most sensitive test for iron stores in your body)
- thyroid-stimulating hormone (TSH), free T3, and possibly, reverse T3
- cortisol
- fasting insulin and glucose
- testosterone (I prefer total and free testosterone in women with hair loss)
- antinuclear antibody (tells you whether the hair loss is related to an autoimmune condition)

Remember, when it comes to your hair loss and prescription therapies, we want to reproportion your hormones, not search and destroy.

The Solution: The Gottfried Protocol for High Androgens

Step 1: Targeted Lifestyle Changes and Nutraceuticals

Lifestyle reset, consisting of targeted nutrition and exercise, for a period of twelve to twenty-four weeks helps women with excess androgens. The *most effective strategy* for reducing the levels of androgens in the blood is losing weight by eating a low-glycemic-index and high-fiber food plan, decreasing stress, and practicing yoga.

Lose weight and exercise. We know that weight loss reduces insulin resistance and excess androgens; an exercise program designed to help need not be dramatic: one program of a brisk walk twenty minutes per day resulted in a 7 percent weight loss.[21] Even in adolescent girls with PCOS, weight loss corrects irregular periods, normalizes androgens, and improves cardiovascular risk factors.[22]

Eat for lower androgens. The glycemic index (GI) is a measure of how much the carbohydrates in a food raise your blood sugar. A low GI is less than 55 (out of 100). To put this in perspective, a baguette has a glycemic index of 95; grapefruit, a glycemic index of 25. Eating a low-GI food plan reduces androgens by up to 20 percent.[23] In one study, volunteers fed a low-glycemic diet—25 percent protein, 30 percent fat, 45 percent carbohydrate—had lower levels of insulin-like growth hormone (IGF-1) after seven days. That was good news, because IGF-1 is known to affect three important aspects of acne: growth of skin cells, skin-cell production of androgens, and rate of oil production.

Fiber! Scientists agree that for women with PCOS, a low-GI, high-fiber diet is best.[24] That's because unless you have sufficient fiber to remove it, most testosterone is secreted into the bile and then reabsorbed in the gut and used again. Fiber increases excretion of testosterone in the stool. Foods that contain fiber include fresh fruits and vegetables, certain whole grains, and beans. Just a tiny sampling of fiber content to give you an idea: 1 cup of raspberries contains 8 grams, 1 cup of adzuki beans contains 17 grams, 1 ounce of oat bran contains 12 grams, and 2 cups of cooked chard has 8 grams. Once you get familiar with the amounts of fiber in foods, you can keep loose track to make sure you are getting enough each day. I recommend 35 to 45 grams of fiber per day.

Eat foods containing zinc. Zinc plays an important role in sexual development, menstruation, and ovulation. Zinc deficiency is associated with higher androgens and acne. If you have acne, eat foods with zinc, such as green beans and sesame and pumpkin seeds. It's better to get zinc from food sources, since cases of zinc toxicity have been found among people who supplement to excess.

Avoid dairy. Milk, cheese, and eggs have been shown to increase matrix metalloproteinase (MMK), which then drums up inflammation, which leads to higher androgens and acne. You can take antibiotics to block MMK, but I suggest removing dairy for six weeks to see if it helps your symptoms.

Eat more protein. To lower your androgens, eat organic chicken and turkey, low-mercury fish, and grass-fed beef. Most of us don't get enough of the lean stuff. I recommend eating 0.75 to 1 gram of lean protein per pound of lean body mass. A 125-pound woman with 20 percent body fat (or 25 pounds of fat) has a lean body mass of 100 pounds. She needs to eat 75 grams of protein per day if she is relatively sedentary. She needs 100 grams of protein per day if she exercises intensively. Recreational exercisers should eat 80 to 90 grams of protein per day. I count myself as a recreational athlete and eat about 85 to 90 grams per day. Here's a typical protein lineup: breakfast, 4 ounces of tempeh (6 grams of protein/ounce, for a total of 24 grams); lunch, 4 ounces of chicken or turkey breast meat (9.5 grams/ounce, total 38 grams); dinner, 4 ounces wild Alaskan salmon (7 grams of protein/ounce, for a total of 28 grams)—grand slam total of 90 grams of protein.

Omit sugar. Sugar, that irresistible substance reviled by nutritionists but loved by the rest of us, is a big factor in excess androgens. Significant levels of sugar increase serum insulin and IGF-1, both of which raise androgens and cause excess-androgen symptoms. Advice? Sorry for all of you sweeth-toothers. Avoid it altogether.

Get your oil changed. You've probably heard that omega-3, long-chain polyunsaturated fatty acids (such as fish oil) are the most proven supplement on the market for improving health. We evolved as human beings with a good balance between omega-3 and omega-6.[25] But our modern diet has led us to eat too many omega-6s, which are found in processed food, corn and safflower oils, and farm-raised fish. Not all omega-6s are bad, but they tend to cause more inflammation in the body, whereas omega-3s are anti-inflammatory. Here's more data on PCOS: women with too much omega-6 compared with omega-3 have higher circulating androgens.[26] Women with more omega-3s in their blood have lower androgens in the blood plus a better cholesterol profile, and as a result, less risk of cardiovascular disease, one of the risks of excess androgens. You get good sources of omega-3s from eating wild Alaskan salmon and taking a daily fish oil supplement that's been shown to be low in mercury.

Take up yoga. Yoga was shown recently to be more effective than other forms of exercise at improving insulin resistance in PCOS.[27]

FROM THE FILES OF SARA GOTTFRIED, MD

Patient: Casey

Age: Twenty-nine

Plea for help: Pimples, irregular periods, trouble losing weight, an increase in hair on her arms and face.

Casey wants to try getting pregnant soon. She exercises five days a week and eats what she believes is a healthful diet, but the scale wouldn't budge, and she really wanted to lose 15 pounds. She had a body mass index of 27 (normal BMI is 18 to 25).

Recently, she moved to San Francisco from Boston, where she had an ultrasound that showed the Pearl Sign (several cysts in a row) on her ovaries. Her doctor suggested taking a birth control pill to regulate her periods and help with weight loss. When I met her, she was still getting her period every thirty-eight to forty-five days. When Casey showed me her lab test, it revealed a total testosterone level of 156, which is high.

Remember the criteria of the Androgen Excess and PCOS Society? It doesn't take a detective to note that Casey has all the criteria: high testosterone and hirsutism, multiple cysts on her ovaries and oligomenorrhea (fewer than nine menstrual cycles a year), and no other reason for her high testosterone. When I checked Casey's glucose:insulin ratio, we found she had insulin resistance.

Treatment protocol: I put Casey on a low-GI food plan, with 45 percent carbohydrates, 30 percent fat, 25 percent protein. For breakfast, she ate eggs with chopped spinach or kale. For lunch, she ate lean protein such as chicken or beans with a large serving (6 ounces) of steamed vegetables and a small serving (2 ounces) of whole grains, such as brown or black rice. Her dinner was similar, with the addition of a large salad (8 ounces) with 2 tablespoons of dressing. Casey gave up dairy products and grew to love eggplant, bell peppers, carrots, and avocado. She started a yoga practice.

Results: Within six weeks, she had lost 8 pounds and her skin was almost completely clear. She began menstruating regularly (every twenty-nine days). When I retested her GI, I found she no longer had insulin resistance.

Even a 5 percent reduction in weight can normalize your hormone levels—a small lifestyle and nutritional change with a huge impact. I'm looking forward to seeing her future baby pictures.

Chromium. Chromium is a mineral that acts as an insulin sensitizer, which means it helps to reverse insulin resistance and lowers both your serum insulin and glucose levels when they are high.[28] Folks with type 2 diabetes, the type that results from insulin resistance, have lower blood chromium levels compared with nondiabetic people. Chromium levels also decline with age.[29] Chromium is a safe supplement worth trying if you are insulin resistant. I recommend a dose of 200 to 1,000 mcg per day of chromium picolinate.

Inositol. When they want to conceive, many women are given big-gun prescription drugs such as metformin and clomiphene. However, metformin, an antidiabetic drug that lowers blood sugar, can cause serious side effects such as lactic acidosis, which is an excessive accumulation of lactic acid in the body. In addition to diet, nutraceuticals that influence insulin can make a big difference, and may be a better alternative in younger women and girls. Inositol is a naturally occurring B-complex vitamin known to improve insulin sensitivity.[30] Two inositol supplements you can get at the drugstore or health food store show promise in correcting PCOS: D-chiro-inositol (DCI) and myo-inositol (MI).

Women with PCOS appear to be deficient in DCI. New evidence supports that overweight women with PCOS be given the combination of DCI and MI first, prior to any prescription therapy. A while back, the *New England Journal of Medicine* reported the bold news that in women with PCOS, DCI cut free testosterone *by more than half* and lowered blood pressure and triglycerides in eight weeks or less.[31] DCI also works in lean women with PCOS.[32] Recommended dose: DCI 600 mg twice per day (but you can also find DCI in carob, buckwheat, and grapefruit) and myo-inositol at a dose of 2 grams once or twice per day.

Vitamin D. Vitamin D is a fat-soluble vitamin that is present in eggs and fish. It is added to other foods, such as milk, and is also available as a dietary supplement. I recommend about 2,000 IU per day. Vitamin D deficiency is emerging as a factor in the metabolic disturbance of PCOS.[33] In fact, 44 percent of women with PCOS are vitamin D–deficient, compared with 11 percent of controls.

Other Lifestyle Changes

Women with metabolic syndrome and insulin resistance have a *higher tone to their sympathetic nervous system.* In other words, the coveted balance between the sympathetic nervous system, activated by stress into fight or flight, dominates over the parasympathetic nervous system, also known as rest and digest. This may show up as an increased diastolic blood pressure (the lower number of the blood pressure fraction).

Yoga. Yoga has been shown to rebalance the wayward hormones of PCOS, as described earlier.

Acupuncture. Acupuncture induced regular ovulation in one-third of women with PCOS, suggesting that acupuncture is a good

alternative for many women before they turn to prescription medications, such as metformin or clomiphene, to induce ovulation.[34]

BPA. Women with PCOS have higher levels of BPA, and the
amount correlates with both androgen level and insulin resistance.[35]
It's a good idea to minimize your exposure: BPA is a plastic found in
thermal print receipt paper, the plastic lining most canned food, and
flame retardants. See chapter 6, "Excess Estrogen," for a discussion
of BPA.

Step 2: Herbal Therapies

Cinnamon. That innocent-looking cinnamon stick in your hot milk
or sprinkle of cinnamon in Moroccan stew adds more than just flavor. One Cochrane Review of four trials assessing Chinese herbal
supplements in subfertile women with PCOS found increased pregnancy rates when herbs such as cinnamon were added to clomiphene, a medication that may induce ovulation in infertile women.[36]
Cinnamon is a natural insulin-sensitizer—so it acts like metformin,
but in a natural way—stimulating glucose uptake by fat cells, which
lowers both glucose and insulin levels. In a study of people with
diabetes, cinnamon reduced fasting glucose and cholesterol.[37] As a
bonus, cinnamon lowers blood pressure (often elevated in women
with PCOS and metabolic syndrome) and helps correct abnormal cholesterol levels. Cinnamon also increases lean body mass.[38]
You don't even need much—the most effective dose is ½ teaspoon
per day.

Saw palmetto. While it has not been proven in randomized
trials to help women improve hyperandrogenism, saw palmetto is
known to reduce the conversion of testosterone to the more potent
DHT and to block the androgen receptors. In other words, it acts
as an antiandrogen. If you have high androgens, particularly FAGA,
you may want to try a small dose of saw palmetto in a capsule at the
low dose of 160 mg/day.

Tian Gui. In Traditional Chinese Medicine (TCM), PCOS doesn't
fit neatly into a single category. Tian Gui capsule is a composite of

various herbs *proven more effective than metformin* (though less effective than a birth control pill) at lowering androgens.[39]

Step 3: Bioidentical Hormones

I commonly see women on hefty doses of testosterone who are not having their blood levels monitored carefully. Sometimes the result of excessive dosing is cystic acne, head-hair loss, or excessive sweating and body odor. When I measure testosterone levels in women with these symptoms, they are often closer to the normal levels for a man. Once the dosage drops, their symptoms resolve.

If, after meticulous informed consent, you choose to take testosterone, I recommend checking several things in your blood: your free, total, and bioavailable testosterone levels; cholesterol levels (because testosterone can lower HDL, your good cholesterol); and liver enzymes (because testosterone can damage your liver). Part of your informed consent should include that we do not know the long-term effects of augmenting your testosterone levels. The longest duration of the randomized trials of testosterone in women is six months.

Sometimes women read online or in a magazine that DHEA is a good idea for dealing with low energy. They go to their local health food store, buy a bottle of pills, and start taking a dose of 25 mg/day, the level usually recommended for women. But side effects inevitably ensue: greasy skin and hair, acne breakouts. When I lower the dose to 2 to 5 mg/day, the side effects often resolve. If they don't resolve, I strongly suggest stopping the DHEA.

Other than reducing excessive doses of testosterone or DHEA, however, I can't make any recommendations for bioidentical hormones—none are proven to lower your androgens.

Women who take cortisol or adrenal extract—ground-up adrenal gland from animals—can lower their DHEA, the prehormone to testosterone. However, I advise extreme caution with glandular extracts because they are over the counter, with no regulatory oversight. If you take glandular extracts, you do so at your own risk; please consult your local physician.

Signs of Androgen Balance (and Lack of PCOS)

When you have balanced levels of androgens, you feel calm and confident and look your best.

- You exhibit optimal mood and assertiveness.
- Your skin is not excessively greasy or dry, but clear, with minimal to no acne.
- You're neither pumped up like a bodybuilder nor flabby and undertoned, but have the right bone density, muscle size, and strength for your size and weight.
- Your hair is where it should be: on your head, not your chin or nipples or chest, and you have a normal distribution of pubic hair.
- You conceive when you're ready, not held hostage by ovaries that make too much testosterone and prevent ovulation.

CHAPTER 9

LOW THYROID: WEIGHT GAIN, FATIGUE, AND MOOD PROBLEMS?

Many doctors view women who are concerned about their thyroid as if they're suffering from mild hysteria. Don't believe them. *Stand your ground.* If three or more symptoms from Questionnaire Part G feel familiar to you, I urge you to read this chapter and then have a frank yet firm discussion with your doctor.

Introducing the Thyroid

The thyroid gland secretes hormones that regulate the activities of almost every cell in our bodies. It controls the body's sensitivity to other hormones, such as estrogen and cortisol. It regulates how quickly we burn calories and maintains our metabolism, which explains why weight control is such a problem when the thyroid is out of whack. In other words, your thyroid is your very own metabolic thermostat. Sluggish thyroid and metabolism are a setup for poor mood—even, perhaps, the slow downward spiral toward cognitive decline and Alzheimer's disease.

When your thyroid is working properly, you feel energetic, think clearly, and are upbeat. Your weight is easier to manage. Your bowel moves food along at a normal pace, in a transit time from ingestion to elimination of twelve to twenty-four hours. You don't wear socks to bed or outline your eyebrows with a brown pencil. Your cholesterol is normal—not too high and not too low. Your hair stays on your head, your skin is moist and your nails aren't dried out, your sex drive is strong, and your memory is crystal clear.

The Lowdown on Low Thyroid

The symptoms of low thyroid were summarized decades ago on *I Love Lucy,* when Lucille Ball hilariously peddled a sham energy drink called Vitameatavegemin by asking, "Are you tired, run down, listless? Do you poop out at parties?" She could have added, "Do you have a bowel movement less than once a day? Are you gaining unexplained weight, most of which is fluid? Are you cold all the time, achy, slow thinking, or depressed?" Low thyroid can cause these problems.

You may think your sluggishness or poor memory is simply a sign of getting older. Age, however, does not explain a puffy face, high cholesterol, excessive menstrual bleeding, and many other symptoms of low thyroid function. Mary Shomon, a colleague of mine and impassioned advocate for her patients, calls the triad of fatigue, weight gain, and depression *thyropause,* because these symptoms are akin to those that can occur with the ovarian sputtering that characterizes menopause. Oprah was famously diagnosed with thyroid issues in 2007, although certainly her thyroid doesn't explain the entire story of her weight challenges. Oprah isn't alone in this: if you look at women in this country who are forty-two and older, you'll find that 24 percent are taking thyroid medication, and 11 percent are on antidepressants.[1]

In fact, 15 to 20 percent of people with depression are low in thyroid hormones.[2] That's a statistic too big to ignore. In imaging studies, the hypothyroid brain looks remarkably like the depressed brain: both show subtle changes in blood vessels, myelination (fatty insulation around nerves), and neurogenesis (nerve growth).

Why Doctors Underdiagnose Thyroid Issues

It's estimated that about 60 million Americans, both men and women, struggle with thyroid problems. Most don't even know it. Given the depth of suffering, we can no longer ignore that so many people are burned out, confused, and underfunctioning. The medical profession needs an urgent call to action: increase the diagnosis of hypothyroidism.

Conventional physicians often respond with skepticism, derision, and even hostility to women who earnestly ask for thyroid help. Many of their doctors have expressed the belief that "doctors like me" are prescribing thyroid treatment indiscriminately and under the false pretense that it will help with weight problems and fatigue. I'd agree that some alternative medicine providers appear to have a tendency to overdiagnose and overtreat patients. As I've emphasized, the best practice is to apply rigorous science, which I've distilled for you in this chapter.

For women with a thyroid disorder, thyroid treatment *will* help with weight and fatigue issues because it addresses the root cause of women's symptoms. Women respond most effectively when the best of both worlds are combined: thyroid symptoms are *carefully considered* with objective blood testing using the latest scientific guidelines.

Why are thyroid malfunctioning issues often missed or undiagnosed?

I've identified three main reasons:

1. *Doctors are well intentioned but underinformed.* In general, they may
    • have an outdated reference range—doctors treat women using the "normal" reference ranges they learned in medical school, years ago. They don't know that laboratory-based reference ranges are skewed by in-

cluding patients with hypothyroidism, and are unfamil-
iar with new national guidelines for a narrower normal
range.

    • be unaware of current findings. They haven't read
the latest data, which shows improved outcomes in people treated for borderline thyroid function (referred to by
clinicians as *subclinical hypothyroidism*).

    • rely on the myth that numbers don't lie. Too many
doctors rely on a limited lab test such as TSH more than
they believe what the patient is telling them. Ultimately,
this leads to the misconception that thyroid symptoms
must always be accompanied by an abnormal TSH.
Truth? Occasionally, patients endure *abnormal thyroid
function not indicated by TSH,* such as low triiodothyronine (T3) from exposure to thyroid disruptors from the
environment.

2. *Women are disempowered.* "It's just aging." When women
    get patted on the back by their doctors with the remark,
    "You're just getting older," in response to thyroid com-
    plaints, they may be afraid to disagree for fear they don't
    have data to back them up. Or they give up too soon,
    perhaps as another symptom of hypothyroidism. As pa-
    tients, we're conditioned not to fight, and when you are
    also hypothyroid, you've got little fight left. *It's time to
    start demanding more from your team of medical profession-
    als, and if they don't agree, move on to a new team.* Who
    among us wants to end up on antidepressants, sleeping
    pills, or to purchase "fat" clothes and be sent to a psy-
    chiatrist for a biological problem?

3. *The revolution is just starting. Join the movement.* The
    grassroots movement to reclaim thyroid health has not
    yet reached all women. Fortunately, there is a bottom-
    up revolution taking place to change the problem of

underdiagnosed thyroid problems, led by powerful ac-
tivists such as Mary Shomon, arguably the most popular
thyroid advocate internationally, and Janie Bowthorpe,
founder of another popular thyroid patient-to-patient
online tribe. Unfortunately, even the most well-read
women who come to my medical practice have never
heard of either woman. They stare at me, perplexed,
when I tell them their thyroid function is low, and
further (based on the ten or so years of lab tests they
brought in for our first appointment), that it's been low
for a decade but *undiagnosed and untreated*. Together, we
initiate The Gottfried Protocol for Low Thyroid. Within
days they feel renewed ardor and have a sparkle in their
eyes.

Getting someone on your team isn't as hard as you think: Empower and educate yourself to have the will and tenacity to get the
best help. Use the strategies described in Appendix B to identify a
doctor who can serve as an informed and compassionate partner for
you. Don't settle for being dismissed. Spread the word, so that we
can amplify this message and help people struggling unnecessarily
due to low thyroid function.

It's Not Just Aging

Chances are you have a friend or two, probably female, who has had
trouble with her thyroid. That's because women face a 20 percent
chance of developing a thyroid problem at some point in their lives.
Unfortunately, too many physicians mistake the *symptom* for the
problem—weight gain and depression, for instance. Or worse: many
doctors believe women try to use the low-thyroid diagnosis as an
excuse to avoid a nutritional and exercise regimen to manage their
weight effectively, but data show that more than 10 percent of the

U.S. population has undiagnosed thyroid problems, and that figure may be as high as 65 percent in people aged forty-nine and older.[3]

Too often, we think the problems we're having are age related, when a simple test would indicate if they are caused by low thyroid. It reminds me of the diagnosis for cataracts. When patients complained of blurry vision, doctors used to joke about how we're all getting older. Now we send them straight to an ophthalmologist for a cataract test.

The Science of Low Thyroid

Skip this section if you struggle with brain fog, a key symptom of low thyroid function. Come back and read it when you've implemented The Gottfried Protocol and are able to concentrate fully again!

One of the largest of the endocrine glands, the thyroid is attached to the front of the trachea, just below the larynx, and consists of two relatively flat ovals connected by a narrow bar in a butterfly shape. The name comes from its resemblance to the *thyreos,* the shield used by ancient Greek warriors. Unlike a shield, however, the thyroid is asymmetric; the right lobe is normally much larger than the left.

For some reason (perhaps fluctuating estrogen levels), the thyroid is larger in women than in men and grows slightly during pregnancy. Some African communities adorn brides with a tight necklace. When the swelling thyroid gland causes the necklace to break, people assume she's pregnant.[4]

Thyroid tissue is made up of millions of tiny baglike follicles that store *thyroglobulin,* a kind of protein. Before its release into the bloodstream, thyroglobulin is converted into thyroxine (T4) and other closely related thyroid hormones. Compared with other markers of metabolism, such as glucose, thyroid hormones circulate in the blood in very low concentrations and, in healthy individuals, remain stable over long periods of time. Certain hormones may change how much thyroglobulin you make, for example, synthetic estrogen pills, which raise thyroglobulin by 40 percent, result in 10 percent less free thyroid hormone (thyroxine, T4) available in the blood.[5]

If your thyroid is healthy, it produces hormones in the correct amounts: mainly thyroxine (T4), triiodothyronine (T3), T2, T1, and reverse T3. The amount of T4 you produce is dependent on iodine and TSH. The main reason people in the United States develop low thyroid symptoms is because they're producing too much TSH, not because they have an iodine deficiency, which I'll discuss later in the chapter. TSH is made by your master gland, the pituitary, which is regulated by the hypothalamus and limbic system. When you are *euthyroid*—blissfully normal, with neither an underactive nor an overactive thyroid, and thyroid hormones to reflect it—you make less TSH (Figure 6), the most basic test of thyroid function. The normal range is debated, but evidence favors 0.3 to 2.5 mIU/L.

When you are hypothyroid—you don't make a sufficient supply of thyroid hormones (T3 and T4) to meet your body's needs—you produce more TSH in the brain. What causes someone to make too much TSH? In the United States, the cause is most commonly Hashimoto's thyroiditis, when your immune system attacks your thyroid, and initially leads to high levels of thyroid hormone in the blood plus antibodies. Over time, the battle causes your weakened thyroid to stop making as much thyroid hormone, and a feedback loop tells your control system to make more TSH. When you make more TSH in your pituitary, it travels to your thyroid in the blood and orders the gland to make more thyroid hormone. You either keep up with the orders from headquarters, or you don't—perhaps because your immune system has destroyed your thyroid, or an environmental toxin is disrupting your thyroid function. Symptoms, such as fatigue, weight gain, and mood changes begin to appear.

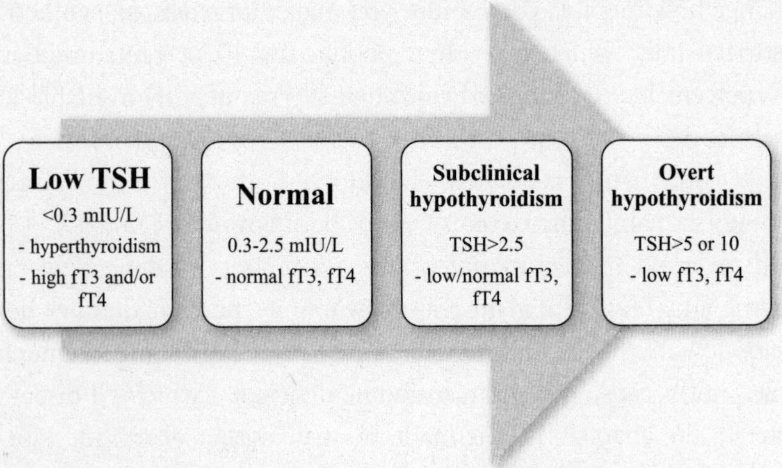

Low TSH	Normal	Subclinical hypothyroidism	Overt hypothyroidism
<0.3 mIU/L	0.3-2.5 mIU/L	TSH>2.5	TSH>5 or 10
- hyperthyroidism	- normal fT3, fT4	- low/normal fT3, fT4	- low fT3, fT4
- high fT3 and/or fT4			

Figure 6. Spectrum of Thyroid-Stimulating Hormone Results. Thyroid-stimulating hormone (TSH) is the most basic test of thyroid function. The normal range is debated, but evidence favors 0.3 to 2.5 mIU/L. When your TSH is lower, subclinical or overt hyperthyroidism is the likely diagnosis. Above 2.5, your diagnosis is hypothyroidism.

Thyroid by the Numbers: It's the *Free* T4 and T3 That Wreak Havoc

Maybe you aren't a numbers person, but I urge you, when it comes to your thyroid, to pay attention. These are numbers you'll want to understand, because chances are that if you recognized yourself in the questionnaire, you have a thyroid issue. T4 is the inactive version of thyroid hormone. Essentially, that means you need it, but it's mostly a precursor of the more important or "active" version, which is T3 (triiodothyronine). T4 is essentially a storage hormone, biologically a lame duck, waiting in the wings to be converted into T3, the catalyst for weight loss, warm limbs, and good mood. T4 makes up more than 90 percent of your thyroid hormones, but it must be converted into T3 before it can be used. Unfortunately, too often women are treated with only T4, with no acknowledgment that T3 should be in the mix.

More than 99 percent of your thyroid hormones are linked

to specific "binding proteins" found in the nucleus of the cells. Most of the T4 in your blood is attached to a protein called thyroxine-binding globulin. Less than 1 percent of the T4 is unattached, or "free"—but it's the free-roaming T4 that causes thyroid problems.

Similarly, less than 1 percent of your T3 is free. Despite being present in such small amounts, free T3 has a greater effect on the way you use energy. It is the primary influence on your weight, cholesterol, energy, memory, menstrual cycle, skin, hair, body temperature, muscle strength, and heart rate.

About Reverse T3

Reverse T3 (rT3) is an inactive metabolite of T4, and provides a mechanism to slow down metabolism in order to save energy. Generally, if you are healthy, T4 gets made into T3, and a small portion of T4 gets converted into reverse T3. Put another way, reverse T3 provides a feedback system to keep you in balance under normal conditions. But occasionally this plan backfires, and what was designed to be adaptive for your body becomes disadvantageous. Here's why: if your body is stressed or on a calorie-restricted diet, a signal is sent to change the ratio, and you produce more reverse T3. When faced with stressors such as the flu, extreme cold, a car accident, hospitalization, or a vow to lose weight with calorie restriction, for example, your metabolism will slow down by raising production of reverse T3. When that happens, you may become thyroid resistant: you don't respond properly to thyroid hormones, either your own endogenous hormone or prescription medication, which means you may continue to have hypothyroid symptoms even if your thyroid blood tests, such as TSH, are normal. Most mainstream doctors claim this is a rare condition, and they often miss it—mostly because they don't check for it. Furthermore, mainstream doctors believe that high reverse T3 is mostly found in hospitalized patients and chronic disease. Yet I commonly find high reverse T3 in my clients, who are neither sick nor hospitalized but coping with stressful, ordinary lives. Repeat this mantra ten times: stress makes TSH less reliable.

My decision to test reverse T3 in women with persistent symptoms of thyroid insufficiency in the face of normal TSH is not simply expert opinion. The science comes from the most esteemed journal on the topic, *The Journal of Endocrinology and Metabolism,* which documented that the thyroid hormones I was taught to measure routinely—namely, TSH and T4—do not adequately reflect what's happening *inside your cells.* One study found that normal reverse T3 predicted survival and physical functioning better than other thyroid blood tests, and that people with low serum T3 and high reverse T3 had worse physical performance associated with aging (such as difficulty arising from bed, dressing, eating, walking, hygiene, grip, and other common activities of daily living) than those with normal levels.[6]

Hypothyroidism: More Risk After Babies?

Even if you're not middle aged, you could be at risk for hypothyroidism. After giving birth, about 7 percent of women develop what's called postpartum thyroiditis, when the immune system attacks the thyroid, causing mood swings, lethargy, thinning hair, and difficulty with weight loss. Women with baseline thyroid antibodies before pregnancy are much more likely to develop postpartum thyroiditis. Of course, lots of women experience postpartum blues, sleep deprivation, and struggles with weight and hair loss. Since many doctors never think to check a woman's thyroid after she's given birth, too many new mothers suffer from an unrecognized thyroid condition.

Here's the single most common scenario I hear in my integrative medicine practice among mothers with thyroid problems: "Dr. Sara, I was doing just fine until I had my first baby. I couldn't get the weight off, despite serious portion control and exercise. I'm talking Baby Boot Camp five days per week! I was bone tired, and it was more than just sleep deprivation. My hair fell out, and it was more than the crazy postpregnancy hair loss. I couldn't even think about sex, as in: 'Don't you come near me! Are you insane?' Heart palpitations. Joints of an old person. Yet my doctor kept looking at me with that knowing glance that said, 'Oh, honey, you just had a baby. It's hard,' but never checked my thyroid."

Low Thyroid: Do You Have It?

When you have low thyroid function, you make more TSH. It's your body's way of trying to get your thyroid back in balance. It's a bit counterintuitive, but hang with me while I explain why—TSH is not made in your thyroid, it's made in your pituitary, the manager of your thyroid. When your thyroid gland is not making enough thyroid hormone, your brain senses this. Your hypothalamus, the pituitary's boss, tells the pituitary to crank out more TSH and whip that thyroid into shape by stimulating greater production of thyroid hormones. As a result, the hormone factory in the thyroid (if it has the necessary resources and cortisol isn't interfering) manufactures more thyroid hormones, which are then sensed by the brain. Often the thyroid will adjust sufficiently, and TSH settles back down to normal, which is an example of one of the hormone feedback loops in the body. How high your TSH levels climb usually correlates with the severity of the problem.

Here's how mainstream medicine defines the problem:

- **Overt hypothyroidism**: TSH levels are high, but total and free T3 and T4 are below normal. This affects less than 1 percent of the adult population.
- **Subclinical hypothyroidism**: TSH levels are high, above 2.5, but total and free T3 and T4 are in the normal range. This affects 9 percent of the population.

In more than twenty years of practice, I've observed *gradations of thyroid imbalance*. More women than we recognize brave thyroid imbalance because of old reference ranges for thyroid imbalance. That's a lot of sluggish, uncomfortable, and unhappy people roaming around. Many doctors prefer not to treat subclinical hypothyroidism because they believe treatment hasn't been shown to be helpful. To be fair, most of the reviews recommend against treatment.[7] Research supports a balanced approach somewhere between no treatment and aggressive treatment.[8] That's the middle ground that I advocate.

The Magical Reference Range

Leading medical facilities use a reference range of TSH that is outdated and consider a normal TSH range to be between 0.5 and 5.5 mIU/L. In 2002, the American Association for Clinical Chemistry issued new guidelines, recommending that the upper limit of normal TSH be considered 2.5 mIU/L. In 2003, the American Association of Clinical Endocrinologists changed its recommended normal target range for TSH to 0.3 to 3.0 mIU/L. Furthermore, we have robust evidence to narrow the optimal range for TSH even further—some even suggest an upper limit of 1.5 mIU/L.[9] We should adhere to the revised, lower normal ranges for TSH levels, which will ensure that people get the treatment they need for low thyroid issues.

I like to believe that people are inherently good—your doctor might not be intentionally hiding something from you; he or she just might have completed medical training prior to these new guidelines and may still be using the old reference range when monitoring your medication, symptoms, and lab tests. That's why the task falls on you to become an educated healthcare consumer. Demand a blood test and review the results, comparing them to the optimal ranges that I've provided. Note that the time of day your blood is drawn can make a difference: TSH levels tend to be in the midrange in the morning, to drop at noon, then rise at night. To keep your results consistent and comparable, take the test in the morning.

FROM THE FILES OF SARA GOTTFRIED, MD

Patient: Linda

Age: Fifty-two

Plea for help: "*I don't feel at home in my body anymore. I'm exhausted most of the time, and my periods are irregular with flooding (bouts of heavy bleeding). I feel cold all the time, and my weight seems to increase alarmingly by several pounds per week despite regular exercise and eating the same food for years.*"

While working at the HMO, I met Linda, who came in for a Pap smear. I was a newly minted gynecologist. She told me her saga. Her bowel movements had slowed significantly. She also reported that her hair was dry, and her fingernails were chipped and cracking. Her internist brushed off her concern about a possible thyroid problem, relegating it to aging.

I checked her TSH: 4.2 mIU/L (too high), indicating that her body was depleted of thyroid hormone. While she got dressed after my exam, I called Linda's internist. Since I was new and didn't want to step on a senior doctor's toes, at least not during my first few weeks, I thought this was prudent. "Dr. Gottfried, we treat when TSH is higher than 5.0, or even 10.0 unless there's significant symptoms of full-blown hypothyroidism. I don't believe in treating subclinical hypothyroidism." Nevertheless, I still thought she needed treatment and went ahead anyway.

Treatment protocol: I wrote Linda a prescription for levothyroxine, the cheaper generic form of T4. This was a case in which T4 alone was needed to boost her metabolism.

Results: Linda called two months later to tell me that she had a renewed zest for life, had shed 10 pounds, and was delighted to feel like she was getting her body back.

Perimenopause, Thyroid, and How Health Unravels

Women in perimenopause and older are more likely to suffer from thyroid problems. From the scientific literature, we know that women in this age range are the most likely to develop Graves' disease, the top reason for an overactive thyroid (hyperthyroidism). Over time, this disease can burn out the thyroid gland and cause hypothyroidism.[10]

Additionally, 25 percent of women over the age of sixty have antibodies against the thyroid. It's unclear if this is clinically significant, but it's an important risk factor for future thyroid problems, as 11 percent of women with thyroid antibodies have hypothyroidism.[11] Plus, when TSH is greater than 2.0, the long-term low levels of thyroid hormone in hypothyroidism are associated with delayed reflexes and a greater risk of developing Alzheimer's disease.[12]

Looking for a link between women's thyroid function and cardiovascular risk, one study found that *subclinical hypothyroidism*—defined at the time as a TSH greater than 4.0 mIU/L—predicts heart attack and atherosclerosis.[13] Women with a TSH greater than 4.0 had more than double the risk of heart attack. When you treat borderline low thyroid function in women, you improve the heart (notably, the left ventricle), as measured by cardiac output and cardiac index, measures of how efficiently your heart pumps blood. In other words, the women treated for subclinical hypothyroidism for one year had more cardiac efficiency.[14] Perhaps this and similar studies will get more women the treatment they deserve.

Even when doctors treat women, I find they don't go far enough. In a typical day in my office, I see patients with fatigue, mood issues, hair loss, and reduced midlife zest—many of whom have been treated with the same dose of T4 for decades. I check their T3, and it's low. We add a small dose of T3, and it helps a lot, similar to what we find in treatment-resistant depression.

Thyroid Disruptors: Are Environmental Toxins to Blame for Rising Rates of Hypothyroidism?

Environmental pollutants, termed *endocrine disruptors,* affect not just the estrogen receptor as xenoestrogens, but also disrupt normal thyroid function. Chemicals that affect either the hypothalamic-pituitary-thyroid axis or thyroid receptors are called *thyroid disruptors,* and include more than 150 industrial chemicals. Examples are polychlorinated biphenyls (PCBs), dioxin, and bisphenol-A.[15] Some thyroid disruptors, such as PCBs, dioxin, and FD&C red dye #3, uniquely affect T3 levels. TSH measurement may not reliably identify altered thyroid hormone production, so unfortunately testing does not necessarily uncover the presence of these disruptors. Given the growing rates of thyroid insufficiency in the United States coupled with increasing exposure to thyroid disruptors, my recommendation is that we apply the precautionary principle and severely limit our exposure.

COLLECT MORE DATA: TAKE YOUR BASAL TEMPERATURE

Using your humble bathroom thermometer is a simple way to assess your thyroid. That's because low body temperature is sometimes correlated with low thyroid. Your temperature is normally lower in the morning and evening and higher in the afternoon, so I recommend checking your basal temperature, under your arm, first thing in the morning. If you're still menstruating, check between Day 2 and Day 4 of your cycle. Make sure you get a basal body thermometer that measures temperature at the lower scale, between 96 and 99 degrees F. Normal is between 97.8 and 98.2 degrees, but temperature can vary significantly and should be considered in the context of symptoms and blood testing. Nevertheless, if your basal temperature in the morning is consistently below 97.8 degrees, this is further evidence of low thyroid function.[16]

What Causes Low Thyroid?

Hashimoto's thyroiditis. In North America, the most common reason for low thyroid is the burned-out phase of Hashimoto's thyroiditis, named for the Japanese specialist who discovered it in 1912. With this disease, also known as autoimmune thyroiditis, your body's own immune system attacks the thyroid gland, causing inflammation and an *overproduction* of thyroid hormones. This is followed by *underproduction* of the thyroid hormones. Many women have "flares" of increased immune attack. It is diagnosed with a blood test to check for antibodies against the thyroid, thyroid peroxidase antibodies, and anti-thyroglobulin antibodies.

Burnout occurs when your thyroid is unable to produce adequate thyroid hormone, and your thyroid cells are destroyed. Hashimoto's typically progresses slowly, over the course of several years, and the signs can vary widely, depending on the severity of the hormone deficiency. Although Hashimoto's can occur in women of any age as well as in men and children, women in middle age are diagnosed up to twenty times more often than men.

Goiters. Another common cause of hypothyroidism is goiter, a noncancerous enlargement of the thyroid gland that occurs in more than 700 million people throughout the world. Iodine deficiency is the leading cause worldwide for hypothyroidism. Approximately one-third of the world's population lives in areas of iodine deficiency, and the prevalence of goiter in areas of severe iodine deficiency is 80 percent. The problem can occur almost anywhere, particularly in regions far from the sea. Iodine deficiency can cause miscarriage and stillbirth, severe mental impairment, deafness, and dwarfism. Recently, we've learned that despite widespread salt iodization for the past twenty years, endemic goiter and hypothyroidism remain serious problems for nearly 7 percent of the world's population.[17] You're unlikely to see people with a goiter from iodine deficiency in the United States, because the table salt we use comes fortified with iodine, although iodine deficiency still exists. For all you foodies out there, note that the artisanal sea salt you may favor usually contains negligible quantities of iodine. Seafood and sea vegetables are, of course, fine sources of iodine, but they tend to have small amounts; 3 ounces of shrimp, for instance, contains 21 to 37 micrograms of iodine. The recommended dose for adults is 150 micrograms/day, but if you have autoimmune thyroiditis, use extreme caution as iodine may worsen your thyroid function.

Stress. As I described earlier, *long-standing stress is the enemy of a balanced hormonal system.* Tenacious stress causes you to make less free T3, the active thyroid hormone, and too much reverse T3, which blocks thyroid-hormone receptors. The adrenal glands secrete hormones—the most important of which is cortisol—that regulate your response to stress. As countless studies have shown, chronic adrenal stress affects the proper functioning of your hypothalamus and pituitary glands, which direct the production of thyroid hormone.

Previously, I explained how the hypothalamic-pituitary-adrenal (HPA) axis controls cortisol levels. Similarly, the hypothalamic-pituitary-thyroid (HPT) axis is modulated by levels of cortisol and melatonin (and their circadian rhythm), which then affect thyroid levels.[18] Too much stress throws off this delicate balance; in folks with excess cortisol, there's a proportional decrease in thyroid function.[19] When you have excess cortisol, your body does not respond appropriately to TSH. That may weaken your gut's ability to absorb the micronutrients—including copper, zinc, and selenium—that you need most to make thyroid hormones.

Environment. Bisphenol-A (BPA), a known endocrine disruptor, slows thyroid function by blocking thyroid receptors. As noted earlier, BPA is still found in so many products we use every day: it's in the lining of many cans of food and some plastic water bottles, flame retardants, mattresses, and children's pajamas.

Genetics. Genetic problems may cause low thyroid function, including defects in two genes (PAX8 and TSHR, what we call tyrosine kinase genes), which interfere with normal development of the thyroid gland prior to birth. Defects in five other genes (DUOX2,

SLC5A5, TPO, TG, and TSHB) lower your ability to produce thyroid hormones even if the thyroid gland is normal. Genetic testing is becoming increasingly easier, but tests for these genetic problems associated with the thyroid are still not widely available.

Goitrogens. Yes, soy may slow down your thyroid function. Goitrogens are compounds (found in soy, millet, and certain vegetables such as broccoli and Brussels sprouts) that suppress the thyroid by interfering with the cells' uptake of iodine, which is key to normal thyroid production. Several drugs prescribed in cases of excess thyroid, or hyperthyroidism, are designed to block the thyroid; two examples are propylthiouracil and lithium (used to treat bipolar disorder). If you take one of these, make sure your doctor checks your thyroid function. Cooking renders most goitrogens inactive, except with soy and millet. You need not avoid goitrogens; just make sure you are getting the right amount of iodine and track your thyroid levels.

Cancer treatment. Low thyroid function is increasingly recognized to be a consequence of cancer therapy, particularly with newer anticancer therapies.

Vitamin D deficiency. We know that vitamin D deficiency is more common in folks with autoimmune thyroiditis, as well as in people who harbor antithyroid antibodies.[20]

Thyroid, Gluten, and Gluten Sensitivity

Here's a fascinating angle on a common reason for hypothyroidism: *celiac disease* and *gluten sensitivity*. Celiac disease is a permanent intolerance to eating gluten, and it triples your risk of problems with low thyroid function. In people genetically predisposed to this disease, eating gluten results in inflammation and damage to the lining of the small intestine, preventing this twenty-foot section of the gut from absorbing nutrients crucial to your health. Symptoms include diarrhea, abdominal pain, fatigue, and bloating.

One percent of Americans have celiac disease, although many more—an estimated six out of one hundred—suffer from gluten sensitivity. Many struggle for years with "irritable bowel syndrome," until a good medical detective helps them figure out the root cause of their long-standing bowel problems. Many people don't know they suffer from gluten intolerance because they have no symptoms at all. They don't know they aren't absorbing crucial nutrients until they start to develop symptoms of hypothyroidism, or perhaps signs of osteoporosis, such as bone fractures. If you're interested in testing for celiac disease, here are the main genes found in families of people who suffer from celiac: about 90 percent of celiac patients are positive for DQ2, the gene for celiac, and 7 percent have DQ8.

Too often, doctors don't think of celiac as a root cause for such vague and nonspecific symptoms as fatigue and bloating. This wasn't a sexy topic in medical school, and U.S. board-certified doctors aren't really on the lookout for this common problem. Fortunately, knowledge is spreading, and more people are getting diagnosed prior to the onset of symptoms. If you have celiac disease, you may be missing out on key nutrients, such as the fat-soluble vitamins A, D, E, and K; you may not be absorbing iron, vitamin B_{12}, and folate, and some of these nutrients impact your thyroid function as well.

If left untreated, celiac disease can cause ulcers in your small intestine, or intestinal stricturing, which is when the internal opening narrows as a result of inflammation and scarring. Celiac disease increases the risk of bacterial overgrowth of the small intestine—an imbalance between the good and bad bacteria in the gut that favors the bad. Even worse, celiac disease puts you at greater risk for cancer of the small bowel, including adenocarcinoma and lymphoma. Fortunately, the cancer risk reverses with a gluten-free diet.

People with a sensitivity to gluten develop something known as leaky-gut syndrome, or increased intestinal permeability, when the tight junctions between the cells lining the small intestine become disrupted.[21] We also see increased intestinal permeability in the healthy relatives of celiacs, which is not surprising given that celiac disease is genetically transmitted, as described in greater detail in chapter 7, "Low Estrogen." Symptoms of leaky gut include bloating, food sensitivity, and weight gain. If you have autoimmune thyroiditis, consider testing for leaky-gut syndrome with a blood or urine test ordered through your doctor.

Celiacs are much more likely to have antibodies against the thyroid.[22] It's not definitive whether a gluten-free diet can slow progression of the auto-attack, but the best data show that eating gluten-free normalizes hypothyroidism and prevents progression.[23]

I believe that since celiac patients are more likely to have hypothyroidism, the corollary is true as well: all patients with hypothyroidism should be tested for celiac and gluten sensitivity, particularly since removing gluten may reverse the thyroid problem. Ask your doctor for a test.

————COULD YOU HAVE HYPERTHYROIDISM?————

Sometimes it's too much thyroid that causes the problem. Some of my patients initially have hyperthyroidism, or excess thyroid, when the thyroid produces too many hormones. With overt hyperthyroidism, you have low TSH but elevated levels of free T3 or T4. With subclinical hyperthyroidism you have low TSH, but normal levels of T3 and T4.

Hyperthyroidism affects only 2 percent of women (and 0.2 percent of men), but rates increase as you age; 15 percent older than sixty have hyperthyroidism.[24] Symptoms include palpitations, shortness of breath, weight loss, tremulousness or shakiness, and proptosis (eyes bugging out).

It's not hard to treat an overactive thyroid, but it's important to do so. If you don't, the symptoms can become more severe over time. Untreated, hyperthyroidism can lead to cardiovascular problems such as a potentially dangerous type of arrhythmia called atrial fibrillation, cardiomyopathy (a disease of the heart), and congestive heart failure. When you have hyperthyroidism, you are more likely to have increased bone turnover, which over time may lead to bone loss and fracture. Another serious consequence is thyrotoxicosis, also known as thyroid storm, which has a significant risk of mortality.

IODINE AND RADIATION EXPOSURE

After the meltdown of the nuclear power plants in Fukushima, Japan, in early 2011, authorities distributed potassium iodine to the evacuation centers. The U.S. Surgeon General suggested that Americans have some on hand, in case nuclear radiation came our way in significant amounts. (Keep in mind that it's important not to take potassium iodine as a preventive measure—use it only if you are about to be exposed.) As I mentioned, iodine is important for normal metabolic and thyroid functioning and for the production of thyroid hormones. Nuclear accidents release radioactive iodine (I-131), which your body can't distinguish from the iodine you get in seafood and iodized salt. This is bad, because the thyroid absorbs and concentrates iodine, and a relatively small dose of radiation can increase your risk for developing thyroid cancer even ten or twenty years later. Potassium iodine can come to the rescue by saturating the thyroid gland, crowding out the radioactive iodine, and preventing it from being absorbed for up to twenty-four hours. The CDC recommends that you take the pills as quickly as possible after radiation exposure. It may be dangerous to take it prior to exposure, particularly if you have Hashimoto's thyroiditis.

THE HORROR OF HAIR LOSS

For many people, rapid hair loss is an early sign of a thyroid problem, often first diagnosed in the beauty salon. In addition to thinning and shedding, your hair can become coarse, dry, and easily tangled.

If the cause of your hair-loss woes is low thyroid, it's likely this kind of general hair loss will slow and eventually stop once your hormone levels are stabilized. But sometimes the problem continues even after treatment, especially if you're taking levothyroxine, a synthetic hormone often used to treat hypothyroidism. Excessive or prolonged hair loss is a known side effect of this drug. You'll want to look into this if you're still losing hair despite what your doctor calls sufficient treatment. Some people find their hair loss diminishes if they take Thyrolar, a synthetic combination of both thyroid hormones, T4 and T3.

Sometimes the problem is male-pattern hair loss, on the temples and top of the head, seen in women with high testosterone. The problem may be exacerbated in some patients treated with drugs for thyroid problems.

The nutritional supplement evening primrose oil inhibits the conversion of testosterone to dihydrotestosterone. And it is a good source of essential fatty acids—the symptoms of hypothyroidism are quite similar to those for insufficient essential fatty acids. I generally recommend that women suffering from hair loss take 1,000 mg per day.

In one study, 90 percent of women with thinning hair were deficient in iron and the amino acid lysine.[25] Lysine helps transport iron, which is essential for many metabolic processes. Good sources of lysine are foods rich in protein, such as meat and poultry, eggs, and some fish (cod, sardines). Because grains contain small quantities of lysine but legumes contain lots, meals that combine the two—Indian dal with rice, beans with rice and tortilla, falafel and hummus with pita bread—are a good way to get complete protein in your diet and keep hair on your head.

The Solution: The Gottfried Protocol for Low Thyroid

Step 1: Targeted Lifestyle Changes and Nutraceuticals

Several micronutrients, required by your body in small quantities for optimal physiological function, can alter your thyroid balance. Additionally, certain heavy metals and endocrine disruptors from the environment can harm your thyroid function. For more information, go to http://thehormonecurebook.com/HormoneDisruptors.

Copper. The thyroid gland is quite sensitive to copper and zinc, which must remain in proportion; an imbalance in these two elements can result in hypothyroidism. Additionally, thyroid hormone regulates blood levels of copper by adjusting the copper transport protein ceruloplasmin, and thereby changing the level of copper inside and outside of cells. Meats, poultry, and eggs are the best dietary sources of copper, which means vegans need to supplement their diets with an abundance of nuts, seeds, and grains, other good sources of copper.

Even with sufficient copper in your diet, you may be like me: I have trouble absorbing copper and consistently measure low on blood tests. For this reason, I take a multivitamin containing 2 mg of copper to augment the amount of copper I get from my food. As discussed earlier in this chapter, your serum levels of both copper and selenium may indicate thyroid resistance.

Zinc. Zinc is important for the conversion of T4 to T3, and supplementation has been shown to raise free T3 (fT3), decrease reverse T3 (rT3), and lower TSH.[26] It is necessary to stimulate the pituitary and make the proper amount of TSH, and it must be taken in the correct proportion with copper, since taking too much zinc may interfere with copper absorption. Generally, more than 50 mg/day is too much. I take 20 mg of zinc each day with my 2 mg of copper.

Selenium. Selenium is important to the enzymes that protect your thyroid from damage by free radicals, which are the molecules with odd or unpaired electrons that may damage your DNA and accelerate aging. Selenium supplementation appears to reduce immune overactivity, as measured by autoimmune antibodies to the thyroid, and to improve mood and well-being in selenium-deficient people.[27]

There is limited evidence that supplementing with selenium in healthy individuals makes a difference.[28] However, in older people living in nursing homes, selenium helps to optimize thyroid hormones.[29] Take selenium only if you're deficient and have autoantibodies to the thyroid. As I've mentioned, you want the appropriate amount for you: not too much and not too little. Many multivitamins contain the recommended amount of 200 mcg/day.

Vitamin A. Your thyroid depends on sufficient quantities of vitamin A, so I encourage you to get the recommended daily allowance of 5,000 IU. Evidence is good that vitamin A supplementation has a beneficial impact on thyroid function.[30] However, taking more than 10,000 IU per day may be associated with toxicity, heralded by symptoms such as night blindness, nausea, irritability, blurred vision, and hair loss. Toxicity does not occur when you get vitamin A from food; excellent sources include chicken livers (11,000 IU), raw carrots (½ cup has 9,000 IU from beta-carotene), and dandelion greens (5,000 IU).

Iron. In addition to iodine, selenium, copper, zinc, and other micronutrients, iron is also key to normal thyroid function. Low iron levels correlate with both hair loss and hypothyroidism.[31] In fact, many of the symptoms of low iron—such as weakness, fatigue, brain fog, low sex drive, and palpitations—overlap with hypothyroid symptoms. If you don't have enough iron, it may affect several of the steps of thyroid-hormone production by reducing the activity of the enzyme thyroid peroxidase, which is iron dependent. Iron deficiency may also reduce conversion of T4 to T3.

The most sensitive way to measure your iron level is to ask your doctor for a serum-ferritin level, and to keep your level between 70 and 90. Too much iron may cause overload, resulting in problems with your liver. I recommend iron from food sources, such as leafy greens and grass-fed beef. If those fail to keep your ferritin in your target range, you may need to find out why you aren't absorbing it well.

Some women also need to take a supplement, such as ferrous sulfate or ferrous fumerate. However, many women find that iron supplements cause constipation and dark, hard stool. If that is the case, I recommend magnesium, probiotics, and a decreased dose of iron. I usually recommend 50 to 100 mg per day of elemental iron with careful monitoring of your progress through serum ferritin. Vitamin C increases absorption. Taking iron within four hours of thyroid medication may lower absorption of the thyroid medication. It is generally not necessary to take iron after menopause, since you are no longer losing blood each month.

MERCURY

Alice in Wonderland's Mad Hatter was based on nineteenth-century hatmakers, who often became mentally ill from the mercury rubbed on felt to soften it. Mercury also gets into our bodies by way of fish, particularly large fish and shellfish; medications, such as thiazide diuretics, prescribed for high blood pressure; vaccines, which may contain thimerosal, a mercury compound used as a preservative; and dental fillings. I recommend starting a mercury-free campaign that includes eating only fish with low levels of mercury, replacing your old metal fillings, and reducing your exposure in a reasonable way. If you're pregnant, ask your doctor about how much and what kinds of fish you should eat. You can find numerous websites that will give you information on mercury levels in fish, such as the Centers for Disease Control or the Monterey Bay Aquarium seafood watch site.

Soy isoflavones. As mentioned earlier, soy foods or isoflavones have either little or no effect on thyroid function if you are getting sufficient iodine. You don't need to avoid soy foods (unless you have a food intolerance), but keep an eye on your thyroid tests if you have a fondness for regular soy consumption. Limit to two servings per week.

Raw brassica. Certain foods, such as Brussels sprouts and kale, are good for your estrogen metabolism but, if eaten raw, may decrease thyroid function. Fortunately, cooking seems to lessen the blow.

Vitamin D. With the bad rap the sun's rays have been getting lately, some people have been covering up or staying out of the sun too much, and not getting enough vitamin D. It's difficult to gain a sufficient amount through your diet, which is why some food products, such as milk, are fortified with vitamin D. The best food sources are liver and low-mercury fish such as herring, sardines, and cod. Sunshine is still the best way to get vitamin D, but my advice is not to overdo it.

Step 2: Herbal Therapies

For thousands of years, practitioners of Ayurveda, the ancient system of medicine from India that I sometimes find helpful in treating metabolic problems, have prescribed several botanical therapies to help with thyroid. One is kanchanar guggulu; another is bladderwrack. Despite folkloric precedent and use in Asia, these have not been supported by solid scientific evidence. Similarly, at least one health site suggests coleus, guggulu, and bladderwrack for low thyroid function, but there is insufficient data to warrant any of these recommendations.[32]

Step 3: Bioidentical Hormones

There are several options for augmenting thyroid function if the recommendations I've made above don't provide the lift you need. When it comes to bioidentical hormones, I prescribe the smallest doses possible and for the shortest duration, with the intention to never rise above the physiological range—that is, the normal range that occurs naturally and is considered optimal.

I tell my patients that finding the right thyroid prescription is similar to shoe shopping—sometimes you nail it with the first pair of shoes that you try on, but other times you need to try various pairs before you find the best fit. I was taught in medical school and residency to use synthetic T4 in all cases, but I've found over the past few decades that hypothyroid symptoms are more likely to resolve—the shoe is more likely to fit—when I start with desiccated or glandular thyroid prescriptions. Overall, I achieve better results for a wider range of symptoms when I use desiccated thyroid rather than synthetic T4. Just as conventional physicians question the validity of the hypothyroid diagnosis, many also question the benefit of desiccated thyroid, and consider it obsolete. My experience tells me otherwise.

There are several different options to consider when you need thyroid augmentation or replacement. Here's a shopping list; except for Tirosint, which is a liquid soft gel, the first three are oral tablets.

- Glandulars or Natural Desiccated Thyroid (Armour, Nature-Throid)
- T4 (L-thyroxine,* Synthroid,* and more recently, Tirosint*)
- T3 (Cytomel,* liothyronine,* or compounded)
- T3/T4 combinations (Thyrolar* or compounded)

Glandulars, you'll recall, are ground-up endocrine glands from animals. Several companies make natural thyroid-hormone replacement products; the one I generally prescribe is Armour Thyroid. This is made by Forest Pharmaceuticals from the desiccated thyroid glands of pigs and is available by prescription. Forest states that only grain-fed, USDA-inspected pigs are used. Nature-Throid, from Western Research Laboratories, is another glandular made from porcine thyroid glands.

---

* Approved and regulated by the Federal Drug Administration.

Since these products replace or augment thyroid hormones, the most common side effects are similar to the symptoms for either too much (hyperthyroidism) or too little (hypothyroidism). You'll know when you have the right dose by how good you feel.

How to Choose Your Thyroid Medication

All of the medications mentioned above require a prescription. Over-the-counter thyroid treatments (besides those mentioned in Steps 1 and 2) are not worth your time or money, and may be harmful. Here are my recommendations based on the best evidence:

1. *Start with natural desiccated thyroid.* Desiccated thyroid has been available since the early 1900s, in Armour Thyroid and Nature-Throid. Neither is FDA-approved, but that's not as bad as it sounds. Many prescription drugs have not been approved because their use predated formation of the FDA, and they were "grandfathered" into practice. (Phenobarbital, a seizure medication, is an example.) Such common thyroid medications as levothyroxine and Cytomel were not FDA-approved until recently.

   Armour and Nature-Throid contain "USP" thyroid, which means the manufacturer has prepared them according to the formulation of United States Pharmacopoeia (USP, a nongovernmental organization). In other words, both Armour and Nature-Throid meet USP potency and consistency standards.

   Regarding the substantial controversy about the best treatment for hypothyroidism, the evidence is mixed (and documented elsewhere, so I will not take up valuable space here rehashing the studies). As I described at the beginning of the chapter, there are grassroots, patient-to-patient movements and books devoted to women who never felt their hypothyroid symptoms were resolved by taking only T4 yet felt astonishingly better on desiccated thyroid.[33] And there is evidence that desiccated thyroid is safer and more stable than synthetic T4.

If your physician is open to it, I recommend that you begin with the smallest dose of desiccated thyroid, either Armour or Nature-Throid. Check out the best-selling books by Mary Shomon and Janie Bowthorpe to learn more about why I recommend this medication. Personally and professionally, I believe desiccated thyroid is the most effective treatment for the broadest spectrum of women with a sluggish or absent thyroid. I take it myself. After starting or making any change in your thyroid medication, homeostasis takes six weeks, so you must wait this long before assessing your biochemical progress or your labs, and then reconcile your labs with your residual symptoms and with your clinician.

2. **Move on to T4.** If your physician is not open to desiccated thyroid or you are uncomfortable that the FDA hasn't approved its use, or perhaps have an ethical or religious objection to consuming porcine products, or even a gluten sensitivity or celiac disease, choose Tirosint. However, I recommend that you get monitored closely by a knowledgeable clinician who can track your symptoms, free thyroid levels (free T3 and free T4), and reverse T3, as well as TSH. Keep in mind that Tirosint has a shorter track record than any other medication on the list.

3. **Assess for progress and add T3 as needed.** If Tirosint does not abolish your symptoms, you may need to add T3. I prefer Cytomel as it is regulated by the FDA and often paid for by insurance, at least in part. Be cautious with taking T3 because it is four times more potent than T4, and some women taking T3 get anxious, tremulous, or suffer heart palpitations, which may be quite

serious and require urgent medical attention. Some of my patients cannot tolerate Cytomel even at the minimum dose (5 mcg), and need either to cut the tablet into a smaller dose or to use a compounded version that releases more slowly. For free T3, I recommend levels 2.5–3.4 ng/dL, and pay attention to how a person feels.

4. **If symptoms persist, consider thyroid resistance.** This is where you may require the A team—a clinician who understands and routinely tests people for thyroid resistance with one of the three tests covered earlier in this chapter: TRH stimulation test, fT3/rT3, or copper/selenium. See Appendix D for how to find doctors knowledgeable in this field.

You may wonder why most of my patients do better with natural desiccated thyroid or a combination of T3 and T4. I'm not certain, but I suspect their response relates to the fact that desiccated thyroid contains about 80 percent T4 and 20 percent T3, plus a tiny amount of T2 and T1, whereas levothyroxine contains solely T4.

FROM THE FILES OF SARA GOTTFRIED, MD
Patient: Mom
Age: Sixty-seven
Plea for help: "*My thyroid function is low. Topping it off would slow down aging? OK, I'll try it, if you think it's safe.*"

It's my mom who taught me daily about healthy eating. At school, I was the four-eyed geek with the dense, dark-brown bread with local honey and natural peanut butter, plus an apple, for lunch. No sugary Hostess Ho Hos for me. She called it brain food. Mom is gorgeous and is aging slowly, but she has put on a few pounds over the years, and she has seen her share of hair loss.

Treatment protocol: I suggested we run a thyroid panel, and we found her free T3 was low and her TSH was 3.4. I recommended taking ¼ grain of Armour Thyroid.

Results: "I feel more bounce in my step. I found myself running up the stairs in my house! I haven't run up the stairs in our home in fifteen years!"

How to Manage Treatment with Thyroid Hormone

Once you and your doctor determine that it's a good idea for you to start thyroid medicine, you've made it through the hurdle of the underdiagnosis of thyroid problems, but now you've got the next hurdle of getting the appropriate dose. I strongly encourage you to adjust thyroid medication only under the care of a knowledgeable clinician, ideally board certified, who has worked for at least ten years in a busy practice. Never sell yourself short.

Here's how one patient described it: "Why does my doctor read my numbers and not listen to how I feel instead? That is my question." I have found that it is essential to both listen to a patient's residual symptoms and to review the appropriate laboratory tests, particularly when you consider the potential issue of thyroid resistance. In general, I am looking for the main symptoms along with any other hormonal imbalances (such as high cortisol; see chapter 11 for a more thorough discussion of this common hormone combination) to be resolved—plus thyroid hormones improved to the optimal range. But doctors shouldn't look just at the numbers. To forge an effective strategy for the right treatment, it's just as important to listen.

Thyroid in Balance

I believe every woman can correct her thyroid, boost her metabolism and mood to levels that are her birthright, and manage her weight both sensibly and sustainably. Here's what you can achieve:

- Stable weight. You look at a piece of cake and it doesn't land on your hips.
- Comfortable-temperature hands. People don't recoil in horror at your cold hands when you extend a handshake.
- Your hairdresser is in awe of your silky hair since your last visit.
- That longed-for zip back in your step (and sex life).

CHAPTER 10

COMMON COMBINATIONS OF HORMONAL IMBALANCES

As we all know, life doesn't always fit into perfect categories. More often than not, life is messy and disorganized. The same is true for hormones. Just as your health does not exist in a vacuum but is a vast interconnected web of influences and functionality, the same applies to your neuroendocrine system. While some people have one hormonal imbalance, the majority of us have some kind of combination. The point of this chapter is to provide guidance for those who have multiple hormone issues. How do you know? If you answered "yes" in the questionnaires in chapter 1 enough times to be torn between which chapter to visit first, then chances are you are experiencing one of the common combinations of hormonal imbalance. I've got solutions to help you optimize your health in a way that is holistic and comprehensive.

The Neuroendocrine System and You

Your hormonal system communicates with your mind and the rest of your body as a complex and sophisticated *neuroendocrine communication network* that encompasses your brain chemicals and hormones. Specific parts of your brain—essentially, your hypothalamus and pituitary, which are part of your limbic system—are the boss of your network.

Here's the problem: One part of your brain tends to exert more influence than any other, and that's your amygdala, where you take in stress, interpret, and then embed news and stimuli from your environment, and manufacture your mental and emotional state. Women aged thirty-five to fifty have a tendency to overrespond emotionally to triggers in an immediate, reactionary, and sometimes overwhelming manner. There's a mismatch between the trigger and the response. I know, because I've been there, and I see many women each day in my office who feel this way. Here's how one woman describes it:

> I'm so up and down with my emotions, Dr. Sara. They're right at the surface. Discernment? Gone. Some days at work, I'm on my game and can keep it together, and other days, I burst into tears for no good reason. It's not cool when that happens at work. It's also not just before my period, although it's certainly amplified. I just can't trust myself anymore to have my act together.

It is very difficult to manage the amygdala, yet it impacts your levels of critical hormones such as cortisol, estrogen, progesterone, and thyroid. The amygdala, hypothalamus, and pituitary organize, integrate, and coordinate what you're interested in: mood, fertility, sexual desire, skin texture, general aging, and weight via neuro-endocrine communication. Your brain determines hormone levels throughout the body, and reciprocally, hormone levels direct brain activity through feedback loops—and the dance between the two determines your ability to feel optimal vim and vigor.

How to Approach Multiple Hormone Imbalances

I've addressed the intercommunication of the main endocrine glands to some extent in previous chapters, but I'd like to devote a whole chapter to this crucial idea. Now that you have a sense of how to apply The Gottfried Protocol for individual hormone imbalances, I want to share with you how to deal with several hormonal issues when they occur simultaneously. As the number of symptoms rises along with the complexity and interconnections of your hormonal problems, I strongly recommend working with a trusted clinician. But here's the good news: when you fix more than one hormonal problem at a time, you amplify both the health benefit and how good you feel.

Find the Root Cause, Especially with Multiple Hormone Imbalances

I was taught, particularly in surgery and other areas of medicine where *triage* is an operative word, to prioritize the most pressing problems facing a patient, and to act on the most immediate and proven solutions. But hormones are not surgery; you are not hemorrhaging or infected. For hormonal balance, especially when more than one system is imbalanced, you need a different and more nuanced method. My patients achieve the best results when they agree to partner with me on a *systems* approach to why their hormones went awry, and to spend the time looking at how it all started. The root cause of your hormonal issues, particularly multiple hormone issues, tends to begin well before symptoms appear. By adjusting the levers that got you out of hormonal balance, you are more likely to experience sustained balance and restore homeostasis. The following case is a great example of what I mean.

FROM THE FILES OF SARA GOTTFRIED, MD

Patient: Jocelyn

Age: Forty

Plea for help: "I'm really tired, and feel like I have no reserve. I'm drinking more coffee to lift me up in the morning but it doesn't seem to help, and then I have trouble falling asleep. I'm easily frazzled and can't concentrate, especially when I'm busy and under deadline. I'm overwhelmed and it's just not like me to feel this way. Every time my kids bring home a virus, I catch it. Exercise doesn't feel good, and I used to be an athlete. This is new in the past few months, and it's bringing me down. I can't handle it! I'm not full-on depressed, but I'd like to feel more human again."

Jocelyn took my questionnaire and checked off five signs of low cortisol: fatigue, loss of stamina, chronic overwhelm, difficulty fighting infection, and poor sleeping. She also noted three signs of low thyroid function: dry skin, brain fog, and mild depression. Given her multiple symptoms, I checked her blood for cortisol—we found that her morning level of cortisol was slightly low at 6 mcg/dL (I believe the optimal range for adults is 10–15.0)—and TSH, which indicated mild hypothyroidism at 2.7 mIU/L (I use 0.3 to 2.5 mIU/L as an optimal range). Her twenty-four-hour urine test for cortisol was normal. Her blood pressure was low normal at 92/61.

Treatment protocol: We applied The Gottfried Protocol for low cortisol and thyroid, Step 1, simultaneously. Jocelyn began a supplement regimen of a vitamin B complex, tyrosine at 1,000 mg per day, and vitamin C at 1,000 mg per day for her low cortisol. For her thyroid, she began a broad-spectrum mineral supplement that included copper 1 mg per day and zinc 20 mg per day, and she increased her vitamin A consumption by eating carrots and dandelion greens. She started a hip-hop class, which I suspect raises cortisol, as found in a 2004 study of African dance published in *Annals of Behavioral Medicine.* Her biggest aha! moment came when she realized that it was the type of exercise that made a difference—she needed to exercise in a way that boosted her cortisol.

After six weeks, Jocelyn felt better but still had half of her symptoms. Her TSH was improved at 2.3 and her morning cortisol was 8, which is still below the optimal range. We added Step 2 of The Gottfried Protocol for her low cortisol, and she began taking licorice as a capsule twice per day. (Check with your doctor before taking licorice, as it may raise your blood pressure.)

Results: After another six weeks, Jocelyn's symptoms resolved on the licorice, plus her TSH was normal at 1.3 and morning cortisol was normal at 12. Her blood pressure was normal at 110/75, which was more typical for her when she was feeling balanced. Jocelyn's main "lever" was enduring stress with low cortisol, and the combination was impacting her thyroid function. When her cortisol was addressed through Step 2, and thyroid through Step 1, we corrected both imbalances without resorting to any prescription medications. This is not just my unique experience with reversible hypothyroidism caused by adrenal dysregulation, but a pattern documented by other clinicians.[1]

Guidelines

Jocelyn's case suggests a few guidelines for multiple hormone imbalances. When more than one hormone is out of whack, things get more complicated, and I recommend additional resources to help guide you.

- **Work with a trusted doctor.** When more than one hormonal system is off, I suggest strongly that you find a collaborative doctor who has the time, knowledge, and interest to tackle your hormonal imbalances with you. If you feel you haven't found the right match, see Appendix D for ideas and resources on how to choose a clinician who will be sensitive to your preferences, and won't jump straight to prescriptions as the only option.

- **Consider testing.** When you have multiple hormone imbalances, blood or other testing (such as urine or saliva) reviewed with your trusted doctor is a good practice, since there is significant overlap between symptom groups. Hormones perpetually interact with one another, so measurement can be a helpful tool.

- **Isolate the primary problem.** Address the primary problem first. If you map your symptoms on a timeline, usually the primary hormone issue will be obvious as a root cause. This was clear with Jocelyn's example: when her adrenal dysregulation was repaired, the thyroid problem resolved. As you may have learned in chapters 2 and 4, the glucocorticoids, most notably cortisol, are the main modulators—the alpha hormones—of the hypothalamus and pituitary, and these in turn control the feedback to the ovaries, thyroid, and adrenals.[2] For most women, I look first to the glucocorticoids in any situation of multiple hormonal imbalances.

- *Identify the antecedents, triggers, and mediators.* In functional medicine, these factors are called the ATM. Typically, when you have a problem such as an overactive hypothalamic-pituitary-adrenal (HPA) axis, you can trace it back to a predisposing factor, known as an antecedent. Here's how one woman in my medical practice described her antecedent: "I was medically boring until age twenty-eight, when my mother was dying of cancer, and I took care of her for six months until she died. Within a year of her death, my periods stopped and I developed fibromyalgia." Recall that fibromyalgia is related to low cortisol, and amenorrhea (when you experience three months without a period) can be caused by several problems—from a faulty control system of the ovaries (the hypothalamic-pituitary-gonadal axis, which is how the brain controls the ovaries) to gluten allergy to premature menopause.

- *Beware of the most common masqueraders.* As you read in chapters 6 and 9, a broad range of chemicals known as endocrine disruptors often can affect more than one hormonal system—for instance, bisphenol-A acts as a xenoestrogen and a thyroid disruptor, and sadly, levels are detectable in the urine of 93 percent of American adults. Awareness of how chemicals in the environment can affect your hormones is essential.[3]

A Word About Evidence and Combinations of Hormonal Imbalances

There's a myriad of hormonal combinations that I identify in my office: high cortisol and low estrogen; low progesterone and low thyroid function; low cortisol and low thyroid; high cortisol, high insulin, and high androgens (plus high LH, low FSH, and PCOS, *oh my!*), to name a few. Here are the most common combinations that I see in my practice:

1. **Dysregulated cortisol (high and/or low) and thyroid problem.** Here I define *dysregulated* to mean that the body's response to chronic stress is poorly modulated, or regulated, such that cortisol is not kept within an optimal range for the body and is either too high or too low, usually at different times within the same twenty-four-hour period.

2. **Dysregulated cortisol and sex hormones**
   a. Estrogen (low)
   b. Progesterone (low)

3. **Low progesterone (estrogen dominance) and low thyroid hormone**

Cortisol Resistance: Is Cortisol Similar to Insulin?

Just as too many doughnuts, excess stress, environmental toxins, and sedentary living collectively lead to *insulin resistance,* where your cells become numb to insulin, there is growing support for the scientific basis for *cortisol resistance,* where your cells similarly become numb to cortisol.[4] As you now know, cortisol is the alpha hormone, and other hormones such as thyroid, estrogen, and progesterone are submissive. When you do not manage optimally or follow healthy lifestyle design, several imbalances may occur at once, such as insulin and cortisol resistance.

Here's the concept: perpetual stress raises blood cortisol levels. Our latest scientific understanding, however, is that the way cells *react* to cortisol—that is, whether the cells are *sensitive* (which is normal) or *numb* (which is not normal, and a sign of hormone imbalance, and in this case, hormone resistance)—may be more important than actual hormone levels in the blood.[5] (This concept also suggests that questionnaires might be more helpful than blood tests for identifying cellular resistance, since we do not currently have a way to test for cortisol resistance.) As I mentioned, cortisol is one of the hormones known as glucocorticoids. We now have evidence that glucocorticoid receptor resistance (GCR) results from chronically high cortisol levels in the blood. That leads to low cortisol inside the cells of your body, which makes you feel as if you have the symptoms of low cortisol, despite your high blood levels. In other words, your glucocorticoid receptors for cortisol become unable to respond to cortisol. Using the lock-and-key analogy, your "lock" (glucocorticoid receptor) becomes jammed, and cortisol can no longer open the door. The final result is inflammation, which we learned is not good—it creates the *bad neighborhood* that tends to alienate the other happy hormones and neurotransmitters and makes you more susceptible to illnesses and disease, such as cancer and diabetes.

Several trials document this new theory of cortisol resistance.[6] Persistent stress results in cortisol resistance, which makes you more likely to get sick with a cold and to produce more inflammation. Bottom line? Prevent cortisol resistance (and insulin resistance) by applying the health-promoting lifestyle design of The Gottfried Protocol.

Imbalance and Age

In my practice, I've seen some distinct patterns when it comes to age and hormonal imbalances. Here's what I've discovered:

WOMEN UNDER THIRTY-FIVE

Most often, the younger women who come to my integrative medicine practice have only a single hormonal problem, such as high cortisol, low progesterone, high estrogen, or high testosterone. These are the most common imbalances that I see and treat with The Gottfried Protocol. And although these younger patients come to me with symptoms, at this age the fix is often stunningly simple. Remember the theory that those of us who are aged thirty-five to fifty have the lowest psychological well-being of any age group? Before age thirty-five, there's less stress and better resilience to meet it; there's usually less hormonal upheaval from pregnancy; and there's more organ reserve, longer telomeres, and a generally superior ability to roll with the punches. Women under the age of thirty-five are less likely to have multiple hits to their homeostasis, so it's simpler to find the original cause for their hormonal problem.

Occasionally I see multiple hormonal issues in this age group. When I do, it's most frequently women who have both cortisol problems and a thyroid issue, or high androgens together with wayward cortisol. I find that infertility is related to low progesterone, or sometimes low thyroid function. As women get closer to age thirty-five, the combination of the two hormonal imbalances appears more frequently. The most common hormone combination of this age group is dysregulated cortisol along with changes to thyroid, progesterone, or testosterone.

Why is this? Because cortisol is the most essential hormone that you make—you need it *no matter what* to deliver fuel to cells, which is the most basic task of a hormone in your body—and the nonessential sex hormones (progesterone, testosterone, thyroid) will be the first to get imbalanced when cortisol is the top priority. In other words, you will make cortisol, sometimes at very high levels, at the expense of your other hormones.

WOMEN IN PERIMENOPAUSE AND EARLY MENOPAUSE: AGE THIRTY-FIVE TO FIFTY-PLUS

Women from thirty-five to fifty tend to have more than one problem at a time, probably because of the chain reaction of ovarian aging and chronic stress. In fact, how you age is profoundly influenced by how you navigate stress.[7] Sometimes we can identify the primary issue and correct that first. Then, as a result, the secondary hormonal imbalances can be addressed and cleared up. But sometimes you have to address more than one hormonal problem at a time and treat them simultaneously for best results.

That's when the concept of Charlie's Angels becomes increasingly important—you want the entire team of estrogen, thyroid, and cortisol working for you, not against you. You always want to first address the root cause, particularly when you have more than one hormonal issue. And all roads, not surprisingly, usually lead back to the limbic system, amygdala hijack, and the adrenal glands.

In other words, *adrenal function is the first place to look* when you have multiple symptoms of hormonal imbalance, which is due to hormonal intercommunication—that is, there are classic patterns of hormonal and neurotransmitter consequences. When you're stressed at twenty-five, you go to a yoga class, sleep it off, or call a good friend or maybe even your mother. When you're forty-five, chronic and repetitive stress cranks up your cortisol until your adrenals can't make enough, then your thyroid slows down and your joints get cranky, and as a result, your knee may hurt too much to go to yoga. When you're stressed, your thyroid abruptly slows down production of the key thyroid hormones—and you feel cold and achy and your hair falls out. Then you develop extreme PMS because high cortisol from stress blocks your progesterone receptors, and perhaps you develop progesterone resistance. You rage and may want a divorce. Next month, because your ovaries are semiretired, you don't ovulate and then your estrogen is low. Serotonin levels fall, and because serotonin (Nature's Prozac) manages sleep, appetite, and mood, you become an insomniac, which worsens your depression and ramps up your appetite. You get the idea.

In other words, one imbalance (chronic stress and wayward cortisol—initially high, and then low) begets a cascading crescendo of hormonal problems. Dysregulated cortisol is linked to thyropause, low progesterone, and eventually, as you get closer to menopause, low estrogen.

Keep in mind that the key differentiator for ages thirty-five to fifty is that the ovaries are sputtering and this makes many women feel like they are under siege: one day you want another child and feel blissed out, and the next day you want to run away from home to become a forest dweller. As I described in chapter 2, the boss of your Charlie's Angels—your adrenals, ovaries, and thyroid—is in the brain, the hypothalamus. In other words, the hypothalamus is your Charlie. If your hypothalamus *ain't* happy, Mama *ain't* happy. You want the boss, your hypothalamus, to be your ally since it controls the orchestra of your hormonal symphony, and the symphony can get extremely out of tune starting sometime between age thirty-five and forty-five.

Your hypothalamus tells its neighbor, the pituitary, to make more or less of the control hormones for your adrenals, ovaries, and thyroid. Several important factors determine how much hormone your endocrine glands should make, including how much stress you perceive, changes in weight, light/dark cycles (especially how much light you are exposed to at night), quantity and quality of sleep, and medications (such as birth control pills), to name a few.

WOMEN AFTER MENOPAUSE

Unlike women under age fifty, who demonstrate lower psychological well-being (probably because they are focused on being all things to all people and trying to appear as if they have it all together), your hormones quiet down again after fifty. Some women rather enjoy getting their crone on. Those hideous (and sometimes hilarious) dark corners of perimenopause are behind them. Women past menopause often no longer feel a need to endure the sacrifices and occasional masochism of selfless service. Have you noticed that women after fifty are more stress resilient, and seem to have more choices and actions to express their authentic needs and values? That's not just anecdote—it's well documented.[8]

Stress diminishes during this time after childrearing and prime career-building years, and this translates into a calmer neuroendocrine system so the chain reactions don't take hold. You come more fully into your own, and learn not to give a damn about other people's opinions of you. Yes, there's the unforgiving metabolism to contend with, but at least you are of relatively sound mind as you check your thyroid, take on a Paleo diet (see page 174), and make time for yoga. There's more sanity and choice.

You get down to business. You can no longer put off the important stuff that you postponed while you were busy tending a family and career or running a household. There's a planet to save, some other underdog that needs your voice, or a garden to water.

Even with less stress among women over fifty, there might be more cortisol resistance. We know that certain biomarkers change after age fifty: cortisol rises, DHEA and other androgens decrease, and thyroid autoimmunity increases to a peak at ten years after menopause.[9] More women are diagnosed with insomnia, probably related to increased cortisol, and as a consequence, they experience more disrupted sleep and lower melatonin levels. And that can make you feel lousy and foggy brained the next day.

FROM MAIDEN TO CRONE

Here's one woman's experience over her hormonal arc from her thirties through her sixties:

> When I was in my thirties, I never had any clue that the stress of
> an adrenaline-fueled job and a difficult marriage had an impact
> on my hormones, and on my inability to conceive and to carry a
> fetus to term.

When I hit my forties, I found myself in a pressure cooker of a job just as I was—totally unknowingly—about to go through perimenopause. I had three teenagers. Juggle-R-Us. I did a very good job of leaving my emotional self at the door before I went to work, but my body rebelled. I began to suffer from migraines. I never lost a day of work because of migraines, but some days I had to prop up a cardboard likeness of myself at my desk and just soldier on. My periods became heavy, when they had normally been quite manageable—and so painful that I was awakened at night (great for a hard day's work and a long commute). It was as though my emotions spent every day at the amusement park, on the roller coaster. Finally my doctor prescribed a low dose of birth control pills, which smoothed over my emotional life, but did nothing for my migraines (in fact, it probably exacerbated them).

In my fifties, as my periods became more erratic and I lumbered on toward menopause, the first sign that something was terribly amiss was my inability to sleep. My doctor tinkered with hormones, to little avail. Finally she suggested I try an acupuncturist at the college where she was studying. Yeah, right, someone's going to stick me with needles and I'm going to be able to think again? It took a few months, but between weekly sessions of acupuncture and a daily dose of Chinese herbs, I was able to sleep well enough that my brain worked.

Charlotte, whom you met previously, in chapter 4, articulates the interconnection of stress and her other hormonal symptoms, including infertility, migraines, unstable emotions, and sleep problems.

Stress and Downstream Hormonal Imbalances

As you read through my explanation of the common hormonal imbalances I see in my practice, you might notice that most of them have one feature in common: dysregulated cortisol. This is no coincidence. Women respond to excess stress in a predictable manner. Left unchecked, unremitting stress has important consequences—

including infertility, a "fried" control system (the hypothalamus), fatigue, and moodiness—for women who are largely neglected by mainstream medicine. Your organ reserve gets depleted along with your natal chi, according to Traditional Chinese Medicine, and your telomeres may shorten. You age prematurely, and so do your ovaries (diminished ovarian reserve) and thyroid (thyropause).

Recap of Cortisol Interdependence with Other Hormones

Let me repeat: cortisol bosses around production of several major and minor hormones. Cortisol regulates blood sugar, immune function, and blood pressure, plus it inhibits or stimulates many other hormones. When stress is excessive or perceived to be excessive, initially cortisol (a member of the glucocorticoid family) rises in the blood, saliva, and urine. This is accompanied by increased androgens, including DHEA and testosterone. High cortisol blocks or lowers the production of thyroid hormones, sex hormones (such as estrogen and progesterone), growth hormone, and melatonin. Ultimately, high cortisol impacts the glucocorticoid receptor, leading to glucocorticoid resistance (GCR). Over time, if the adrenals can no longer continue the high output, cortisol levels will decrease.

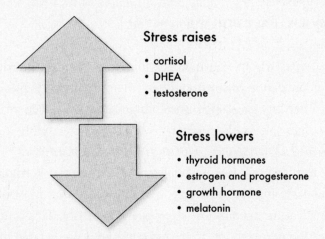

Stress raises

- cortisol
- DHEA
- testosterone

Stress lowers

- thyroid hormones
- estrogen and progesterone
- growth hormone
- melatonin

Figure 7. Effect of Stress on Hormones.

A New Approach to Hormone Imbalance
THE STRESS FORMULA

One of my husband's Stanford friends, Chip Conley, wrote a brilliant best-selling book, *Emotional Equations,* about emotions and the mathmatical formulas that describe them.[10] His simple formulas describe complex yet universal truths about emotions and triggered the idea that I could similarly describe hormonal combinations in the form of equations. I've included several hormonal formulas in this chapter to help you understand the interactions among the variables, which are hormones and actions that affect hormones, such as physiological stress. Here's one applicable to adults to get us started:

$$Stress = \frac{(adrenal\ dysregulation)}{(sleep)\times(exercise)\times(healthy\ food)\times(meditation)}$$

This simple equation shows that stress goes up when your adrenals are off kilter and make too much cortisol. Stress levels go down with restorative sleep, regular exercise, nutrient-dense food, and contemplative practice, such as meditation.

Stress and Dysregulated Adrenals: Common Hormonal Combinations

Referring back to the questionnaires in chapter 1, if you answered "yes" to three or more of the questions as in either Part A or Part B (or collectively, more than three in both Part A *and* Part B), plus three or more in another part, you have a problem with the cross talk between the adrenal glands and either the thyroid or the ovaries. Allow me to explain.

1. Dysregulated Cortisol and Thyroid Problems

Here's the typical scenario. Your local doctor diagnoses a slow thyroid. Relief! Finally, you've got an explanation for the crushing fatigue, poor mood, lack of libido, and climbing weight—you're not going crazy. It's biology, not an invitation to search for neuroses. You begin taking medication, usually a synthetic T4 such as Synthroid or levothyroxine as a tablet by mouth. You feel like a million bucks the first few days and weight starts to fall off. You've discovered the holy grail. Then, BAM! After a few more days or a couple of weeks, you're tired again. Your weight climbs. The honeymoon is over. You're desperately seeking a *course correction*.

There are many women who are properly prescribed thyroid hormone and do not experience the party-crashing adrenal on their thyroid honeymoon. But if your symptoms are atypical, or you feel better but then backslide, or if you answered "yes" to three or more questions in chapter 1, Part A and/or Part B and Part G, I suggest you take into account the important chain reaction between the thyroid and adrenal systems, because an adrenal problem will cause your thyroid issue to be much worse and harder to correct, and vice versa.

THE SCIENCE

Your thyroid reacts to stress and high blood levels of cortisol by slowing down production of thyroid hormones. High adrenaline, the short-acting neurotransmitter that rises in response to stress, is linked to lower thyroxine (T4), which results in high thyroid-stimulating hormone (TSH) and symptoms of a sluggish thyroid. Cortisol, when it is deficient or excessively high for prolonged periods of time, can slow down thyroid function.[11]

We know that the amygdala, the part of the limbic system that perceives stress, contains high numbers of thyroid receptors and type 2 deiodinase, which mediate thyroid hormone production.[12] When your stress is high, and your body is flooded with glucocorticoids such as cortisol, this slows down the hypothalamic-pituitary-thyroid (HPT) axis and thyroid hormone production, and thyroid hormone has a similar effect on the hypothalamic-pituitary-adrenal (HPA) axis.[13] That is, when the amount of glucocorticoids (the fancy term, as you know, for the hormone cortisol and its cousins) in your body goes up, the amount of thyroid hormones produced goes down, and vice versa. Folks with dysregulated cortisol and thyroid problems document this finding, showing that both high and low cortisol can impair thyroid function, although the relationship is not linear.[14]

Both extremes of cortisol can drag down your thyroid. Women who have too much or too little cortisol, plus an underperform-ing thyroid, *get a double dose of fatigue,* yet often neither condition is typically recognized in conventional medicine nor believed to be properly documented by existing biomarkers.[15] Yet fatigue and burnout remain epidemic in our culture. Not surprisingly, 78 per-cent of women report fatigue.[16]

Another way to interpret the interdependence of stress and limbic hijack, together with thyroid function, is to consider the relationship between thyroid and cortisol as nonlinear—and parabolic—which means when cortisol is too high or too low, you make less thyroid hormone. When cortisol is just right, and in the normal range, the thyroid performs best and generates optimal levels of hormones.

THE SOLUTION

I recommend that you put into place The Gottfried Protocols from both chapters 4 and 9. Start with Step 1 for both chapters. Reassess your symptoms six to twelve weeks after you've implemented the changes of Step 1. If you are still not feeling that your hormone is-sues are improved, add in Step 2 from both chapters. If you still are experiencing five or more symptoms from both chapters 4 and 9, see your doctor to consider further testing and a prescription for bi-oidentical hormones. Keep in mind that your thyroid medication re-quires adequate cortisol to work best: not too high and not too low.

2. Dysregulated Cortisol and Dysregulated Sex Hormones (Estrogen and Progesterone)

High cortisol is the single most common hormonal problem I see in my practice, and high cortisol with low estrogen and/or progesterone is another common combination. This varies by age: low progesterone coupled with high cortisol is the most common hormone combination that I see in women younger than thirty-five years of age. If you answered "yes" to three or more of the questions in chapter 1, Part A and/or Part B (the high and low cortisol questionnaires), together with three or more from Part C, Part D, and Part E, this is your hormone combo. Among women over age forty-five, I more commonly see cortisol either high or low together with low estrogens. If you answered "yes" to three or more of the questions in chapter 1, Part A and/or Part B together with Part E, adrenal dysregulation combined with low estrogen is your issue.

THE SCIENCE

Low sex hormones are inextricably linked to the prevalence of stress in the lives of modern women, and we know that the stress begins early. Tests show that 91 percent of female college students feel overwhelmed, far higher than the rate in men, even though it is documented that psychological well-being doesn't bottom out until age thirty-five.[17] Additionally, college women have higher rates of exhaustion than men (87 versus 73 percent) and more anxiety (56 versus 40 percent in men); and prescriptions for sleeping pills have tripled among college students since 1998.[18]

After college, we've got the usual suspects that raise cortisol: caffeine, sleep deprivation, and certain genotypes related to the important brain fertilizer called brain-derived neurotrophic factor (BDNF, which keeps your brain young, agile, and able to learn, or to be neuroplastic)—not to mention low estrogen, eating disorders, birth control pills, and the stress of working and commuting.[19] Many of these factors either cause or are associated with low progesterone.

For instance, when you lose weight from disordered eating or take a birth control pill, you block ovulation and this lowers your progesterone.

Honestly, we all just need more protection from stress, from our wiring to overprovide, and from our tendency toward perfectionism. If you're like me, you need a meditation coach to show up about once per hour to remind you to breathe deeply. While on the subject, I'd love for this coach to help me with detachment parenting and perhaps a reminder to laugh, and to develop an affinity for the simple things, at least until I hit fifty and stop seeking to meet the needs of others full time.

As I mentioned in chapters 2 and 4, your adrenals and ovaries work together in an intricate dance. Estrogens and progesterone are made in both your adrenals and your ovaries, but will be shunted toward the production of more cortisol when a woman is under chronic stress, as shown in Figure 2 of chapter 2. As a result, chronic stress leads to high cortisol levels and lower progesterone levels. You also will be lower in other sex hormones, such as estrogen, testosterone, and DHEA, but let's focus first on progesterone.

2A. LOW ESTROGEN
High cortisol will lower production of both estrogen and progesterone. When stress is long-standing, your body will try to balance the neuroendocrine system by making less estradiol because of Pregnenolone Steal. In women younger than forty, infertility may occur because the combination of amygdala hijack—where you overreact to the normal, daily stressors—and high cortisol makes your ovaries slow down and not ovulate. The balance of ovarian hormones is delicate, and amygdala hijack can take the ovaries offline. During perimenopause, high cortisol and low estrogen worsen symptoms of hot flashes, night sweats, and mood swings. After menopause, low estrogen is depressed further by high cortisol, and may worsen bone loss and cause osteoporosis.

THE SOLUTION

The goal in this situation is to calm the overactivated brain. Apply Step 1 of The Gottfried Protocol from chapters 4 and 7 simultaneously. If symptoms of high cortisol and low estrogen persist, then add in Step 2 from each chapter. Most women are able to regain balance with Steps 1 and 2, but if not, apply Step 3 from each chapter. Women who are treated with estrogen will temporarily lower their cortisol levels, but I recommend normalizing cortisol first before resorting to estrogen therapy because of the significant risks.

2B. LOW PROGESTERONE

In addition to Pregnenolone Steal, high stress will force high cortisol to block progesterone receptors so that you feel low in progesterone on a cellular level, even if blood levels are normal.

Let's take PMS, linked to low progesterone and chronic stress for some women. PMS is a collection of emotional, physical, and behavioral symptoms that affects 40 to 60 percent of women of reproductive age.[20] The cause is not known, but appears to be a multifaceted mash-up of genetics and neuroendocrine vulnerability. Some, but not all, women with PMS have low progesterone.

PMS FORMULA

When it comes to PMS, here is the formula that synthesizes the variables.

$$PMS = Cortisol/Progesterone$$

When stress is high, cortisol rises and PMS worsens. When progesterone is low, PMS also worsens. In other words, there's a dance between cortisol and progesterone in the development of PMS, and you want to address both adrenal function and your production of cortisol as well as your progesterone to minimize PMS.

THE SOLUTION

I encourage you to begin Step 1 of The Gottfried Protocol from both chapters 4 and 5. Retake the questionnaires for both chapters after you've implemented all or most of the recommendations in Step 1 for six or more weeks. Remember that it takes at least this amount of time to reach hormonal homeostasis. After your test period, if you still have more than three symptoms from the questionnaire of one or both chapters, add the recommended strategies from Step 2 for each chapter for another six weeks. If after six weeks of Step 2, symptoms persist, move to Step 3 of each chapter.

3. Low Progesterone (Estrogen Dominance) and Low Thyroid

As you learned in chapter 5, low progesterone is common beginning around age thirty-five and often leads to symptoms of estrogen dominance, whereby too much estrogen is produced relative to progesterone. When this happens, your Lady Justice is not holding the scales in balance, as nature intended. There is some evidence that low progesterone and low thyroid function may be connected.

THE SCIENCE

From chapter 5, you know that the most common reason for low progesterone is aging ovaries. As a woman's ovaries get older, ovulation is less regular, and this lowers your progesterone level.

Here is the evidence that links estrogen dominance, low progesterone, and low thyroid function.

- Subclinical hypothyroidism is associated with a short luteal phase (the second half of your menstrual cycle) and insufficient progesterone.[21]
- Progesterone regulates the expression of thyroid receptors in the uterus.[22]

- Too much estrogen may increase thyroid-binding globulin proteins—meaning that thyroid hormone is more bound and is less available to receptors inside cells—which may lower thyroid hormones and cause symptoms of thyroid insufficiency.
- Hypothyroidism can decrease progesterone receptor sensitivity in animal studies, and perhaps cause "progesterone resistance."[23] (See chapter 5 for more details.)
- Among adolescent girls, selenium and progesterone in the luteal phase have the greatest influence on thyroid function.[24]

Fertility Formula

By now you know that there is a common theme: that stress plays a key role in hormone imbalance. Note that there is a reciprocal relationship between stress and fertility, which can be expressed as follows:

$$Fertility = (progesterone * thyroid\ hormone)/stress$$

THE SOLUTION

Apply Step 1 of chapters 5 and 9 for six weeks, then retake the questionnaire. If three or more of the symptoms from either category persist, then apply Step 2 from each chapter for six weeks. If symptoms continue, move to Step 3 from each chapter for either or both category.

Your Unique Neurohormonal Template

This chapter has provided a sampler of the intricate interconnections between a woman's lived experience and hormonal biochemistry, which often manifest as multiple hormonal dysfunctions. Myriad factors come together and coalesce into a unique hormonal milieu, depending on your body and degree of stress. These factors include your lifestyle, including how you eat, supplement, and move; your genetics and how lifestyle changes the expression of your DNA code; your environmental toxin exposures; and your immunity and infections (both old infections, such as the mononucleosis virus, and current ones).

Awareness is the first step. If you think you have multiple imbalances, take a deep breath. You are on the way to getting the help you deserve, on multiple fronts. If you start to feel overwhelmed, remember: sometimes small shifts can make a large difference for multiple hormonal imbalances, and correcting the problem is easier than living with the consequences. And remember the Pareto Principle: 80 percent of the change comes from 20 percent of the effort.

CHAPTER 11

HORMONAL NIRVANA: STAYING ON COURSE

Congratulations! You've read the book. Your mind must be spinning, a common symptom of women after age thirty-five. Hopefully, you've begun addressing the core hormone imbalances that you classified in the questionnaires by first applying the corresponding lifestyle reset of The Gottfried Protocol. Perhaps you've talked to your girlfriends, your doctor, your therapist. Ready to fix your hormone problems? I bet you now know *what to do* for your hormone cure, but that's only half of the battle. The other half is *compliance*.

Women, weight, and food are a good example. I've observed that most women, myself included, are fat phobic. When I teach about natural hormone balancing in an online course via teleseminar, I often ask women if they know what to do to manage their weight or stress. All the hands fly up. Then I ask how many are doing it, on a daily basis. The hands go down. What's the problem? Compliance, or the act of complying with a desired behavior.

I prefer compliance to other terms such as *self-control*, because I've found, personally and professionally, that self-control is too easily overwhelmed or exhausted, similar to the adrenal glands. Further, working harder at self-control never paid dividends for me as I tried to eat the way I knew I should or to exercise more, and working too hard was probably the main reason for my adrenal burnout in my thirties. Don't get me wrong—self-will got me to important places with my education and medical training, but with age comes wisdom, and sometimes faulty cortisol and progesterone, which limit your will. Paradoxically, when I turned to ancient traditions such as Traditional Chinese Medicine and Ayurveda, I found that surrender suits me more, which is nested in compliance. I find in my own life, and in the mentoring that I provide to women around the world, that the goal of compliance allows more fluid ebb and flow to progress and also allows access to the emotions underneath the experience—for instance, of being stuck habitually with poor eating choices and weight obsession.

Meet Your Cure in the Middle

Commonly in my practice, women want an external solution to solve their every problem. They are hoping for the one medication that fixes everything, with zero side effects. Here's the bad news: I don't believe that medication exists. We want the easy way, but the truth is that hormonal rebalancing, lifestyle management, and sustained improvements are an inside job. Yes, external factors—such as what you eat and which supplements you take—are important, but for even the quinoa and chasteberry to have an optimal effect, you need to meet them halfway. Chasteberry isn't a cure-all. But if you have PMS, and you nourish yourself with healthy foods and the right dose of exercise (instead of bingeing on ice cream the week before your period), the chasteberry is far more likely to help you.

Women, food, and weight are some of my favorite topics, and I don't mean to oversimplify the nuanced and polarizing subject. As a gynecologist, I know that most women are haunted by food and weight, and suffer needlessly. I know because women tell me in my office and online, and sometimes I wonder if food and weight may be the most common *neurotic preoccupation* as well as the greatest sabotage to hormonal balance. I also know because I've been there. I spent years in 12-step food programs, and they helped me understand the right amount of boundaries I need around food. Just as you want the Goldilocks experience of your hormones not too high and not too low, you want your boundaries around food to be just right for you.

Of course there are deeper psychological issues at play when it comes to your relationship to food, exercise, and lifestyle redesign— and they don't lend themselves to quick sound bites. Geneen Roth wrote a great book, called *Women, Food, and God,* about the deeper psychological and spiritual hunger that is beneath a woman's relationship to food. Perhaps your mother restricted food while she was pregnant with you, and you developed a stress response and insatiable hunger. Maybe on a deeper level than simple nutrition, you don't feel fed. I believe weight is archetypal. It's bigger than a number on a bathroom scale.

If you know you have a problem with food, or with sustaining the healthy habits that you know would best serve you, it may be worthwhile to explore this topic further with a therapist who has expertise in food issues, or consider a 12-step program. Indeed, when you feel free to make nourishing choices with food, you meet your hormone cure in the middle and are far more likely to be successful.

What's Next When Hormone Symptoms Improve?

Let's imagine the time has finally arrived: You've reached hormonal balance. You are exercising most days and sleeping eight hours per night. You're eating a nourishing, organic food plan and limiting your alcohol and caffeine, and perhaps you even kicked sugar and gluten. Your libido is teenlike. Your mood is stable. You feel healthy and more alive. The old drudgery has turned to delight. You worry less about your health and you even see beauty in some of life's more mundane moments.

Now it's time to reinforce the right behaviors—your healthful and hormone-friendly behaviors—and to continue to stalk the bad. We've covered how to reset your lifestyle without prescription drugs. We have defined the path of balance. Now it's time to build habits that keep the momentum in a positive direction, and keep you on the path. In this chapter, I'll be both your mentor and your cheerleader, helping you stay on your game once you start to feel fully charged. My mission is to give you the strategies to sustain your hormone balance *for life*.

You know my theme song: it's far easier to get your hormones in balance than to live with the consequences of hormonal craziness. Now that you know that you aren't hopeless or crazy, you have a toolbox that you can bring wherever you go. You have found your personal "hormonal homeostasis." If we define hormonal balance as small deviations from a central axis of normal, the goal is to minimize the perturbations. Now you need to know what to do when you start straying from balance because the perturbations took over.

Keep It Going: The Continuous Gottfried Protocol

By now you've experienced how The Gottfried Protocol translates complex science into an easy-to-follow plan that emphasizes lifestyle redesign. I want to keep you going with my integrative approach so that you continue to optimize eating and drinking, contemplative practice, targeted exercise, supplements, and, as needed, bioidentical hormones.

> *Dr. Sara, you've mentored me to lose 23 pounds in the past year and to maintain the loss. You've helped me get my estrogen, thyroid, testosterone, and cortisol where they need to be. Please keep me on this path. I want to know how to tweak and optimize this process so that I don't get back to that dark place I was in a year ago. (Irene, Sacramento, California)*

Don't look back. You don't have to, now that you have the information you need to keep moving forward. Like many of my patients, Irene loves the benefits of The Gottfried Protocol but needs frequent reminders and support to sustain the changes, and not backpedal into her old patterns. Perhaps she gets too busy to stay on her game, or perhaps it's just the human condition that we all need accountability in order to stay in balance. The only thing that matters is keeping your eye on the prize: the healthiest version of you.

We Are Works in Progress: An Example from My Practice

I first saw Irene, a fifty-four-year-old graphic designer and divorced mother of a teenager, in 2008. With a piercing stare and enviable chunky jewelry, she seemed more fit and energetic than most moms her age. But Irene complained that she didn't feel herself. What bothered her most was feeling flat, sensually and sexually: "I don't want to have my sensual side take a backseat for the rest of my life. I don't want to be fat and prematurely old." Irene's final menstrual period had occurred two years earlier. Once she took my questionnaires, we determined that all three Charlie's Angels—estrogen, cortisol, and thyroid—needed rebalancing. Irene had a slow thyroid and had been treated for twenty years with the same dose of Synthroid, one of the most common synthetic thyroid prescriptions. When I checked Irene's ratio of free T3 to reverse T3, I found the ratio was low, indicating low levels of thyroid hormone in cells throughout her body. She was taking oral estrogen, which lowered her free T3 further.

Irene managed stress well, except when she visited her dysfunctional family in Chicago, or prepared for a tight work deadline. Either circumstance could cause her cortisol to be high at night. We tried the first and second steps of The Gottfried Protocol for High Cortisol. She took fish oil, phosphatidylserine, and rhodiola in the morning. Irene began a strict, hormone-balancing food plan (see Appendix F for samples) and a targeted exercise program of interval training. That worked for the high cortisol but not for her low-thyroid symptoms. We switched her to transdermal estrogen, as a patch. That improved her free T3 but not quite to the vaulted place of thyroid nirvana. Moving to the third step, which is bioidentical hormones in the lowest possible doses, we added Cytomel (a thyroid hormone called T3) to Irene's Synthroid. Within six weeks, Irene reported dramatic improvements. "I feel glorious," she told me. "I lost eight pounds just from the healthy food and exercise. And my chronic need for a nap has totally disappeared."

Recently, however, a crisis with her mother, on top of unexpected financial demands, made Irene feel stressed and under siege: "I've got that not-so-unfamiliar feeling of depression. Not that I can't get out of bed and get my work and mothering done; I'm just drained and treading the old corridors of self-doubt."

From our work together, Irene is now well aware that the root cause is biological, not emotional, when she feels a dip in mood, desire, and energy. These feelings are usually connected to the chronic-stress pattern of not producing enough of the feel-good brain chemicals, such as serotonin and dopamine. When she took the questionnaires again, we found she was low in estrogen and cortisol, so I increased the dose on the estrogen patch and added licorice, which raises cortisol. Within four weeks, Irene had turned the tide of a major backslide. She felt at home in her body again, more confident, energetic, and able to cope.

You too can leverage the neurohormonal feedback loops of your body by using the best evidence to your advantage—applied to your body and unique life context, and congruent with your very specific and reachable goals.

Dr. Sara's Tips for Hormonal Success

There are three essential features of implementing and maintaining your hormone cure. They are goal setting, mind-set, and self-tracking.

SET ULTRACLEAR AND MODEST GOALS

When you hear statistics such as "98 percent of diets fail" or "34 percent of people who lose weight, regain it," it's easy to feel discouraged. Perhaps you've noticed that surgery doesn't solve the weight problem—even 50 percent of people who undergo gastric bypass regain at least some of their weight. It could be that you, like me, were conditioned to eat when you are not hungry, perhaps to placate an emotional need. Here's the good news: you can rewire this conditioning. According to experts in the field of change and my own experience, a more productive approach is to investigate the positive traits that you already have concerning a healthy lifestyle and to amplify those behaviors. This is a fundamental aspect of the burgeoning field of neuroscience and positive psychology.

Conceivably, when you learn that you are low across the board in your hormones—estrogen, progesterone, cortisol, thyroid, vitamin D—you may feel like it's too much to take on the path of the hormone warrior. Yet we know that when you set modest and crystal-clear goals, they are more likely to create sustained change.

We know which modest goals work best, based on rigorous science. Allow me to share a few suggestions as they apply to weight management, since what you eat is heavily linked to hormonal balance. When it comes to sustained weight loss and hormonal balance, some proven goals include the following:

- Modularize. Break a larger goal ("I want to lose twenty pounds") into small, concrete goals ("I will lose a half to one pound per week for the next six weeks").
- Eat like your great-grandparents. Our great-grandparents were eating whole foods before the days of packaged food and fake butter, before McDonald's and *Supersize Me*. Try to eat the way they did. My great-grandmother ate porridge with berries for breakfast, plus lean protein and lots of vegetables for lunch and dinner. She had a big salad every night, and she avoided alcohol. She ate no processed food. We could all benefit by trying to eat the way our ancestors did.

- Cut out the white stuff, including refined carbohydrates, sugar, sugar substitutes, flour, and gluten.
- Track your food religiously, every sip, every bite.
- Shift to less calorie-dense foods, such as apples and celery, instead of rich, sugary, and calorie-dense foods like ice cream.
- Obtain counseling or coaching if needed, for further accountability, to understand the root causes of your eating issues and for emotional support.
- Move more. Walk ten thousand steps per day. Trust me. Setting the goal to walk ten thousand steps will increase your activity level every day, even if you don't make it to ten thousand.

CHOOSE YOUR MIND-SET: FIXED OR GROWTH?

As Carol Dweck, PhD, Stanford professor and author of *Mindset,* puts it, it's not just our abilities and talents that bring us success, but whether we approach our goals with the right mind-set. Professor Dweck describes the "fixed" mind-set as limited, focused on whether you will fail or succeed, and concerned about how you look to others. For instance, we are using a fixed mind-set when we say things like, "I'm not an athlete" or "I'm just not very good at math." When we use a fixed mind-set, we are believing that things will always be as they feel now. Dweck describes the "growth" mind-set as adaptable, eager for a challenge and to engage fully, aware that your talents, temperament, inner landscape, and skill set can be cultivated. When you adopt the growth mind-set, you say things like, "I didn't resist the cake tonight, but next time I'll make sure I drink more water all day to fill up." This is the type of mind-set we try to cultivate in our kids ("I know the math test didn't go well, but next time we'll set up a new study plan and you'll see how much you can improve"), and most of us would do better to apply it to ourselves. In general, I find my patients have a mix of the two, but it's the growth mind-set that sets you up for lasting change.

——READY TO UPLEVEL YOUR HORMONAL HEALTH?—— QUANTIFY WITH SELF-TRACKING

It used to be that keeping a journal was the best approach for tracking your food; then spreadsheets became a more powerful method that allowed measurement of multiple variables. Now we can create a health dashboard on our personal computers, complete with nested classification schemes for our daily habits, and store it in a cloud that synchronizes automatically with mobile phones and other electronic gadgets. There's a name for this movement, the Quantified Self, which is a large collaboration of amateur scientists who track and experiment with their body fat, sleep, exercise, diet, mood, IQ, and DNA for fun and for a more fit life. I love their tagline: "Self-knowledge through numbers." Members identify critical drives to longevity and living a life on point.

Since I've got one foot in science and one foot in the perfect storm of perimenopause, I use dashboards and gadgets to keep me honest and on task. I'm not a Silicon Valley biohacker, but I have blind spots in my field of vision when it comes to behaviors such as mood, sleep, food, and exercise, and I suspect the same applies to you. When a friend asks what I had for dinner two nights ago, it's as if she asked me to recite a T. S. Eliot poem, but with my Fitbit on the waist of my skinny jeans, I can rattle off what I ate for the past week, including the menu and portions. Perhaps like me, you too make decisions based on incomplete and biased information, filtered by your own distractions and flagging memory. Fortunately, a bit of technology allows you to rely on objective, not subjective, data.

The Science of Successful and Sustained Change

Change is hard, but it's not rocket science. We do know that some changes—particularly how you eat and how you move—are harder to maintain than signing up for a monthly massage or tea with your girlfriends. It's valuable to understand the science of behavior change as the foundation for your own hormone cure, both the initial cure as you apply The Gottfried Protocol and the sustained cure as you maintain your progress. The goal is to cultivate the new habits that support your hormone cure.

The factors that best predict successful behavioral change have everything to do with how we sustain that change. Change that's motivated by guilt, fear, regret, or a desire to "fix" a flaw or weakness often leads to a negative and self-defeating cycle in which we try and fail and keep being reminded of what's *not* working. Professor Martin Seligman, of the University of Pennsylvania, describes this as "learned helplessness," which he defined as the tendency of an individual to behave helplessly, and to fail to respond to opportunities for better circumstances. Similar to perception of stress, there is a perceived absence of control over a situation's outcome.

Here's a secret: I observe that women in my practice with learned helplessness have a far more difficult time achieving the hormone cure. Please answer this question honestly: *Do you have the pattern of learned helplessness?* Do you feel you lack the power to change your eating, exercise, and other health habits? In contrast, women who understand the many positive consequences of their lifestyle reset— such as cutting out sugar and flour, and walking most days of the week—achieve the hormone cure much more rapidly and sustain it. The most successful women in my practice also recognize that the locus of control is internal—they understand they have the power to change, and cultivate hope and accountability about meeting their health challenges.

I'm not suggesting that every woman needs to eat gluten-free, meditate every morning, or run a marathon. Perhaps your first step is to stop eating pizza, potato chips, and French fries. Try it: it's hard the first couple of times you're tempted, and then you slowly develop a new identity as a person who doesn't eat French fries. A habit forms. Same with exercise. Perhaps you start exercising when you awaken with burst training for fifteen minutes at home, four days per week. You're sore the first few days, and then you notice that your energy is better during the day. You don't feel as angry and stressed out. You laugh and smile more. Before you know it, you're an evangelist for burst training. The Power of Habit.

HOW WE FORM NEW HABITS

Charles Duhigg, a journalist who wrote the best-selling book *The Power of Habit*, provides the neuroscience details behind how we form new habits. The upshot? Three main tips:

1. Cue. If we want to create a new habit, we need to pick the cue that will signal to us it's time to rely on that new habit. For example, on a bad day, the old version of you might come home, order Chinese take-out, and pour a glass of wine. To create a new habit, you might pick *the same cue* (coming home after a bad day) but instead substitute a new behavior (I'll pick up my favorite salad at Whole Foods and go for a thirty-minute walk after dinner). Hopefully, the immediate reward for both these behaviors would be the same (being able to forget about my awful day), but in the process, you've substituted a new, more hormone-balancing habit for dealing with your bad days.

2. Keystone habits. Have you noticed that when you change certain habits but not others, they snowball into even more positive habits, often without a lot of effort? It's like a sacred pyramid scheme. Many people find exercise or making their bed every morning to be keystone habits. Once you are working out, you feel better about yourself and more energetic—thus, you are less likely to need false energy boosts after lunch, such as sugar and chocolate, and that helps you avoid the late-afternoon slump where you are desperate for caffeine to make it through to the end of the day, helping you fall asleep more easily at night. For some reason, making your bed seems to be a keystone habit that leads people to feel more organized and in control of their lives. The key? Define your own keystone habits. What habits, when you are doing them regularly, seem to have positive ripple effects throughout your life? Target these habits and return to them first, particularly if you find you've fallen off the hormone-cure bandwagon, as the positive cascade is a way to reinforce your progress.

3. Act as if. Yes, it's the slogan of every 12-step program, and I know it sounds hokey, but rigorous science proves that it works. You must believe that change is really possible for you. In other words, you can follow all my advice in this book and get your body humming in perfect hormonal alignment, but if you don't believe it's possible for you to maintain your hormone cure, you won't! The first time you abandon your eating plan on an all-you-can-eat cruise vacation, you'll step on the scale back home and scream. Perhaps you tell yourself, "I knew this would happen. I can't maintain any weight loss. I'm bound to be fat and unhappy forever." And in that moment, by not believing that true change is possible for you, you've actually sealed your fate. Realize instead that it was just a vacation, and get back on board. This might be the hardest tip in this whole book to implement, but *it's crucial;* please keep the faith that hormonal balance is possible for you to both find *and* maintain!

The Stages of Change

We aren't robots who can program ourselves to reach a goal. Successful change comes best in stages. So does maintaining that change. How long it takes and how well it works are another matter, depending on certain factors:

- your daily commitment
- whether the pain of change exceeds the pain of staying the same

- your drive
- your pace
- how high you need to climb
- how you best maintain momentum
- ongoing support and accountability

The Continuous-Improvement Project

Continuous improvement sounds exhausting, but it doesn't have to be. Remember my rocket-science friend who breaks her problems into manageable chunks? Let's use cortisol as an example. Recall that when you're perpetually stressed, you can become low in cortisol, as well as in other hormones that are crucial to your vitality, energy reserves, and mood. Perhaps stress is causing your hormones to become unbalanced again, as Irene experienced. You know from reading this book that persistent stress can rob you of the hormones of vitality, such as estrogen and testosterone, as well as of the neurotransmitters norepinephrine, epinephrine, dopamine, and serotonin.

You don't need to start by giving away your possessions and moving into a monastery. Just take the first step toward putting your cortisol in balance again. If you're not doing so already, you might start by doing one or more of the following:

- taking five minutes twice a day to breathe or meditate
- waking up thirty minutes earlier to walk outdoors
- looking at the top three stressors in your life and seeing what short-term changes you can make. Where's the locus of control? What insights would reduce the stress?
- bicycling or taking public transportation to work instead of driving if possible
- wearing a pedometer to inspire you to walk farther each day
- putting your kids in the after-school program once or twice a week simply to give you some downtime, perhaps

to go to a café to read or meet a girlfriend ("tend and be-friend")

- acknowledging and expressing your feelings in a journal—or better yet, communicating them to someone—instead of repressing them

Finally, when your cortisol levels have stabilized a bit, take on the task of a deeper, longer vision for your health. Is there something else you can do long term to maintain your cortisol levels? Instead of meditating alone, perhaps you can join a local meditation group. Or do what I did, and become a yoga teacher. We teach what we most need to learn. I wrestled with my own emotional overeating for years until I found several 12-step programs, including Over-eaters Anonymous and Food Addicts, where I learned to give up trying harder, surrendered my self-will (a key tenet of most Eastern spiritual traditions), and cultivated a deeper connection to a Higher Power. That worked for me—it doesn't work for everyone, but it helped me achieve and maintain my own hormone cure.

The key to transformation is to start *now* and move forward one step at a time. If you break it down into bite-sized chunks and don't get overwhelmed, change is highly doable. Experts disagree on exactly how long habits take to form, but it is a proven fact that when you perform an action over and over again, eventually it becomes a habit ingrained into your routine. So why not invest a few weeks in developing habits that will make you feel better, now and for the long term?

Four Phases to Continual Hormonal Health

As in any path of merit, the steps along the way are part of a process. When you shift from feeling just OK to feeling vital from your cells throughout your body, you're encouraged to want to stay that way. Sometimes, as with Irene, life will cause you to backslide a bit. Don't kick yourself if that occurs. It happens! The trick is to recognize the backslide as quickly as possible and move to get back on the balanced-hormone path again.

Phase 1. Identify Your Optimal Self, Your Strengths, and Your Weaknesses

Learn which hormones you need to balance and how you do that best.

- **Know your baseline.** The initial questionnaires established which hormones you needed to balance. Keep a record of all of your "yes" responses. To stay on track, take the questionnaires again from time to time, even when you're feeling fine. Have any of the answers changed? What's your percentage of improvement over time? I keep track of my questionnaire results in a spreadsheet (a Google document), which serves as a free health dashboard.

- **Learn your strengths.** Whether you're maintaining your hormone balance or getting back on track, you want to leverage your strengths rather than emphasize your weaknesses. Which assets most help your progress? What has been working and what hasn't? Accentuating the positive works better than dwelling on the negative. Write down your strengths and keep a note tucked into your journal or on your smartphone to remind you during those down days.

- **Explore your liabilities.** What are the things that have dragged or may be dragging you down? What are the behaviors or relationships that may present obstacles to your health improvement? Keep a list of your challenges and liabilities—a health balance sheet—so that you can recognize them when they pop up. The more you understand your social and psychological downfalls, the more strategically you can prevent them from pulling you off the path. We know that just as certain friends may augment your positive behaviors, such as my girlfriend with whom I run every Sunday, there are also relationships that are toxic.

- **Celebrate your success.** Even when you're doing everything right, beautifully maintaining that all-important hormonal rhythm, make sure to stop and give yourself a pat on the back. Share it with your friends who are cheering you on—friends can be the most important advocate for change. Take yourself out for a kombucha, splurge on that necklace in the window, or just revel in the knowledge that you are doing it, girlfriend!

AMPLIFY: A STRENGTH-BASED APPROACH TO CHANGE

Want a road map for applying positive psychology to your process of reclaiming and maintaining hormone balance? Last year, I became more aware, often awkwardly aware, that I was missing the mark as a mom—too busy and too distracted to mother my kids the way I wanted. As usual, when faced with a painful realization, *I designed an experiment.* I committed to discovering my signature strengths and applying them to mothering.

I identified my own major strengths through a questionnaire available to you at psychologist Martin Seligman's website, Authentic Happiness. Professor Seligman, the father of Positive Psychology (the scientific study of strengths and virtues that enable people and communities to thrive), is an inspiring scholar of *what can go right,* as opposed to what can go wrong. His questionnaire indicated that my top strengths are creativity, love of learning, appreciating beauty, curiosity, and hope. I need to draw on these signature strengths when, for instance, I want to engage with my children as a resourceful and happy mom. Instead of ordering them around like a drill sergeant, I sought to connect with them in ways that reinforce my creativity, love of learning, and appreciation.

You'll notice that "patience" didn't quite make it on my list of strengths. My old methods of willful effort (which worked superbly during my years of medical training) to be a more patient and even-tempered mom hasn't worked for me, and believe me, I've given it plenty of chances. Instead of radical vows each night to be more tolerant, now I plan activities with my kids, such as a hike or a natural-dye workshop, that we can do together and that tap into my signature strengths. When I feel *creative*, engage my *love of learning* and *appreciation of beauty*, I'm more serene and unruffled as a mother, because I'm happy! And you know that when Mama is happy, everyone is happy.

Similarly, when I leverage my *love of learning* and *curiosity* to understand how alcohol raises my cortisol and estrogen beyond the optimal levels for my body, it reinforces my commitment to the changes—both initial and ongoing—that mend my particular hormonal vulnerabilities. What are your strengths? Write a list, ask your friends, take the questionnaire at Professor Seligman's site. You might be surprised at what you find. You can amplify what *you're already good at* to grow in other areas of your life.

Phase 2: Keep on Tracking
Take care not to backslide all the way back to square one. Keep the assessment and refinement going. Select what might work best to help you stay on target. Try to make balanced health a priority.

- **Take hormonal inventory**. Depending on how many hormonal imbalances you have and how serious they are, take a monthly or quarterly inventory by revisiting the questionnaires.

- **Create accountability.**
  - Get a buddy to implement and track The Hormone Cure with you. Compare notes each time you take the questionnaires. Share your successes, as well as the things you've tried that miss the mark.
  - Choose *The Hormone Cure* as a book-club project and download my guide at http://thehormonecure book.com.
  - Go public about your progress. There's evidence that connecting online via social media raises oxytocin, the hormone of love and bonding. Go to http://www .facebook.com/GottfriedCenter and "like" my page where I post daily about new hormone data, women's health, and life as a woman in perimenopause.
- **Make exercise nonnegotiable.** Create an exercise routine so that it becomes a habit, like brushing your teeth. Just do it, and track your progress.
- **Be mindful of your meditation.** If you have incorporated a contemplative practice in your life, notice its effect on your hormones and your day. Remember that effect when you're tempted to let those few minutes a day slide for more pressing duties.
- **Discover what inspires you.** Keep track of what keeps one foot in front of the other for you. Then do it!

Phase 3: Address Behaviors

Research shows that we rarely proceed in a linear fashion from one stage to the next. An integrative approach has room for human foibles—the more realistic view that with change, most of us take two steps forward and one step back. When you're motivated, you rarely relapse to your starting point. If it occurs, a relapse provides an excellent opportunity to learn what didn't work for you and to make adjustments for the next round of change.

- **Forgive yourself.** Most of us would never talk to a friend the way we talk to ourselves. We are overly self-critical. Accept the fact that no one is perfect, including you, and try to remember this.
- **Plan ahead.** Sometimes it seems that just when we get into a smooth routine, we're foiled again! Traveling, illness, work demands, the kids, and so much more can get in the way—in fact, you can plan on it. So prepare for disruptions: Pack some extra supplements of fish oil or chasteberry (depending on your particular hormonal issue) in your glove compartment or in that massive purse of yours. Carve out time to hit the treadmill when you're at that jam-packed conference. You send your body a powerful message when you take the time to care for yourself.
- **Be flexible.** This might sound as if it contradicts the last tip, but it's about attitude. When unanticipated obstacles arise, do your best to apply a calm mind and steady heart. Become skillful at up- and down-leveling your nervous system. Might I even suggest laughing about it? And have confidence that you will get back on track.

Phase 4: Lay the Groundwork for Ongoing Support

Make sure others help you keep the momentum going.

- **Get your doctor on board.** Schedule a follow-up with your doctor and keep him or her informed about what you are doing, changing, and implementing. Your health information will be up to date and available if needed, and who knows, dare I say that your doctor might even learn a thing or two? If he or she hems and haws about doing the kind of testing you want, offer a copy of this book. If that doesn't work, see Appendix D for how to find a physician who's more in tune with an integrative or functional medicine approach.

- **Educate your besties**. Let your spouse, your kids, and your closest friends know what you're doing and why. Instead of interrupting when you're meditating, or complaining that your supplements don't leave room for their gummy vitamins, your kids can become your allies in health. Stranger things have happened. As for your spouse or partner, I know from experience that he or she will be joyful that you have more energy, feel fewer crazy moods, and want more sex.

- **Stay in touch.** You can keep in touch with me virtually on my website, via my newsletters, frequent webinars, and online courses. We are in this together, not just for the duration of this book but also for the long haul. My job is to sit on your shoulder and convey the opportunities for improvement, to help you serve your body even better than you do now.

My great-grandmother understood fifty years ago the idea that food is information for your body, not an emotional panacea and certainly not just calories. You can choose to be like my great-grandmother Mud and eat whole foods while avoiding sugar, exercise regularly and strategically, learn how to hit the "pause" button via yoga or another contemplative practice, and take proven supplements—which I believe are the *pivotal preventive tactics* to reduce the risk of falling prey to hormonal upheaval. You can choose to be empowered about methods to manage stress rather than feeling like a victim. You can choose to change how you eat, move, think, and supplement by following The Gottfried Protocol.

My Wish for You

I like to think that my great-grandmother Mud would be proud of my goals for you. Mud resides in my heart as my first role model. She showed me a healthy path with dignity even into her nineties. While others were feeling depressed and downtrodden, she was noshing on vegetables and stretching. When they were drinking excessive alcohol, she sipped hot water with lemon. As their bodies got fat and sedentary, she chased younger men.

Here are my goals for you:

- to find healthcare that is responsive to and respectful of your preferences, needs, and values
- to have your symptoms and concerns taken seriously
- to find the root causes of your disease instead of just putting a Band-Aid on the problem
- to know that you can exercise, eat healthful foods, manage your stress, and balance your hormones naturally
- to become as dogged, fierce, and clever as Charlie's Angels (you choose which one), never stopping until the last piece of the puzzle is in place

My vision for you is to feel—from the inside out—sparkly, fulfilled, and content. I want you to feel blessed by a hormonally balanced life, full of the spunk, engagement, and buoyancy that are your birthright. Your new life of balance begins with a simple mantra: set goals, track progress, get feedback. *Lather, rinse, repeat.*

In this book, we've reviewed reams of science—we've discussed randomized double-blind trials, obscure brain parts, serotonin transporters, telomeres, epigenomics, little-known endocrine glands, contemplative practice, and the occasionally embarrassing tidbits of female experience. You've read pages of my proven method to correct your hormones, starting with lifestyle tweaks and moving progressively through various supplements, botanicals, and bioidentical hormones. Here at the end, I want to bring the focus back to what truly matters when it comes to health: your personal and comprehensive hormone cure. You now know *what to do to return to hormonal balance,* and in this final chapter, we've covered the *compliance* side of the equation—the science of successful change, and how to improve health by leveraging positive psychology and health habits.

When I was a thirty-something woman who felt miserable and stressed out, I was astonished that conventional medicine had no answers for me. As I looked around my own medical practice, I noticed an epidemic of women who felt similar symptoms, wanted help, but had trouble finding what they most needed. Doctors simply don't learn this material in mainstream medical schools. It's not your doctor's fault—we simply were never taught to approach health in this way. It was only through my own health and hormonal struggles, combined with taking care of women in my practice, that I figured out how to move the needle on stress, and that changed everything. Ultimately, you have tremendous power to change your hormones, reclaim your body, and get Charlie's Angels working for you, not against you. You understand the importance of root-cause analysis and have a clear sense of your own root cause from the questionnaires. You know the tactics to resist constant temptations to eat poorly and become sedentary. You have the information you need to support your hormonal biochemistry. Follow my great-grandmother's advice: find the internal solution rather than resorting to external prescriptions. My greatest hope is that the information in this book provides a drugless road map that will lead you systematically to increased health and vitality—and that when you achieve this goal, you'll be able to reach your fullest potential.

EPILOGUE

"All truth passes through three stages.
First, it is ridiculed.
Second, it is violently opposed.
Third, it is accepted as self-evident."
—*Arthur Schopenhauer*

When I turned forty, I had an epiphany: *Hormonal balance was taken from us in the past century.*

The theft occurred gradually and beneath the radar. Synthetic hormones were not just suggested but proselytized to unsuspecting American women prior to 2002, as most baby boomers can attest. The food industry changed our kitchens—instead of stocking our homes with broccoli and pastured eggs, we were convinced that it was healthy to eat packaged and convenience food. Sugar consumption rose dramatically. We got exposed to hundreds of toxic chemicals, many of which are endocrine disruptors. We sit more, which slows down metabolism and accelerates aging. We have an obesity epidemic, and 70 percent of the costs of our failing healthcare system are for preventable conditions. We commute more on clogged highways and breathe unhealthy air. These insidious factors behind hormonal imbalance affect not just women but also men and children. We're more stressed and wired, both with electronic gadgets and from the adrenal fallout, than ever before.

What's even more painful to me is that solutions are known and proven. *Lifestyle redesign,* as systematized in The Gottfried Protocol, is extremely effective and grounded in robust science, but not yet part of mainstream medicine.

I had another epiphany ten years ago: *U.S. doctors are not educated to identify and correct the root cause of women's suffering—the epidemic of hormone imbalance.*

After I started medical school in 1989, I was appalled when I became aware of the vast uncontrolled medical experiment that was being performed on American women. It seemed that hormonal imbalance was approached as a business endeavor by pharmaceutical companies, and that most doctors blindly went along, trusting what they heard. Although I was taught to offer women synthetic estrogen and progestin, most commonly Prempro, for their perimenopausal and menopausal symptoms, I realized that the evidence wasn't there to support the recommendation. In my experience, excess stress is the central story at the root of hormonal imbalance for women over thirty-five. The effects of adrenaline and cortisol have a profound ripple effect on other endocrine organs such as the ovaries and thyroid, yet few practitioners of mainstream medicine seemed to take the female stress response seriously.

There are proven methods to preventing and treating hormonal imbalances that originate with stress and cortisol, which typically disrupt hormonal cross talk between your thyroid and ovaries. As I've described, chronic stress affects glucocorticoid regulation, which is controlled by the hypothalamus, pituitary, and adrenals. If you've been on the path of repair for a while, you know that correcting the adrenals and their control system takes the longest amount of time. As my friend Lisa Byrne, founder of the online community The Well-Grounded Life, says, "It's a process, not a prescription."

I struggled for many years to heal my own hormonal problems naturally and by using the best science, and then brought my carefully crafted protocols to the women I served. As a gynecologist, teacher, wife, mom, scientist, and yoga teacher, I spent years formulating, synthesizing, and testing a comprehensive plan for hormonal problems. It's my life's mission to bring the fruits of my years of study, inquiry, and obsession with neuroendocrine optimization to other women, and to help them feel balanced again.

You can choose a vital life and join The Hormone Cure Revolution. For more information and to see the schedule of meetups in your town, go to http://thehormonecurebook.com/revolution.

PART III

APPENDIX

APPENDIX A:

THE GOTTFRIED PROTOCOL, BY HORMONE IMBALANCE

HORMONE IMBALANCE	DOSE	NOTES
HIGH CORTISOL		
Vitamin B₅ (Pantethine)	500 mg/day	Low risk — best evidence for people with high cholesterol and heart disease
Vitamin C	1,000 mg three times/day (total daily dose of 3,000 mg)	Low risk, but in some people, may cause loose stool
Phosphatidylserine (PS)	400 to 800 mg/day	Reduces cortisol levels and improves mood under stress
Fish or krill oil (Omega-3)	1,000 to 4,000 mg/day	Increases lean body mass
L-theanine (γ-glutamylethylamide)	250 to 400 mg/day	Reduces anxiety and other bio-markers (blood and saliva tests) of stress, such as salivary immunoglobulin (SIgA, an indicator of stress in the gastrointestinal tract)
L-lysine combined with L-arginine	2.64 grams of each/day	Combination reduces salivary cortisol levels as well as anxiety
L-tyrosine	1,000 mg/day	Improves response to stress and improves working memory
Asian ginseng (Also known as Panax ginseng)	200 to 400 mg/day	Improves quality of life; reduces fatigue and stress; improves immune function; helps lower blood sugar; and improves cognition, working memory, and calmness

Korean red ginseng	250 to 500 mg/day	Decreases menopausal symptoms and significantly lowers the ratio of cortisol to DHEAS
Ashwagandha	300 mg twice/day	Reduces anxiety
Rhodiola	200 mg twice/day	Reduces stress-related fatigue, improves mental performance and concentration, decreases cortisol levels and depression
LOW CORTISOL		
Combination of vitamins B_1, B_6, and C	Vitamin C at 600 to 1,000 mg/day plus a good vitamin B complex	Restores cortisol production and diurnal rhythm when given intravenously but less risky to take orally
Licorice root extract	600 mg, standardized to 25% (150 mg) glycyrrhizic acid	Take with caution; can alter HPA function in fetuses and high doses can cause high blood pressure; when taking licorice, make sure to have your blood pressure checked
Bioidentical cortisol in Isocort, an adrenal-support pill from Bezwecken	One or two pellets up to three times/day — no more than six/day — taken with a meal	Use after having tried Chapter 4's Steps 1 and 2 of The Gottfried Protocol
LOW PROGESTERONE		
Vitamin C	750 mg/day	Very safe, even though recommended allowance is 75 to 90 mg/day
Chasteberry, available as capsules or liquid tincture	500 to 1,000 mg/day	Very safe — there are few reports of adverse effects
Fertility blend (chasteberry formulation)	3 pills/day	Proprietary blend, so dose of chasteberry is not provided

Agnolyt (chasteberry formulation)	Tincture contains nine grams of 1:5 tincture for each 100 grams of aqueous alcoholic solution	Few reports of adverse effects
Bladderwrack, a form of seaweed	Dosage in one study was 700 to 1,400 mg daily	Few reports of adverse effects but may worsen autoimmune thyroiditis because it contains iodine
Saffron	15 mg twice/day	A safe option for depression, painful periods, and PMS
Calcium, magnesium, and vitamin B_6	• Calcium carbonate or citrate, 600 mg taken orally twice/day • Magnesium at 200 mg/day • Vitamin B_6 at 50 to 100 mg/day	Higher-than-recommended doses of Vitamin B_6 can cause nerve toxicity. Ideally, I prefer you obtain calcium from food sources given recent controversy over supplements.
St. John's wort	300 mg three times a day	Relieves both behavioral and physical symptoms of PMS
EXCESS ESTROGEN		
Di-indolemethane (DIM)	200 mg/day in a capsule or tablet	Favors the production of protective estrogens and reduces bad estrogens
Seaweed (Alaria is a type of brown alga)	5 grams/day	Significantly lowers estrogen levels
Resveratrol	Recommended only from food sources, such as grapes and blueberries, not from wine	Also acts as an antioxidant
Turmeric	• Sprinkle a teaspoon of organic turmeric on your lunch or dinner. • In supplement form: Integrative Therapeutics' Curcumax at one tablet twice/day following meals; or Pure Encapsulations' CurcumaSorb at one 250 mg capsule, up to six times/day between meals	Counters the proliferative effect of estrogen on cancer cells

Hops	• Integrative Therapeutics' Revitalizing Sleep Formula contains 30 mg of hops. • Integrative Therapeutics' AM/PM Perimenopausal Formula contains 100 mg of hops. • Tori Hudson's Sleepblend and Julian Whitaker's Restful Night Essentials are sleep formulas containing hops.	Hops is active against breast, colon, and ovarian cancer cells; however, hops supplements are unregulated by the FDA.
Melatonin	0.5 to 3 mg at night	Maintains the body's circadian rhythm and may prevent breast cancer. Ideally, minimize light at night and expose yourself to daylight in the morning rather than relying on a supplement.
LOW ESTROGEN		
Vitamin E	50 to 400 IU/day taken for at least four weeks	Decreases hot flashes and other low-estrogen problems by increasing blood supply to the vaginal wall and improving menopausal symptoms
Magnesium oxide	400 mg/day for four weeks escalating to 800 mg/day if hot flashes persist	Higher doses can cause loose bowels, so check with your doctor before going beyond 400 mg/day
Maca	2,000 mg/day	Increases estradiol in menopausal women, and helps with insomnia, depression, memory, concentration, energy, hot flashes, and vaginal dryness, as well as improved body mass index and bone density
Pueraria lobata (PL) or *Pueraria minifica*	Brewed as a tea	Traditional Chinese herbal remedy for menopausal symptoms
Rhubarb	Available in the United States as rhaponticin, brand name Phytoestrol	Reduces hot flashes

St. John's wort	300 mg three times a day	Consult your doctor first if you are taking an antidepressant.
Black cohosh	• 40 to 80 mg/day • One to four 2.5 mg tablets/day of Isopropanolic extract of black cohosh for six months	Very rarely, higher doses may be associated with liver damage (signs include nausea, vomiting, dark urine, and jaundice), so you should discuss first with your doctor and should take the lowest dose that helps your symptoms.
Red ginseng	6 grams/day	Improves cortisol-to-DHEA ratio and quality of life in women with postmenopausal symptoms of fatigue, insomnia, and depression
Asian ginseng (Panax ginseng)	200 mg/day taken as an oral pill	Known to improve mood and add to a general sense of well-being in postmenopausal women
Hops	100 mg/day	Hops may be best as an in-between treatment while you are waiting for other, more lasting measures to kick in.
Valerian root extract	300 to 600 mg, usually taken as a pill, or two to three grams of dried herbal valerian soaked in a cup of hot water for 10 to 15 minutes, taken 30 minutes to two hours before bedtime	Do not combine with alcohol because of a theoretical concern that it may make alcohol more toxic. Side effects, including migraines, dizziness, and gastrointestinal disorder, are rare.

EXCESS ANDROGENS		
Zinc	It is best to get zinc from food sources such as green beans and sesame and pumpkin seeds.	Plays an important role in sexual development, menstruation, and ovulation
Omega-3	Good sources of omega-3s are wild Alaskan salmon and an omega-3 supplement that's been shown to be low in mercury and other toxins.	Women with more omega-3s have lower androgens in the blood plus a better cholesterol profile, and as a result, less risk of cardiovascular disease, one of the risks of excess androgens
Chromium picolinate	200 to 1,000 mcg/day	Chromium is a safe supplement worth trying if you are insulin resistant.
Inositol: *d-chiro-inositol* (DCI) or *myo-inositol* (MI)	• D-chiro-inositol (DCI): 600 mg twice/day, or 0.6 grams twice/day • Myo-inositol: 2 grams once or twice/day	Inositol is a naturally occurring B-complex vitamin known to improve insulin sensitivity.
Vitamin D	2,000 IU/day	I prefer to personalize the recommendation of 2,000 IU/day depending on your measured blood level.
Cinnamon	Half a teaspoon/day	Cinnamon also lowers blood pressure, helps correct abnormal cholesterol levels, and even increases lean body mass.
Saw palmetto	160 mg/day by capsule	Acts as an antiandrogen
Tian Gui capsule	Dosage depends upon formulation	Tian Gui contains more than eleven herbs.

LOW THYROID		
Copper from food sources and multivitamin containing copper	Multivitamin containing 2 mg of copper is recommended	Meats, poultry, and eggs are the best dietary sources of copper.
Zinc	Up to 50 mg/day	Zinc must be taken in the correct proportion with copper, since taking too much zinc may interfere with copper absorption, i.e., 20 mg of zinc with 2 mg of copper.
Selenium	200 mcg/day (many multivitamins contain this recommended amount)	There is no evidence that selenium supplementation in healthy individuals makes a difference — take it only if you're deficient and have autoantibodies to the thyroid.
Vitamin A	Recommended daily allowance is 5,000 IU	Taking more than 10,000 IU per day may be associated with toxicity, indicated by symptoms such as night blindness, nausea, irritability, blurred vision, and hair loss. Toxicity does not occur when you get vitamin A from food.
Iron	50 to 100 mg/day of elemental iron, with careful monitoring of your progress through testing of serum ferritin; iron is also available from food sources such as leafy greens and grass-fed beef	Too much iron may cause overload and problems for your liver. Many women find that iron supplements cause constipation and dark, hard stool.
Vitamin D	From sunshine and supplements, and through diet. Dose according to serum level. Typical dose is 2000 I.U. per day.	The best food sources are liver and low-mercury fish, such as herring, sardines, and cod.

APPENDIX B:

GLOSSARY OF TERMS

ACTH—A hormone released from the anterior pituitary gland in the brain. ACTH levels in the blood are measured to help detect, diagnose, and monitor conditions associated with excessive or deficient cortisol in the body. See Appendix C.

Addison's disease—A disease caused by insufficient production of hormones by the adrenal glands, causing decreased cortisol production and adrenal failure.

Adrenal dysregulation—Refers to the hypervigilance that has insidiously inserted itself into your life and hijacked your hypothalamic-pituitary-adrenal (HPA) axis. Under prolonged stress, the HPA axis can cause chronically elevated cortisol levels that may be linked to overweight, high blood pressure, and diabetes or prediabetes. Over time, cortisol production can't keep up with demand, which can lead to chronic fatigue syndrome, fibromyalgia, anxiety, insomnia, depression, and more.

Adrenal glands—Glands that produce hormones that you can't live without, including sex hormones and cortisol, which help you respond to stress and have many other functions. Your adrenal, or suprarenal, glands are located on the top of each kidney.

Agnolyt—Considered one of the best extracts of chaste tree vitex, an herb that improves PMS symptoms.

Allostasis—The process by which the body responds to stressors in order to regain homeostasis.

Amygdala—The part of the temporal lobe of the brain that is the center of vigilance, worry, and fear. It is involved in the assessment of threat-related stimuli and is necessary for the process of fear conditioning.

Anabolic hormones—These hormones, such as testosterone and DHEA, build the body. They are the hormones that influence muscular growth; they are sometimes known as anabolic steroids.

Androgen—The class of sex hormones that stimulates male characteristics by binding to androgen receptors on cells. Women, even though we have far lower levels of androgens than men, are exquisitely sensitive to androgen levels at the proper amount for vitality, confidence, and maintaining lean body mass. Ovarian overproduction of androgens is a condition in which the female ovaries make too much testosterone, and which is linked to polycystic ovarian syndrome. This condition can lead to the development in a woman of male characteristics, such as rogue hairs, acne, and sometimes hair loss.

Anovulation—A lack of egg production in the ovaries, which in turn leads to estrogen dominance.

Anti-thyroglobulin—An antibody directed against thyroglobulin, which is a key protein in the thyroid gland essential to the production of thyroid hormones.

Apoptosis—Programmed cell death; it is necessary to regulate cell growth and differentiation.

Armour (desiccated thyroid hormone)—Individuals with low thyroid function, or hypothyroidism, often benefit from thyroid-replacement therapy. There are many symptoms of low thyroid function, but the top three are weight gain, fatigue, and mood changes such as low-grade depression. In some folks, use of natural desiccated thyroid hormone, such as Armour or Nature-Throid (both bioidentical to human thyroid hormone), results in marked improvement in chronic symptoms that may fail to respond to a wide array of conventional and alternative treatments.

Ashwagandha (*Withania somnifera*)—A popular Ayurvedic herb, often used in formulations prescribed for stress, strain, fatigue, pain, skin diseases, diabetes, gastrointestinal disease, rheumatoid arthritis, and epilepsy. Ashwagandha is also used as a general tonic, to increase energy and improve health and longevity.

Ayurveda—The ancient Hindu medical system of India, based on the use of food, movement—such as yoga and meditation—and botanicals. The Sanskrit term literally translates as "scripture for longevity."

B vitamins—Naturally occurring vitamins formed by microorganisms and found in some foods, including meat, fish, shellfish, and liver. B vitamins are used for treating anemia and depression, preventing cervical cancer, elevating mood, boosting energy, and maintaining fertility.

Bioidentical hormones—Interest in a more natural approach to hormone therapy has focused attention on bioidentical hormones—hormones that are identical in molecular structure to the hormones women make in their bodies. They are not found in this form in nature but are made, or synthesized, from a plant chemical extracted from yams and soy.

Biomarkers—Biological molecules found in blood, other body fluids, or tissues that are a sign of a normal or abnormal process, or of a condition or disease. A biomarker may be used to see how well the body responds to a treatment for a disease or condition.

Botanicals—A botanical is a plant or plant part valued for its medicinal or therapeutic properties, flavor, or scent. Products made from botanicals that are used to maintain or improve health may be called herbal products, botanical products, or phytomedicines.

Burnout—A chronic stress state characterized by fatigue, headache, disturbed sleep, pain, attention deficit, feelings of apathy and meaninglessness, and detachment from work.

Catabolic dominance—The predominant breaking down of more complex substances into simpler ones in living organisms, often resulting in a release of energy.

Catabolic hormones—These hormones break down tissue in order to liberate energy.

Chasteberry tree—An herb used for menstrual irregularities, symptoms of menopause, premenstrual syndrome (PMS), female infertility, preventing miscarriage in patients with progesterone insufficiency, controlling postpartum bleeding, aiding in expulsion of the placenta, increasing lactation, and treating fibrocystic breasts.

Chronic fatigue syndrome—A serious and complicated disorder defined by profound fatigue that is unimproved by rest and worsens with activity. Symptoms may include weakness, muscle pain, sleep problems, and impaired memory and concentration, and may result in reduced participation in daily activities.

Chronic stress response—This reaction is caused by long-term activation of the stress-response system—and the subsequent overexposure to cortisol and other stress hormones that can disrupt almost all of your body's processes—putting you at increased risk of numerous health problems.

Circadian rhythms—Physical, mental, and behavioral changes that follow a roughly twenty-four-hour cycle, responding primarily to light and darkness in an organism's environment. They are found in most living things, including animals, plants, and many tiny microbes.

Clomiphene citrate (also known as Clomid)—A fertility prescription that may increase the number of eggs released at ovulation. It is prescribed for women who do not ovulate regularly.

Computerized axial tomography (CAT or CT)—This scan combines a series of X-ray views taken from many different angles to produce cross-sectional images of the bones and soft tissues inside your body.

Congenital adrenal hyperplasia (CAH)—A rare condition in which you inherit from a parent the tendency to make too much cortisol or one of the other sex hormones because you lack the enzyme that helps you make the normal amounts of all hormones.

Cortisol—A steroid hormone produced by the adrenal glands. It plays a role in bones, the circulatory system, the immune system, the nervous system, stress responses, and the metabolism of fats, carbohydrates, and proteins. See Appendix C.

Cortisol awakening response (CAR)—The salivary cortisol measurement sampled immediately after waking up. This response can serve as a reliable marker of hypothalamic-pituitary-adrenocortical activity.

DHEA—One of the androgens, along with testosterone, used for mild depression by women in their forties. It is used by men for erectile dysfunction, and by healthy men and women who have low levels of certain hormones, to improve well-being and sexuality, as well as for slowing or reversing aging, improving thinking skills in older people, decreasing the symptoms of menopause, and slowing the progress of Alzheimer's disease. See Appendix C.

Diabetes—High blood sugar, present when the body cannot move sugar into its fat, liver, and muscle cells to be stored for energy. This is because the pancreas does not make enough insulin or cells do not respond to insulin normally.

Di-indolemethane (DIM)—An extract from cruciferous vegetables that increases the metabolism of bad estrogens.

Diurnal cycle—A recognizable daily cycle.

Dopamine—A neurotransmitter that helps control the brain's reward and pleasure centers. It also helps regulate movement and emotional responses, and it enables us to not only see rewards but also to take action to move toward them.

Double-blind trials—A drug trial in which neither the researchers nor the patients know what they are getting. The computer gives each patient a code number and the code numbers are allocated to the treatment groups so that neither the patient nor the doctors know whether the treatment is medicine or a placebo.

Eczema (Atopic dermatitis)—A long-term skin disorder that involves scaly and itchy rashes.

Endogenous—Caused by factors within the body, resulting from conditions within the organism.

Endometriosis—A female health disorder that occurs when cells from the lining of the womb (uterus) grow in other areas of the body. This can lead to pain, irregular bleeding, and problems getting pregnant (infertility).

Epidemiologists—Scientists who investigate and describe the causes and spread of disease, and develop the means for prevention or control. They respond to disease outbreaks, determining their causes and helping to contain them.

Epigenetics—Refers to modifications to gene expression other than changes in the DNA sequence itself, such as addition of molecules to the DNA and altering how a gene interacts with important interpreting molecules in the cell's nucleus.

Epigenomics—Refers to the study of external factors that influence the genome, or the full set of an individual's DNA—that is, the epigenetic effects on gene expression.

Epinephrine—A hormone with neurotransmitters made in the inner core of the adrenals that help you focus and problem-solve. It creates amounts of glucose and fatty acids that can be used by the body as fuel in times of stress or danger when increased alertness or exertion is required.

Estradiol—The most commonly made estrogen in women who are still cycling. It is responsible for the growth of the womb (uterus), breast development, fallopian tubes, and vagina, and plays a role in the distribution of body fat in women. See Appendix C.

Estrogen—A hormone that affects libido, mood, joints, and mental state. It is used to treat breast tenderness, cysts, cancer, fibroids, endometriosis, endometrial cancer, hot flashes, and symptoms in women who are experiencing or have experienced menopause. See Appendix C.

Fibromyalgia—A common syndrome in which a person has long-term, body-wide pain and tenderness in the joints, muscles, tendons, and other soft tissues. Fibromyalgia has also been linked to fatigue, sleep problems, headaches, depression, and anxiety.

Follicle-stimulating hormone (FSH)—FSH functions with luteinizing hormone and stimulates the release of eggs from the ovaries. It is controlled by the hypothalamus and pituitary gland. See Appendix C.

Free T3 (Free triiodothyronine)—A free T3 (fT3) test is used to assess thyroid function. It is ordered primarily to help diagnose hyperthyroidism and may be ordered to help monitor the status of a person with a known thyroid disorder.

Free T4 (Free thyroxine)—The free T4 (fT4) test is thought by many to be a more accurate reflection of thyroid hormone function and aid in the diagnosis of female infertility.

Gastroesophageal reflux disease (GERD)—A condition in which the stomach contents leak backward from the stomach into the esophagus (the tube from the mouth to the stomach). This action can irritate the esophagus, causing heartburn and other symptoms.

Genome—The complete set of a person's genetic code.

Glandular therapy—A technique that is useful to treat hormonal problems by alternative healers but lacks randomized trial data. Generally the historical motive was to support the weak gland of the patient with an analogous animal gland rich in specific nutrients.

Glucocorticoids—Made in the outside portion (the cortex) of the adrenal gland, glucocorticoids regulate the metabolism of glucose and are chemically classed as steroids. Cortisol is the major natural glucocorticoid.

Hawthorne effect—The phenomenon in which subjects in behavioral studies change their performance in response to being observed.

Hippocampus—The main home for memory formation and storage in the brain, found under the frontal part of the cerebral cortex. It is the brain region responsible for memory, with its high number of cortisol receptors.

Homeostasis—Maintaining stability in a biological environment during change.

Human chorionic gonadotropin (hCG)—A pregnancy hormone made by cells that form the placenta, which nourishes the egg after it has been fertilized and becomes attached to the uterine wall. Medications containing hCG are often used in fertility treatments.

Hyperarousal—The scientific term for "stressed out," meaning that the body's alarm system never shuts off.

Hypercortisolism—Known as Cushing's syndrome, hypercortisolism is a disorder that occurs when your body is exposed to high levels of the hormone cortisol. It can also occur if you take too much cortisol or other steroid hormones precursors.

Hyperplasia—Increased cell production in a normal tissue or organ. Hyperplasia may be a sign of abnormal or precancerous changes, particularly atypical hyperplasia of the endometrium. Hyperplasia of the adrenals may also occur in response to chronic stress and overactivation of the hypothalamic pituitary adrenal (HPA) axis.

Hypertension—The term used to describe high blood pressure. Blood pressure is a measurement of the force against the walls of your arteries as your heart pumps blood through your body.

Hypervigilance—Abnormally increased arousal, responsiveness to stimuli, and scanning of the environment for threats.

Hypocortisolism—Also known as low cortisol, hypocortisolism occurs when your adrenal glands are unable to make a normal amount of the main stress hormone, cortisol.

Hypoglycemia—The depletion of feel-good neurotransmitters that occurs when your blood sugar (glucose) is too low.

Hypopituitarism—When the pituitary does not make normal amounts of some or all of its hormones—including the hormones that control the ovaries, thyroid, and adrenals—as a result of head injury, brain surgery, radiation, stroke, or a problem called Sheehan's syndrome, which is when a woman bleeds severely during childbirth.

Hypothalamic-pituitary-adrenal (HPA) axis—A feedback loop by which signals from the brain trigger the release of hormones needed to respond to stress. Because of its function, the HPA axis is also sometimes called the stress circuit.

Hypothalamus—An area of the brain that produces hormones that control body temperature, hunger, moods, sex drive, sleep, and the release of hormones from many glands, especially the pituitary gland.

Hypothyroidism—An underactive thyroid, characterized by fatigue, weight gain, and mood problems.

IFN—A marker of immune function.

Isocort—A plant form of cortisol available as a nutritional supplement. Used for waning adrenal glands.

Kanchanar guggulu—A substance used for the thyroid but not supported by the best evidence (randomized trials).

Leptin—A hormone that controls hunger, metabolism, and the utilization of food as fuel or fat. See Appendix C.

Limbic system—The region of the brain involved with emotion.

Luteal phase—Second half of the menstrual cycle.

Luteinizing hormone (LH)—Functions with follicle-stimulating hormone and stimulates the release of eggs from the ovaries. LH is controlled by the hypothalamus and pituitary gland. See Appendix C.

Maca (*Lepidium meyenii*)—Grown in central Peru in the high plateaus of the Andes mountains, maca is used for female hormone imbalance, menstrual irregularities, enhancing fertility, menopause symptoms, impotence, and as an aphrodisiac.

Magnetic resonance imaging (MRI)—Used to diagnose health conditions that affect organs, tissue, and bone. Scanners use strong magnetic fields and radio waves to produce detailed images of the inside of the body.

Mastalgia—Breast pain generally classified as either cyclical or noncyclic.

Mastodyna—Pain occurring in the female breast.

Melatonin—A hormone secreted by the pineal gland in the brain that helps regulate other hormones and maintains the body's circadian rhythm. Melatonin also helps control the timing and release of female reproductive hormones. See Appendix C.

Neuroplasticity—The ability of the brain to change, stretch, and learn by forming new neural connections throughout life. Neuroplasticity allows the nerve cells in the brain to adjust in response to new situations or changes in their environment.

Neurotransmitters—Chemicals, such as serotonin and norepinephrine, used to communicate between brain cells. Improving the balance of these chemicals seems to help brain cells send and receive messages, which in turn may boost mood.

Norepinephrine—A neurotransmitter made in the inner core of the adrenals that helps with focus and problem solving. It acts as a neuromodulator in the nervous system and as a hormone in the blood.

Osteopenia—The term used for bones that have become somewhat less dense than normal, but not as severely as in osteoporosis. A person with osteopenia is at risk for getting osteoporosis.

Osteoporosis—A problem in which bones are less dense and more fragile than usual and thus at greater risk for fracture, even with a small amount of trauma. This disease often affects bones in the hip, spine, and wrist.

Oxytocin—The hormone of love and bonding that helps to buffer stress. It also acts as a neurotransmitter in the brain. See Appendix C.

Perimenopause—Also called the menopausal transition, the interval in which a woman's body makes a natural shift from more-or-less regular cycles of ovulation and menstruation toward permanent infertility, or menopause.

Phosphatidylserine—A fatty acid that has been shown to reduce cortisol levels, phosphatidylserine has received some interest as a potential treatment for Alzheimer's disease and other memory problems.

Pituitary—The gland in the brain controlling hormones, such as estrogen, progesterone, thyroid, and oxytocin.

Polycystic ovary syndrome (PCOS)—A condition in which there is an imbalance in a woman's female sex hormones. This hormone imbalance may cause changes in the menstrual cycle, skin changes, trouble getting pregnant, and other problems.

Pranayama—The breathing technique of yoga that is said to increase physical and psychological performance.

Pregnenolone—The mother hormone (see Figure 2 in chapter 2) or precursor to other sex hormones. It keeps memory and vision acute, and anxiety at bay. It is used for slowing or reversing aging, for arthritis, depression, endometriosis, fatigue, fibrocystic breast disease, memory enhancement, menopause, premenstrual syndrome (PMS), and stress. See Appendix C.

Premarin—A synthetic extract of several estrogens, also known as "conjugated equine estrogens," derived from horse urine.

Prempro—A commonly prescribed hormone replacement pill that contains estrogens from horse urine and is a synthetic relative of the hormone progesterone (a combination of Premarin and Provera).

Progesterone—Released in your ovaries, this hormone can be converted into other hormones such as cortisol in the adrenals. A low amount of progesterone can cause anxiety, night sweats, sleeplessness, and irregular cycles. See Appendix C.

Prometrium—A pill containing bioidentical, micronized progesterone.

Puberty—The stage of life when females become fertile.

Relora—An herbal combination that has been shown to reduce evening cortisol and stress-related eating, but only in overweight and obese women. Relora also reduces anxiety in premenopausal women.

Reverse T3 (Reverse triiodothyronine)—A molecule that has the same molecular formula but different structural formula from triiodothyronine, a hormone made by the thyroid gland. It has three iodine molecules and is derived from thyroxine.

Rhodiola—Used for increasing energy, stamina, strength, and mental capacity, and to help the body adapt to and resist physical, chemical, and environmental stress.

Secondary adrenal insufficiency—This insufficiency occurs when the pituitary gland fails to produce enough of the hormone adrenocorticotropin (ACTH) to stimulate the adrenal glands to produce cortisol.

Serotonin—A chemical substance found in the brain, intestinal tissue, and blood platelets. It functions as a neurotransmitter; changes in its concentration are associated with several mood disorders.

Sex hormone binding globulin (SHBG)—A protein that binds free testosterone and may make it biologically inert. When you take oral hormones such as estrogen pills or birth control pills, SHBG rises, which may diminish sex drive and cause persistent irritation in the vulvo-vaginal area. In Polycystic Ovary Syndrome, low SHBG may cause higher levels of free testosterone to cause rogue hairs and acne.

Taurine—An amino acid that supports neurological development and helps regulate the level of water and mineral salts in the blood. Taurine is also thought to have antioxidant properties.

Telomeres—The caps on chromosomes, emerging as a new biomarker of biological aging; telomeres are specialized structures that are essential for protecting chromosome ends and ensuring chromosome stability.

Thyroid—A gland that keeps the metabolism balanced, giving you energy, comfortable warmth, and manageable weight. See Appendix C.

Thyroid antibodies—The presence of thyroid antibodies in your blood may suggest that the cause of thyroid disease is an autoimmune disorder.

Titer—A measurement of the amount or concentration of a substance in a solution. Titer usually refers to the amount of antibodies found in a patient's blood.

Transdermal estrogen—A prescribed hormone patch or cream proven to improve mood and libido.

Tryptophan—An amino acid needed for normal growth in infants and for nitrogen balance in adults. It is an essential amino acid, which means your body cannot produce it—you must get it from your diet.

TSH (thyroid-stimulating hormone)—A hormone produced by the pituitary gland at the base of the brain in response to signals from the hypothalamus gland. It tells the thyroid gland to make and release the hormones thyroxine (T4) and triiodothyronine (T3).

Tumescence—A swelling or an enlargement. I use the word in descriptions of female sexual energy and of how ancient traditions, such as Taoist sexual methods and tantra, direct and build sexual energy.

Tyrosine—An amino acid that serves as a precursor to important neurotransmitters depleted by stress, such as norepinephrine and dopamine.

Vagus nerve—A nerve that originates in the brain stem and supplies nerve fibers to the lungs, heart, esophagus, and gut.

Vivelle dot—A form of bioidentical estrogen patch.

APPENDIX C:

HORMONES AND THEIR FUNCTIONS

HORMONE	JOB	COMMENT
ACTH	ACTH levels in the blood are measured to help detect, diagnose, and monitor conditions associated with excessive or deficient cortisol in the body.	Released from the anterior pituitary gland in the brain
Adiponectin	Adjusts how you burn fat	Secreted by fat cells
Aldosterone	Controls the level of electrolytes in your blood and urine, mediating water retention and blood pressure	Can be low in adrenal dysregulation, stage 3 exhaustion, which is associated with low cortisol because aldosterone and cortisol are produced in the same location of the adrenal gland—the outer layer or cortex
Allopregnanolone	Calms and neutralizes stress	Daughter (derivative or metabolite) of progesterone
Cortisol	The main stress hormone; governs blood sugar, blood pressure, and immune function; member of glucocorticoid family	Produced in your adrenal glands under most conditions, stressful or otherwise
Dehydroepiandrosterone (DHEA) and DHEAS (sulfated version)	Affects mood and sex drive, can convert into testosterone when needed; member of androgen family	Too much DHEA has been associated with depression in menopause, acne

Dihydrotestosterone (DHT)	May shrink hair follicles; three times more potent than testosterone; member of androgen family	Testosterone can be converted to dihydrotestosterone (DHT). DHT is the main cause of male-pattern hair loss (in men and women).
Estradiol	Responsible for the growth of the womb (uterus), breast development, Fallopian tubes, and vagina; plays a role in the distribution of body fat in women; member of estrogen family	Most common estrogen in women who are still cycling
Estriol	Main estrogen of pregnancy	Used topically for vulvovaginal dryness
Estrogen	Regulates menstruation; builds uterine lining to prepare for pregnancy; keeps women lubricated, from joints to vagina	The estrogen family are sex steroid hormones produced primarily in the ovaries to promote female characteristics such as breast growth and menstruation.
Estrone	Least abundant of the three estrogen hormones in reproductive-aged women; predominant estrogen in postmenopausal women	
Follicle-stimulating hormone (FSH)	Functions with luteinizing hormone, both stimulating the release of eggs from the ovaries	Controlled by the hypothalamus and pituitary gland
Insulin	Drives glucose into cells as fuel and deposits fat	Chronically high insulin increases estrogen, and estrone, specifically, increases the cells' resistance to insulin.
Leptin	Regulates appetite and adiponectin, which adjusts how you burn fat.	
Luteinizing hormone (LH)	Functions with follicle-stimulating hormone, both stimulating the release of eggs from the ovaries	Controlled by the hypothalamus and pituitary gland

Melatonin	Regulates our sleep/wake cycle	Helps control the timing and release of female reproductive hormones
Oxytocin	Both a hormone and a neurotransmitter, which means it acts as a brain chemical that transmits information from nerve to nerve; called by some "the love hormone" because it increases in the blood with orgasm in both men and women	Oxytocin is also released when the cervix dilates, thereby augmenting labor, and when a woman's nipples are stimulated, which facilitates breast-feeding and promotes bonding between mother and baby.
Pregnenolone	This lesser-known matriarch of the sex-hormone system is responsible for maintaining a facile memory and vision in vivid Technicolor.	Pregnenolone is the "mother" hormone (or "prehormone") from which other hormones are made.
Progesterone	Counterbalances estrogen by helping regulate uterine lining (i.e., keeps the lining from getting too thick), emotions, and sleep	One of the sex hormones made in the adrenals
Testosterone	Hormone of vitality and self-confidence, and producing too much is the main reason for female infertility in this country. Also involved in sex drive; producing too little is linked to low libido in women and men.	One of the sex hormones, also an androgen. Although it is often thought of as the male hormone, women need to have some testosterone in their bodies as well. The difference between men and women lies in the quantity of testosterone (men produce much higher quantities).
Thyroid	Affects metabolism and energy, weight, mood	Thyroid hormone is essential to the smooth operation of hormone pathways. You need adequate thyroid hormone to make pregnenolone from cholesterol, and then to make progesterone.

| Vitamin D | Synthesized from cholesterol and exposure to sunlight. It can also be ingested from food, but it is not officially an essential vitamin because it can be made by all mammals exposed to the sun. It is considered a vitamin and a hormone. | Present in eggs and fish, is added to other foods such as milk; available as a dietary supplement |

APPENDIX D

HOW TO FIND AND WORK COLLABORATIVELY WITH PRACTITIONERS FOR YOUR HORMONE CURE

I'm a big fan of etiquette scripts when it comes to charged or difficult conversations. Scripts help me with a starting point, with someone *else's* skillful ideas about what might be particularly useful in a given situation. For instance, say you have an acquaintance you don't know well who tells you she just got diagnosed with cancer. You say, "That's big." And *pause*. You listen. You hear what she has to say. You don't rush in with your own brush with cancer, or how you cared for your mom with metastatic breast cancer, or how you can imagine how they feel. Just, rather simply: *"That's big."* In this section, I'll share scripts that my patients have found helpful with their other health providers.

I'm told often by women in my practice that there's something very challenging about asserting yourself with your doctors when they dismiss your hormonal symptoms or decline to perform the tests you've reasonably requested.

I understand the mainstream doctors' beef—I trained in the same system. After getting educated for so many years, and then, finally, having your own medical practice, you want to have a little authority. You recommend smart things, hopefully change lives, and establish caring and long-term relationships. But all day long, in those seven-minute appointments, while American doctors are dispensing advice and rules, there's often not much room for dialogue or partnership.

Here are some of the characteristics of a doctor who works collaboratively and won't treat you paternalistically.

- **Is a keen listener.** Not in a hurry to interject his or her own opinion.
- **Stays current with the literature.** Ask if they know about the latest thyroid guidelines from chapter 9 on what defines a normal thyroid-stimulating hormone.
- **Understands nuance.** Do they hear your symptoms, attune to your narrative, and then consider your labs? Noncollaborative doctors prefer to treat labs only.
- **Has a right-sized ego.** Do they get defensive with your suggestions? Get a bit hot under the collar when you kindly notice they didn't wash their hands in front of you at the beginning of the appointment?
- **Has time to address your concerns.** Or is the hand on the doorknob when you work up the nerve to mention your libido or irritable mood?

Here are some scripts that I suggest as conversation starters.

- "I just read a book about how to fix hormone problems, and I learned a lot. I brought you a copy in case you are interested. I know we don't have much time today, but I would like to discuss it at my next appointment, and what my problems might be. Would you be willing to discuss it next time?" (Note: This is how I first read Dr. Uzzi Reiss's book, *Natural Hormone Balance*. It works!)
- "I've read a lot about hormones and am trying to make myself an educated consumer. I read in a particular book, by a doctor who specializes in hormones, that it's important to look beyond some of the standard tests to really understand what's going on. Because I'm experiencing [insert your symptoms], I wonder if you'd be willing to order a blood test for me."
- "I've been reading a book about hormone imbalance and how it relates to . . . [fill in the blank: cortisol, estrogen,

testosterone, progesterone, insulin, leptin, vitamin D, thyroid]. I have these three symptoms of . . . [fill in the blank: high cortisol, high or low estrogen]. Would you be willing to order a test for me?"

- If your doctor declines to perform testing, stand your ground. Be polite but assertive. "These references show there's a link between . . . I'd really like to pursue testing to get to the bottom of this." Or "Can you explain to me why it's not worthwhile to test? I have seventeen references here that document the link between high cortisol and high blood pressure, high fasting glucose, fatigue, and belly fat, so I'd prefer to test." Then pause.
- If your doctor then says something along the lines of *"I don't believe in adrenal fatigue"* or *"Why don't you just try this antidepressant?,"* you can also recommend the citations I've compiled for practitioners at http://thehormonecure book.com/practitioners.

If your doctor continues to refuse, you might ask if he or she can refer you to someone who'd be willing to order the tests, or, alternatively, you might consider the following websites to find a doctor who practices integrative medicine.

- Graduates of the Fellowship at the University of Arizona Center for Integrative Medicine: http://integrativemedi cine.arizona.edu/alumni.html.
- Members of the Institute for Functional Medicine: http://www.functionalmedicine.org/practitioner_search .aspx?id=117.
- Members of the American College for the Advancement of Medicine: http://www.acamnet.org. (Scroll down to use "Physician+Link" to find a doctor in your area.)

APPENDIX E

RECOMMENDED LABS FOR HOME TESTING

These are the laboratories I use routinely for my patients at http://thehormonecurebook.com/tests. Please note that my preference is to use blood testing for most hormones, but saliva and urine testing are often reliable. For cortisol testing, I prefer a diurnal (4-point) cortisol test.

- **Canary Club** is a nonprofit community with many great resources headed by Richard Shames, MD, esteemed hormone expert, and his team. Membership is free and they have been able to negotiate competitive pricing, often lower than I can offer or you may obtain through other labs: http://www.canaryclub.org.
- **Genova Diagnostics,** http://www.gdx.net, has several tests that I find helpful to unravel hormonal problems, including the Complete Hormones and also the Estro-Genomic Profile. I also find great information for my patients in their "NutrEval" test.
- **Mymedlab.com** provides you with direct access to blood testing of a broad array of tests mentioned in this book. They also offer a Personal Health Record and help with interpretation.
- **ZRT Laboratory** is a pioneer in saliva testing. I like their blood spot testing for thyroid and vitamin D. Great choice if your practitioner declines to test your free T3: http://www.zrtlab.com.

APPENDIX F

THE GOTTFRIED FOOD PLAN

You probably know what to eat. Yet I have many women ask me, in the privacy of my office, to lay out a plan. This is a basic food plan that I've gathered over the years from various sources. I find it is nourishing and easily adapted to the individual, similar to a yoga pose. Most importantly, this food plan balances your hormones, lowers inflammation, and reduces risk of insulin resistance.

One of the key ways to reduce inflammation in your body and lower cortisol is to remove the most common food allergens, as described recently by JJ Virgin in *The Virgin Diet*. She recommends removal of the seven top culprits, including gluten, soy, sugar, and dairy.

The main idea is to calibrate from the basic plan. If you lose weight on this volume of food, add one ounce of whole grain at breakfast or three ounces at dinner. All food should be organic and in season. For more information and recipes, go to http://thehor monecurebook.com.

Breakfast*

1 ounce gluten-free oatmeal or quinoa flakes, measured and then cooked

4–6 ounces low-glycemic fruit, such as berries

8 ounces yogurt or 2 eggs or protein powder for a smoothie (one serving)†

1–3 tablespoons ground flaxseeds or soaked chia seeds (add more depending on bowel function)

Lunch

4 ounces lean protein (organic chicken, grass-fed beef, low-mercury fish, lamb) or 6 ounces tofu, tempeh, or beans‡

6 ounces cooked vegetables (preferably low-glycemic if weight loss is your goal, and steamed)

1 serving fruit (1 apple, 1 banana, or 6 ounces low-glycemic fruit; can be traded once or twice per week for a single 5-ounce serving of wine, depending on your weight, weight goal, sleep, and estrogen symptoms)

Dinner

4 ounces lean protein (organic chicken, grass-fed beef, low-mercury fish, lamb) or 6 ounces tofu, tempeh, or beans

6 ounces cooked vegetables (preferably low-glycemic if weight loss is your goal, and steamed)

8 ounces salad (ideally 2 ounces lettuce and the remainder in raw vegetables of your choice, including radishes, purple cabbage, cucumber, carrots, radicchio, and fennel)

2 tablespoons dressing (but no sugar in the dressing; sugar must not be one of the ingredients), for serving with salad

---

*I encourage women with PMS to have a low-glycemic smoothie for breakfast, containing medicinal fiber, especially in the seven to ten days prior to menses.

†You can also have 6 ounces yogurt plus 2 tablespoons cream or milk in your coffee or morning beverage. Other alternatives are 4 ounces lean meat protein, 6 ounces plant-based protein, or 1 ounce nuts with 4 ounces yogurt.

‡Men get 2 more ounces protein than women.

APPENDIX G

NORMAL AND OPTIMAL RANGES FOR HORMONE LEVELS AND RELATED LABORATORY TESTS*

HORMONE TEST	UNITS	CONVENTIONAL REFERENCE RANGE (FOR WOMEN)	OPTIMAL RANGE (FOR WOMEN)
ALT (Alanine aminotransferase, a liver enzyme)	U/L	7–35 U/L	0–19
Cortisol (serum)	µg/dL	7–28 morning, 2–18 afternoon	Optimal: 10–15 morning, 6–10 afternoon
Cortisol (blood spot, e.g., ZRT/ Canary Club)	µg/dL	8.5–19.8 (morning), 3.3–8.5 (evening/night) according to ZRT labs (may vary at other labs)	Same
Cortisol Morning (saliva)	ng/ml	3.7–9.5	Same
Cortisol Night (saliva)	ng/ml	0.4–1.0	Same
Cortisol Noon (saliva)	ng/ml	1.2–3.0	Same
Cortisol Evening (saliva)	ng/ml	0.6–1.9	Same
DHEAS (serum)	µg/dL	65–380	Top half of normal range: approximately 200–380

* Note that your lab may vary based on the normal distribution. Consult your practitioner for personal recommendations or go to http://thehormonecurebook.com/practitioners/ to find a collaborative clinician.

DHEAS (blood spot)	μg/dL	40–290 (age dependent)	Top half of normal range: approximately 165–290
DHEAS (saliva)	ng/ml	2–23 (Age dependent)	Under 30: 6.4–18.6 ng/ml; 31–45: 3.9–11.4 ng/ml; 46–60: 2.7–8 ng/ml; 61–75: 2–6 ng/ml; on oral DHEA (5–10 mg, 12–24 hours after last dose): 2.8–8.6 ng/ml; transdermal DHEA (5 mg): 3–8 ng/ml
Estradiol (serum)	pg/ml	Premenopause: depends on timing with cycle. Overall 15–350 pg/mL in premenopause. Postmenopause and not on hormones < 32	Day 3: < 80; Day 14: 150–350; postmenopause approximately 50 for bone strength
Estradiol (blood spot)	pg/ml	43–180 premeno-luteal or ERT	A normal range for estradiol on day 14 for women in their twenties is 350 pg/ml, and less than 32 after menopause.
Estradiol (saliva)	pg/ml	1.3–3.3 premenopausal (luteal phase, usually day 21–23)	In premenopause, I believe salivary estradiol of 1.3–1.7 is optimal.
	pg/ml	0.5–1.7 pg/ml postmenopause	In postmenopause, I believe salivary estradiol of 1.0–1.7 is optimal.
Fasting Blood Glucose	mg/dl	60–99	70–86
Free T3 (blood spot)	pg/ml	2.5–6.5	Top half of normal range (varies by lab), for ZRT 4.5–6.5
Free T4 (blood spot)	ng/dL	0.7–2.5	Top half of normal range (varies by lab), for ZRT 1.45–2.5
FSH (blood spot)	U/L	0.6–8.0 premenopausal-luteal	Day 3: < 10, but women still conceive when higher than 10
HDL	mg/dL	40 mg/dL or higher	> 55
Hemoglobin A1c	%	< 6%	< 5%
hsCRP (blood spot)	mg/L	< 3	< 0.5

IGF-1 (blood spot)	ng/ml	100–300 (age dependent)	Top half of normal range (e.g., 200–300) depending on age
Insulin (blood spot)	mIU/ml (μIU/mL)	1–15 μIU/ml	2–6 μIU/mL
LDL Cholesterol	mg/dl	<130 mg/dL	I assess based on particle size: you want to minimize small dense LDL particles
Progesterone (serum)	ng/ml	Luteal phase: 8 to 33	Luteal phase (day 21–23): 15–33
Progesterone (blood spot)	ng/ml	3.3–22.5 premeno-luteal or PgRT	Luteal phase (day 21–23): 15–23
Progesterone (saliva)	pg/ml	75–270 premenopausal (luteal); 12–100 postmenopausal or follicular (before ovulation)	Age dependent — discuss with your practitioner
Ratio: Pg/E2 (blood spot)		100–500	Top half of normal range: 300–500
Ratio: Pg/E2 (saliva)	pg/ml	100–500 when E2 1.3–3.3	Top half of normal range: 300–500
Serum Ferritin	ng/ml or mcg/L	11–307 nanograms per milliliter (standard units) or 11 to 307 micrograms per liter (international units)	70–90, especially if hair loss
Free Testosterone (serum)	pg/ml	0–2.2	Top half of normal range: 1.1–2.2
Testosterone (blood spot)	ng/dl	20–130 premeno-luteal or TRT	75–130
Testosterone (saliva)	pg/ml	16–55 (age dependent)	Top half of normal range: 36–55
TPO (blood spot)	IU/ml	0–150 (70–150 borderline)	<70
Triglycerides (blood spot)	mg/dL	< 150 mg/dL	< 50

TSH (blood spot)	uU/ml	0.5–3.0	The normal range is debated, but evidence favors 0.3 to 2.5 mIU/L. In women who still feel symptoms or have a diagnosis of autoimmune thyroiditis, I will optimize to 0.1–2.0. Ideal is to know the baseline TSH from an earlier age when client feels great and in balance.
Vitamin D, 25-OH, D_2	ng/ml	< 4 if not supplementing (< 10 nmol/L)	Same
Vitamin D, 25-OH, D_3	ng/ml	32–100 ng/ml (80–250 nmol/L)	75–90
Vitamin D, 25-OH, Total	ng/ml	32–100	75–90

APPENDIX H

FERTILITY AND CONCEPTION, PREGNANCY, AND LACTATION PROTOCOLS

It's thrilling, and *exhausting*. It's maddening and marvelous. It's everything and more. Yes, it's time to dish on pregnancy and how it forces you to meet your limitations and your greatest power as a woman. While I promise not to go *Women's Studies* on you, I want to separate the truth from the myth when it comes to your body on hormonal rocket fuel, also known as the fertility matrix.

First, let's get the not-fun stuff out of the way. Modern medicine has helped millions of couples conceive, but it is typically with the use of expensive and sophisticated techniques such as fertility drugs and in vitro fertilization (IVF). There are also many natural ways to upgrade your fertility that aren't often discussed within the confines of a doctor's office. These methods that I recommend target the complex system of hormonal cross talk that plays a pivotal role in helping you to get pregnant, carry a healthy child to term, thrive when you're home postpartum, and if you choose to do so, breast-feed your precious baby. I am often asked about all aspects of women's lives, from the role of stress preconception to the safety of supplements when a woman is pregnant or lactating. My hope is that this new appendix will answer most of those questions!

Fertility and Conception

It is truly a mindbender when you shift from preventing pregnancy at all costs to encouraging pregnancy, embracing pregnancy, and stepping into the grace and mayhem of motherhood. I've gone through it twice, and let me tell you, the hormonal ride is fierce and furious for many women. The good news is that pregnancy is the most effective cure for PMS. The bad news is that we live in a culture that unfairly projects so much junk onto pregnant women—from the politics of reproductive choice to one's judgment about weight and food choices. Let's just say that my hormones in pregnancy made me want to eat everything in sight, and the regular documentation and humiliation of my public weighing was enough to send my cortisol through the roof. It's as if you are pronounced guilty of child abuse—by a medical assistant—based on whether your weight gain is acceptable or not.

At the same time, many women find it difficult to get pregnant, and it can create an internal pain that is unfathomable. The trust that you developed over years in your female body suddenly comes into question, and most women have to cram the equivalent of medical school into their nights and weekends as they research the options available to them. While in vitro fertilization and other high-tech reproductive assistance is commonplace, I believe it can be helpful to assess the elephant in the room before heading to a doctor's office: stress hormones, particularly cortisol, and how they pull other hormones out of balance.

Stress

The pressure to get pregnant has affected most women at one point or another. Maybe the timing is good, maybe your parents are pushing for grandkids, or the ticking of the biological clock has gotten a bit louder, or maybe you just desperately want to have a baby (even if the timing isn't good). However, it's a cruel trick that society plays on us when baby stress ramps up, because stress is one of the most detrimental forces to your fertility.

Anyone who wants to conceive needs to navigate stress (and cortisol, the main stress hormone) so that cortisol is in the sweet spot, not too high and not too low. Why? High cortisol blocks progesterone receptors. Progesterone is a must-have for baby-making; not only do healthy progesterone levels improve your fertility, but upgraded molecular sex between progesterone and its receptor is needed for feelings of gratitude and joy during pregnancy and post-partum. Progesterone will make your pregnancy experience easier, happier, and healthier for you and your child.

Dr. Tori Hudson recommends that women who want to increase their fertility and reduce their stress take rhodiola (*Rhodiola rosea*). Not only does it provide a boost to thyroid function, but research shows that it may improve egg maturation. Rhodiola also lowers cortisol levels and increases serotonin.[1] Women have half the serotonin of men, so we tend to need help in this department, as I learned from my colleague and friend Dr. Daniel Amen.[2] Even athletes perform better with rhodiola. Recently, a randomized trial showed that athletes rode a bike faster, harder, and more efficiently after taking rhodiola compared to a placebo.[3]

Age

Women are having children later in life. I love this, because it means most of us are going to college and having careers, but conception past 40 comes with some extra health considerations, including a greater risk of some genetic problems. I'm supercareful to use language that feels welcoming yet tells you about the risks.

- Make sure you are taking L-methylfolate in your daily multivitamin, starting three months prior to conception. Folic acid (vitamin B_9) has been shown to reduce anemia in pregnancy and prevent neural tube defects, which is a structural abnormality in the fetus. Many women, particularly in the United States, need L-methylfolate, which is the more active form of folic acid, to prevent problems in pregnancy.
- Especially if you haven't previously had a child, you may want to genetically test yourself and your partner. To learn more about the genetic tests that I recommend, go to http://thehormonecurebook.com/genetics.

- Consider checking egg quality—day 3 estradiol and FSH. You want, ideally, for FSH < 10 and estradiol < 80. Women still get pregnant when FSH is above 10, but it's less likely.
- Be aware that some clinicians perform a Clomid Challenge Test—clomid is a synthetic estrogen blocker.

If you've been trying to get pregnant for less than six months, you're considered subfertile, not infertile. On the other hand, if you are aged 35 or older, infertility is diagnosed after trying to conceive in earnest for six months. If you are subfertile, estradiol and FSH levels can predict an important root cause, and again, help you determine how to proceed.

Nutrition

Many women look forward to "eating for two," but in reality, nutrition and dietary tweaks should be made well before that pregnancy test comes back positive. It is possible—and highly recommended— to eat a diet that up-levels your hormonal balance and fertility *before* you become pregnant. The right foods and supplements will reduce inflammation, balance your hormones, and improve your chances of getting pregnant. Here are my four main rules for a preconception diet:

1. Consume more omega-3s, whether in the form of fish (low in mercury, always wild, not farmed!), omega-3–enriched eggs, walnuts, or a high-quality omega-3 supplement.
2. Get methylated folate (also known as L-methylfolate). Foods that are rich in folic acid include dark leafy greens, asparagus, broccoli, citrus (oranges, lemons), and beans. White kidney beans have been shown to help you slow down the metabolism of carbohydrates, which is good for your entire metabolic system.
3. Eat fewer high-glycemic carbohydrate and gluten products. Pizza, pastries, and processed food can lower your

chances of conception. Many women have a problem with digesting gluten or have an autoimmune response to it, and gluten consumption may affect fertility and menstruation. It's not yet clear how many women are affected by gluten issues, but it's prudent to limit consumption.

4. Eat as much organic, local, and seasonal produce as possible. I recommend one pound per day of vegetables. They'll also improve your metabolism, which leads to improved insulin sensitivity and healthier progesterone receptors.

Other general guidelines include reducing your caffeine and alcohol intake (both raise cortisol) and aiming for 35 to 45 grams of fiber daily.[4] The average American woman gets only 14 grams of fiber per day—measure your baseline fiber intake by going to http://sparkpeople.com.

Women experience a lot of bloating in pregnancy, and part of the problem is that we have 10 feet more colon than men. Instead of a horseshoe like the guy's have, our intestines are more like a Six Flag's roller coaster. Check out Georgetown gastroenterologist Robynne Chutkan's new book *Gutbliss* to learn more.[5]

Pregnancy tends to be constipating, and you need to slowly increase the fiber by no more than 5 grams per day to avoid discomfort before and during pregnancy.

Supplements

It took me a full nine years of medical training to feel confident discerning the safe from the unsafe, the known from the unknown, when it comes to advising women about medications and supplements when they are pregnant and nursing, so I encourage you to come armed with research and questions when you visit your own ob/gyn. Even with all of my training as a doctor, board-certified in all things that can go wrong with a woman's body, I find that many drugs and supplements lack sufficient data to prove safety and efficacy during pregnancy and lactation.

Studies show that multivitamin use can reduce chances of ovulatory infertility as well as birth defects.[6] I recommend adding a prenatal vitamin to your daily regimen for at least three months before you want to get pregnant. Some studies have shown a link between low vitamin D and difficulty with conception, so add a vitamin D supplement if your levels are low.[7]

A Stanford University School of Medicine study shows that in women with low progesterone, fertility rates are higher among those taking chasteberry. After six months of treatment, 32 percent of the women taking chasteberry became pregnant, compared with 10 percent of the group taking a placebo.[8] Supplementing with chasteberry increased progesterone and fertility, and the American Herbal Products Association recommends chasteberry in pregnancy to prevent miscarriage. Other studies have shown that there may be only minimal risk in pregnacy.[9] I can't give you a strict rule on whether to continue it during pregnancy—that decision is best left to a woman to discuss with her practitioner—but my standards are high and I advise against it once pregnant.

GMOs

In my mind, *GMO* stands for Get Me Out! The more data that surfaces about the long-term effects of eating GMO (genetically modified organisms), the more I warn my patients to go 100 percent organic. GMO crops have been associated with rising numbers of autism, leaky gut, asthma, allergies, and reproductive issues.[10]

Dr. Stephanie Seneff performed a study on the effects of glyphosate, the active ingredient used in Roundup weed killer and on nearly all GMO crops, and found that "glyphosate's adverse effects on the gut microbiota . . . can remarkably explain a great number of the diseases and conditions that are prevalent in the modern industrialized world."[11]

A GMO-free diet is well within your grasp. For many, the high price of organic produce has turned into a GMO-buying habit, but I encourage those GMO buyers to reconsider. In the long haul, the benefits of buying organic far outweigh the medical bills and suffering caused by the effects of GMO on the body. Farmers' markets are popping up with ever-increasing regularity across the country, and the affordability may surprise you! In many urban areas, you can also sign up for a CSA (community-supported agriculture) box to be delivered right to your doorstep. I also encourage people to try growing their own food—even a windowsill herb garden is a healthy, toxin-free way to supplement your pantry.

Phthalates and Bisphenol-A

Phthalates—compounds used in plastics—and bisphenol-A are two more chemical compounds to avoid at all costs. The risk of certain chemicals in plastics, particularly to reproductive health, comes from their effect on the hormones. Phthalates are xenoestrogens, and I think of them as a "toxic mimic of estrogen" or "fake estrogen." Phthalates are true imposters: because their construction is so similar to that of estrogen, our bodies readily absorb these toxic substances, only to experience drops in fertility and endocrine disruption when we can't process them like normal hormones.

Most studies on phthalates and their effects on reproduction have been conducted on males.[12] However, recent research into how phthalates and xenoestrogens impact female fertility shows that they disrupt levels of estrogen—the hormone crucial to women's fertility and reproductive cycles. They have been linked scientifically to endometriosis, infertility, and allergy rate increases.[13] In one study, researchers found that odds of implantation failure in women with the highest level of phthalates was double that of women with the lowest level of phthalates, that fewer eggs were retrieved in women with the highest level of phthalates, that a dose-response occurred, and that as phthalate levels rise, egg production and implantation drop.[14]

Here's what you can do to reduce your exposure to phthalates:

- Beware of anything with the word *fragrance* in the title. Lower your exposure by reducing the use of scented personal care products, including baby products and air fresheners.
- When buying plastic products, remember this: "1, 2, 5: Stay alive." Plastic products with the recycling codes 3 and 4 are far more likely to contain endocrine-disrupting BPA or phthalates.
- Never heat food in plastic containers.
- Avoid buying food packaged in plastic, especially meats and cheeses, which are prone to chemical leaching.
- Do your homework. If you see DPB, DEHP, BzBP, or DMP, all phthalates, in the ingredients section, find a different product.
- A nano-filtration system for your drinking water is the best way to cut down your exposure to DEHP, a phthalate found in water pipes. Carbon filters are better than nothing, but may still allow microscopic amounts of DEHP to get through.
- Keep your kids safe: read the ingredients label, and be wary of plastic toys or products made before 2009—that was the year laws were passed banning phthalates in children's goods.[15]
- Eat organic foods, which will be freer of the phthalates found in pesticides and sewage sludge that are used in conventional agriculture.

Pregnancy

Exercise

Along with maintaining a healthy diet and supplement routine, it is also important to figure out the right exercise plan for each stage of your pregnancy. Exercise helps prevent gestational diabetes and improves mood, energy, muscle tone, and sleep quality.[16] Here are the basics:

- If you aren't very active now, work with your physician to develop a gradual, safe workout plan for the duration of your pregnancy.
- ACOG (the American College of Obstetrics and Gynecology) recommends thirty minutes of moderate exercise per day. So do I, but I may change that recommendation based on your prepregnancy level of physical conditioning and your medical condition during pregnancy. Overall, exercise makes you feel better and, in my opinion, helps you create a stronger, healthier baby. As always, consult your doctor for specific recommendations. The old rule was to keep the heart rate at less than 140 beats per minute when you exercise in pregnancy, but this has been debunked in recent years in favor of the "talk test," where you want to be able to speak three- to five-word sentences while exercising. Aim to exercise four to five days per week and listen carefully to the messages your body sends you.
- I know this is almost insulting because it's common sense but I still need to mention it. Avoid contact group sports as well as exercise at high altitude, and do no scuba diving or downhill skiing whatsoever.
- Since hormones released during pregnancy make your joints looser, you are at an increased risk of back or pelvic pain and may experience instability or a greater chance of falling. So if you are suddenly klutzy, blame it on the pregnancy.
- Walking, swimming, cycling, and aerobics are all recommended forms of movement.
- Avoid supine exercise after the fourth month because the enlarging uterus can squish the vena cava (the biggest vein in your body) and limit circulation.

Beginning in the second trimester, the official party line is that you must avoid exercises done on your back. The theory is that you can start to squish your vena cava with your uterus—the vena cava sends blood to your heart to get oxygenated. While this rule of no-more-lying-on-your-back isn't conclusively proven, it's wise to obey it until we know better.

As you progress through your pregnancy, the best thing you can do is listen to your body. If anything feels painful, if you can't perform at the same speed or level that you could before, or if you suspect you're pushing yourself too hard . . . ease off. Yes, it's simply the voice of reason. Speak with your ob/gyn about any concerns you have. Shorten and simplify your workouts as your pregnancy progresses and your symptoms change.

Stop exercising and visit your ob/gyn if you experience any of the following:

- vaginal bleeding
- dizziness
- headache
- chest pain
- muscle weakness
- calf pain or swelling
- preterm labor
- decreased fetal movement
- amniotic fluid leakage.

The Gottfried Protocol for Pregnant and Postpartum Women

As you probably know, there is a much higher safety standard for what we'll recommend for pregnant and postpartum women. It's very expensive to perform the type of safety trials that are needed to put a supplement in the "safe" category for pregnant women. When it comes to The Gottfried Protocol while breast-feeding, I recommend omega-3s and to continue a high-potency multivitamin as you gradually increase your exercise.

Pregnancy

Once you're pregnant, stick to the preconception diet I recommended earlier, and make sure you have plenty of nutrients, lean proteins, and healthy fats. When you're pregnant, you want to make sure you get enough slow carbs such as sweet potatoes and quinoa.

In pregnancy, I strongly encourage you to get your cute self to yoga. There are so many benefits for you and your baby, and the latest evidence shows that yoga even helps prevent high-risk complications such as high blood pressure (both pregnancy-induced hypertension and preeclampsia), gestational diabetes, and intrauterine growth restriction, which is a problem that can lead to your baby not growing as intended. Yoga has also been shown to be supportive in making a healthier baby, as measured in weight and Apgar score.[17]

For medications, drugs are rated A, B, C, or X. Benadryl is a "B" drug, which means it's "probably safe." In general, when it comes to "natural medicine," I recommend that you consult the Natural Medicine Database (http://naturaldatabase.therapeuticresearch.com). Sadly, most of the supplements, such as phosphatidylserine and rhodiola, have this warning: Insufficient reliable information available. Avoid using.

I imagine you are frustrated to hear this, but the truth is that it's just not black and white when it comes to safety in pregnancy and nursing. It's best to use common sense. For women who are pregnant and have morning sickness, most doctors recommend Unisom . . . yet it says on the label it should not be used during pregnancy. This is a great example of how confusing it is to recommend treatments to women. The American College of Obstetricians and Gynecologists states that the recommendation of "taking Vitamin B_6 or Vitamin B_6 plus doxylamine is safe and effective and should be considered a first-line treatment," which is based on consistent scientific evidence. In fact, 33 million women have taken it safely, yet the bottle advises against it. That's just one example of how the standard is much higher for pregnant and postpartum women, and I cannot give blanket statements about whether one supplement is safe or not. Your best bet is to discuss any supplement, over-the-counter medication, and/or prescription with your clinician.

I recommend you find a practitioner who shares your values and with whom you can speak openly. Then you can rely on her advice about what will be safest and what will work best for you individually.

Postpartum

When it comes to women's hormonal health after pregnancy, postpartum is a menopausal state. You enter the birth experience with sky-high hormones, especially estrogen and progesterone, and when you deliver your placenta, your hormones drop to the floor.

I recommend continuing most of the food and lifestyle changes you implemented before and during your pregnancy, but you can now push yourself harder with exercise once you pass your six-week checkup with your clinician. I still recommend hormone testing if pregnant or postpartum mamas feel "off." Postpartum depression is often hormonal in origin, and you need to make sure your hormonal Charlie's Angels are in the optimal zone (see Appendix G). In fact, I work with a psychiatrist who prescribes an estrogen patch as a first line of therapy. The tricky part of being a new mom is the sleep deprivation—lack of sleep alone can tip the best of us toward the blues, even depression. If mood is an issue for you, I urge you to seek professional help.

Because supplementation is a bit of a minefield and the quality of safety data is sparse at best, I encourage new mothers to focus on food-based nutritional healing. We know that women under stress do best when they are with their girlfriends, so I suggest very strongly that new moms join a postpartum yoga class or baby boot camp. Additionally, I recommend essential oils for pregnant and nursing women, and all of the stress reduction techniques listed below.

- yoga, chanting, and other forms of mindfulness
- acupuncture

- HeartMath techniques, such as GPS for the Soul and Inner Balance (see Chapter 4)
- weaning off caffeine and cutting out booze
- massage
- dark chocolate

While some women lose pregnancy weight quickly while breast-feeding, others (like me) don't lose it until they stop breast-feeding. Science hasn't yet nailed down the exact reason for this gap, but there are about two hundred genes involved in your metabolic set point, and the hormones that determine whether you have more "thrifty" genes, which are the genes that allow you to survive a famine, are complex. These hormones include thyroid, leptin, insulin, cortisol, and testosterone. I imagine that women who lose weight rapidly have more of the "skinny" genes than "thrifty" genes. Overall, most of us have about 100x more thrifty genes than skinny genes, which can make all the difference. You can learn more about your genotype and the optimal food plan for your DNA right here: http://thehormone curebook.com/genetics. Following a low-carb, high-fiber, and veggie diet mixed with moderate exercise and hormone-balancing supplements will keep your metabolism running at a healthy speed.

PAPERBACK Q&A

From Dr. Sara: I was absolutely thrilled by the reception to my first book, *The Hormone Cure*. I heard from thousands of readers who found the balance, energy, and vitality they were seeking by following The Gottfried Protocol to balance their hormones naturally and effectively. Nothing gives me greater joy than helping people feel their best! I also heard from many readers who had more questions and wanted more help. We've decided to put the most frequently asked questions here, in the paperback edition of *The Hormone Cure,* because I am committed to getting you the answers you deserve.

1. I am in total hormone chaos. Everything seems off. I don't just have one hormonal imbalance. I love your book, but where should I start?

It's always best to start with the root cause. You can find out what the root cause of your multiple hormone imbalances is by completing my questionnaire either in *The Hormone Cure* or online at www.thehormonecurebook.com/quiz. My quiz will decode the messages your body is sending to you. Here's a hint: start with the issue that has been plaguing you the longest and shows up with the greatest number of symptoms.

If you're still unsure where to start, know this: all roads lead to cortisol. If cortisol is one of your problems, then begin there with Gottfried Protocol Step 1 (see page 17). Start taking phosphatidylserine 400 mg per day and omega-3s 4,000 mg per day, get off caffeine, and download the "GPS for the Soul" or "iPromise" app (which you can find at www.thehormonecurebook.com/destress) for the iPhone or iPad, and practice for seven minutes per day.

Once your hormones are back on track, I recommend assessing yourself at least two to four times per year to make sure you're maintaining that balance. Simply checking in and measuring your own progress will cause improvement because you're paying attention to your body and its needs. You can monitor yourself quantitatively with my questionnaires, lab testing, or both.

I recommend performing a laboratory test for certain hormones if you have three or more symptoms (based on my questionnaire on page 24—look for the pages with a gray color on the edges) or as identified by my online quiz. I recommend checking a thyroid panel and your progesterone-to-estrogen ratio. I encourage younger women to perform a baseline test in their twenties or thirties, and for women aged 35 or older to track these symptoms with lab tests at regular intervals.

Some hormones are more variable, such as cortisol, and others are relatively stable, such as the thyroid panel that I recommend (TSH or thyroid-stimulating hormone, free T3, free T4, and reverse T3). Ideally, perform the tests with your local clinician (see Appendix D, page 335), but if your doctor declines your request or wants more information, you have several options:

- Work with one of the three-hundred-plus collaborative and smart practitioners that I have trained personally in the Hormone Cure. Visit www.thehormonecurebook.com/prac titioners/. Even if you've visited the practitioner page before, go again, because we keep adding new practitioners. We offer training twice per year and keep the Web page current.
- If your doctor is ambivalent, unconvinced, or wants further scientific justification, hand him or her my book! Because of space limitations in this book, we offer the complete list of references for your doctor (and you) to review at http:// thehormonecurebook.com/practitioners/.

- If at any time you are confused or having trouble, see your local practitioner for expert advice.

2. I have high *and* low cortisol. Can you give me a clear plan for what to do?

If you're experiencing symptoms of high and low cortisol, don't stress (pun intended): I've got a plan for you. Learning to manage your stress response, tweaking your diet, and getting the right kind of exercise will get you back on track to hormonal harmony.

It's not uncommon for women to experience symptoms of high and low cortisol simultaneously, but it is a major red flag that you need to manage your cortisol as if your life depends on it—which it does!

Here's my three-step action plan (and see the "Why" explanation following):

- Start first with targeted lifestyle changes: yoga, meditation, or some other way to observe yourself and improve your perceived stress. Even when a scary situation arises, your goal should be to process and deal with the issue without letting it take over your body and mind. At the same time, cut out coffee and alcohol because they tax your adrenals— and your poor, cute adrenals need a break. Getting rid of these two faves is a crucial part of returning to a healthy cortisol pattern, because caffeine and alcohol rob you of restorative sleep. See details below. Then add the supplements I mentioned in the previous Q&A—phosphatidylserine (400 mg per day) and omega-3s (4,000 mg per day). Finally, eat a small square of dark chocolate, have an orgasm, and call me in the morning. Am I your favorite doctor yet?
- If you're not feeling better in four weeks, move on to the targeted botanical therapies. I only recommend supplements that have serious science backing up their effectiveness. When it comes to cortisol, ginseng and rhodiola have been shown to help with stress-related fatigue.[1] When you have

both high and low cortisol within the same day, I recommend ashwagandha. Check the index to find out how much to take.

- Bioidentical hormones: if none of the lifestyle changes and herbal remedies help you bounce back, it's time to speak with your doctor about starting a low dose of DHEA. Make sure you take it with your doctor's guidance.

When you have symptoms of high and low cortisol, what's typically happened is that chronically high cortisol (or some other traumatic event or condition) has maxed out your adrenals, causing your cortisol to drop. This means that you're suffering the effects of high and low cortisol, maybe even on a daily basis. Right now, if you're experiencing symptoms of hypocortisolism—such as fatigue, burnout, low blood pressure, loss of stamina—you're probably suffering from constant stress but not producing enough cortisol to deal with it. This is no fun whatsoever and can lead to more serious health issues, such as depression, memory problems, weight gain, fibromyalgia, rapid aging, bone loss, and even post-traumatic stress disorder (PTSD). It's crucial that you get your cortisol levels balanced as soon as possible—and you'll start to feel better right away.

3. I've had a hysterectomy. Is hormone balancing relevant?

Yes, and I especially recommend that you read the chapters on cortisol, low estrogen, low thyroid, and multiple hormone imbalances.

If the ovaries are removed at the time of a hysterectomy, the natural sources of progesterone and estrogen are gone and the body immediately goes into premature menopause. Ovarian hormones play important roles in protecting the heart, brain, bones, and breasts.[2] In fact, even if the ovaries are kept, it is common for ovarian hormone production to decline after a hysterectomy, resulting in premature menopause. It's going to make a big difference in energy levels, mental acuity, and sex drive to keep the hormones in the sweet spot.

4. What about women after menopause? Shouldn't we be past all that hormone stuff? And why do we still experience some symptoms of hormone imbalance? Is it still helpful to apply The Gottfried Protocol to correct some symptoms, such as memory issues?

Even if you've gone through menopause, you can still improve your hormonal balance—especially when it comes to cortisol and estrogen. Symptoms of hormonal imbalance related to menopause and postmenopause include fatigue, insomnia, brain fog, lower sex drive, and depression; women suffering from these symptoms tend to have higher stress and anxiety scores as well.[3] Using The Gottfried Protocol to maintain hormonal balance will keep your metabolism humming, your libido luscious, and your outlook rosy well past menopause.

Put down the chardonnay! Consumption of alcohol raises estrogen levels and slows fat burning. In postmenopausal women, drinking one or two servings of alcohol a day raises estrone and DHEAS, another hormone that can be converted into estrogen.[4] Excess estrogen can increase your risk of breast cancer. In a vicious cycle, excess fat after menopause is more likely to produce estrogen out of testosterone, a process called aromitization.[5]

With regards to memory, brain-derived neurotrophic factor (BDNF) is a brain chemical that encourages growth of nerve cells and neuroplasticity, especially in the parts of the brain associated with learning, long-term memory, and higher thinking. Estrogen increases BDNF, as does exercise. Not surprisingly, cortisol reduces production of BDNF. Keeping your estrogen level healthy and your cortisol in control will keep you sharp as a tack. And here's another great reason to manage your stress response: extensive research shows that prolonged, elevated cortisol constricts blood flow to the brain. This negatively affects your brain function, decreases your emotional intelligence, and accelerates age-related cognitive function.

Progesterone, estrogen, and serum testosterone—the hormone of confidence and vitality—all decline after menopause as well; these important hormones keep you mentally sharp, upbeat, and calm. I recommend using bioidentical hormones in the lowest possible dose, but check with your doctor if you think you need hormone replacement therapy. Other postmenopausal issues that lead to serious health problems such as insulin resistance, PCOS, and diabetes can also be addressed with The Gottfried Protocol.[6] Keeping your hormones balanced is a vital part of staying slim, sexy, and sassy no matter the number of candles on your birthday cake.

5. I want to work with a practitioner like you. Where do I find one?

You can find a list of practitioners trained in The Hormone Cure and The Gottfried Protocol at http://thehormonecurebook.com/practitioners/. If there isn't a practitioner or coach in your region, get in touch with one of the talented practitioners who offers online consultation.

6. How can I have both high and low estrogen? I'm trying to understand what protocol to follow?

An estrogen imbalance often results in symptoms of both high *and* low estrogen, which may sound like I've lost my mind (and estrogen), but honestly, you can simultaneously experience both. Here's the deal—symptoms of estrogen excess are relative to progesterone, but symptoms of low estrogen are simply relative to your own personal baseline (which is established when you're in your twenties and thirties). So you can have low estrogen—indicated by low sex drive, vaginal dryness, flat mood, pancakelike breasts—but relative to a low level of progesterone, you may still have symptoms of excess estrogen (cystic breast tenderness, abnormal Pap smears, difficulty with weight loss).

If you're not sure what is going on, you can always get your levels clinically tested.

It's much more common to have high estrogen than low estrogen, and many of the symptoms are difficult to differentiate. Excess estrogen suppresses your thyroid activity, which can lead to signs of low thyroid . . . some of which, like fatigue, are confusingly similar to the symptoms of low estrogen. Too much estrogen can also reduce the quality or frequency of orgasm, and because it lowers your testosterone levels, it also diminishes sex drive.

Once you know whether you're high or low in estrogen (whether that's determined by lab testing or through a deeper dive into the self-assessment [pages 24–31] to find the root cause of your problems), you can start following The Gottfried Protocol to treat it.

Hops appear to address symptoms of both high and low estrogen. You can find hops in beer (obviously), but also in herbal form. I recommend 100 mg daily. Another one of the supplements that I highly recommend is DIM (diindolemethane), as it cuts down on the production of bad estrogens and increases production of good ones. Maca, in capsule or liquid form, has been shown to improve libido and to lower anxiety and depression, all of which are symptoms of low estrogen.[7]

7. Does your protocol work for men?

The Gottfried Protocol (find the root cause, treat first with lifestyle changes, then herbal remedies, then bioidentical hormones) does work for men, but the advice and treatment strategies in *The Hormone Cure* are geared toward women. A book (or app!) on male hormone management is on the horizon, so keep your eyes peeled!

In the meantime, another excellent source of information on balancing male hormones is http://thehormonecurebook.com/men. The site includes my recent interviews with a few male health experts, including Abel James ("Fat Burning Man") and Dr. Jonny Bowden. Go here to get the goods!

8. What foods boost serotonin, the brain chemical that helps my mood, sleep, and appetite?

Serotonin is the feel-good neurotransmitter, and you want her in your life. If you want to increase your serotonin production through diet, there is no one "magic bullet" food. As always, a high-fiber diet that includes lots of organic veggies is the best way to love up your hormones.

You can start to improve your serotonin situation by reducing your daily intake of sugar, refined carbohydrates, and caffeine. All of these foods make you feel good in the short term—they give you a quick boost, but then your serotonin levels will begin to drop just as quickly. Instead, aim for a pound of veggies per day, and consider a daily fish oil and vitamin B_6 supplement—both are important precursors to healthy neurotransmitters. A fiber-and-nutrient-filled diet will not only help your serotonin but it will also boost your maxed-out adrenals, your insulin sensitivity, and your cortisol levels.

The supplement 5-HTP has also been shown to improve serotonin levels; what's wonderful about 5-HTP is that it only needs to be taken for a short time, after which serotonin levels should stay elevated. I offer a high-quality version in my online store: http://thehormonecurebook.com/store.

You may also want to consider an evaluation with a functional psychiatrist. My favorite is Dr. Hyla Cass. If you go to http://thehormonecurebook.com/, you can get a free recording that I did with Dr. Cass about how to use 5-HTP while weaning off antidepressants—but due to the risk of serotonin syndrome (too much serotonin), I'd recommend doing this under the supervision of a knowledgeable clinician. Also consider your methylation, as you may be undermethy-lating and may need more methylators (betaine, magnesium, etc.).

9. I don't know what tests to order or what labs to ask my doctor to order.

My recommendation is to work collaboratively with your doctor or to find a new one on my practitioner page (again, http://thehor monecurebook/practiioners/). Test yourself by checking out one of the labs that I recommend in Appendix E—many allow you to order your own hormone tests. I've also added several new labs in addi-tion to those listed in the appendix; for a complete list go to: http://thehormonecurebook.com/labs/.

10. I'm a breast cancer survivor. How can I safely apply The Gottfried Protocol?

The Gottfried Protocol is a wonderful resource for breast cancer sur-vivors who want to improve their hormonal balance, reclaim their vitality, and develop a cancer-preventing lifestyle.

Women with breast cancer often face the issue of low thyroid function, low vitamin D, and energy problems, which can be safely addressed even for people currently on protocols to address hor-mone imbalance such as tamoxifen or aromatase inhibitors. It is completely safe to check your thyroid function and vitamin D, and apply the protocols in my book for these specific problems.

Women on aromatase inhibitors commonly experience joint pain, which I like to address with glucosamine, omega-3s, and other inflammation-reducing strategies. You can find my recommenda-tions about reducing the inflammation associated with breast cancer and read more about cancer and hormonal balance, plus get my interview with breast cancer surgeon and advocate Dr. Susan Love, at http://thehormonecurebook.com/breasthealth. Some of the com-mon issues plaguing cancer survivors include the following.

Estrogen metabolism

In order to maintain a healthy estrogen balance, your body has to break down, convert, and dispose of the estrogen building blocks it naturally produces. Healthy, well-balanced bodies metabolize estrogen by the forms that begin with the number 2: 2-hydroxy-estradiol or 2-hydroxy-estrone. Women who have or are at high risk of developing breast and endometrial cancer have been found to make too much of the bad estrogens, such as 16-alpha-hydroxy-estrone.

Many factors can interfere with normal estrogen metabolism, causing you to produce or accumulate too much of the "less good" estrogens or too much estrogen relative to progesterone. They include the aging ovary, wayward cortisol levels, exposure to xenoestrogens, and nutritional factors such as fat, fiber, and alcohol.

Check your 2/16 ratio, a measure of your good versus bad estrogens. Are you making more of the good, protective estrogens or more of the bad guys that increase your risk of breast cancer? The data support the 2/16 ratio as a key marker of your risk of breast cancer, making it a good one to measure periodically (roughly every three to six months).[8]

Cancer prevention food plan

The cancer-prevention food plan is a simple one. Here's how it works:

- Eat 100 percent organic produce, and aim for seven servings of fruits and vegetables daily. All the antioxidants in fresh, local produce help prevent gene mutation. If seven servings seems out of reach for you right now, order a greens powder to get a head start nutrient-wise.
- Cut out alcohol. One study showed that more than three servings of alcohol per week was linked to an increase in breast cancer risk.
- No sugar. In fact, say "no" to all white foods: white flour, sugar, and simple carbs such as white rice are all on the naughty list.
- Reduce your inflammation with turmeric, and prevent acid-

ity with pumpkin seeds, persimmons, broccoflower, seaweed, and kombucha.

Additionally, there are many other published diets, such as the *Healthy Diet for Women with Breast Cancer* published by Dr. Victoria Maizes, a colleague of Dr. Andrew Weil's at the Arizona Center for Integrative Medicine. Her nutritional protocol is highly regarded and found with a simple Google search.

Vaginal dryness

Sex is no fun when your lady garden is dry, and the health benefits of orgasm are too good to pass up. Luckily, there are quite a few natural, proven ways to reclaim a juicy sex life.

Vaginal dryness is associated with low estrogen, and vitamin E at doses of 50–400 IU per day may be the oldest remedy in the book. According to one study, supplementing with vitamin E was shown to increase blood supply to the vaginal wall and improve menopausal symptoms. Be patient: you need four weeks of vitamin E to experience the effect.

Maca is another magical herb that helps with a variety of issues associated with hormonal imbalance, and one of those is vaginal dryness. No matter how healthy their libido, some women still struggle with dry vaginal walls—and that's the last thing you want when you're trying to achieve a toe-curling orgasm. Add maca, in powder form, to your smoothies for a daily dose of juiciness. You can find it in most health food stores or online.

11. What can I do to revive my libido and to begin to feel juicy again?

Your sex drive is determined by your estrogen levels—when it is low, you'd probably rather go on Facebook than have sex. Luckily, I've got lots of advice for souping up your sex drive. As always, the first step is balancing your hormones. It's easy for your sex hormones—estrogen, progesterone, testosterone—to get thrown off by a hormonal imbalance higher up on the hormone totem pole (think cortisol or thyroid).

Antidepressants and birth control pills are associated with decreased sex drive. If you're on one of these medications for a serious medical issue, don't stop taking anything without speaking with your clinician. But if you're using one of them for a less serious concern (such as acne), it may be time to look into your other options and have a frank discussion with your physician.

Meditation has been shown to improve sex drive, especially Orgasmic Meditation; learn more about that sexy strategy here: http://thehormonecurebook.com/sexy.

As noted earlier, you can combat a dry vagina (how are you supposed to want sex when it hurts?!) with a vitamin E supplement or maca (which improves sex drive and vaginal lubrication). If other strategies don't provide the boost in sex drive you're looking for, you may want to speak with your doctor about a transdermal estrogen treatment.

Low testosterone (yes, even in women) can also contribute to a lagging libido. Here's the The Gottfried Protocol for low testosterone:

Step 1

Nutritional supplements and lifestyle tweaks (you will need to discuss with your practitioner to determine if these are safe during lactation):

- zinc (Napa cabbage 4 mg, oysters 74 mg)
- sprouted grains
- exercise: burst training and if you are not breast-feeding, consider intermittent fasting
- L-carnitine 1,500 to 2,000 mg daily
- vitamin D (data are mixed but it doesn't hurt to try it, plus it helps your thyroid as discussed in chapter 9).

Step 2

I reviewed the botanicals that are marketed as raising testosterone and did not find sufficient data to recommend them.

Step 3

Consider trying over-the-counter DHEA. I usually start at 2 to 5 mg per day, and I'm very careful not to let levels become supraphysiologic by tracking both DHEA and testosterone levels. Men take 25–50 mg and that's way too much for the vast majority of women. Too much DHEA can cause hair loss, greasy skin, greasy hair, and breakouts, so be careful even though it is over the counter. If none of the above work over six to eight weeks, seek out an expert in bio-identical hormones to consider testosterone augmentation. There are many unknown risks of testosterone use beyond six months' duration, so I urge caution with this strategy. I find the methods above work 90–95 percent of the time and raise testosterone.

For more on the risks you need to know before taking testosterone and/or DHEA, go to http://thehormonecurebook.com/sexy.

12. I have been taking antidepressants for years, but now I think some of my problems might be due to hormonal imbalance. What do you recommend for people who want to get off of antidepressants?

Sadly, many doctors prescribe antidepressants and birth control pills for hormonal issues that can be solved naturally. I know, because I was taught to do the same when I was in med school. If you want to get off antidepressants, you must work closely with a trusted doctor to make sure that you do it safely, and for the right reasons. Given the list of adverse effects, antidepressants are worse than placebo if depression is mild to moderate. Don't get me wrong: I'm not suggesting that we discard antidepressants any time soon. I simply believe they're overused.

The first step is to find your pain points. What symptoms does your antidepressant address, and are those issues hormonal? Ask your physician to run some tests on your hormone levels and see what is out of balance. The next step is figuring out a safe and healthy way for you to reduce your antidepressant use and start incorporating treatment strategies from The Hormone Cure.

If you go to http://thehormonecurebook.com/happy and register, you will get several expert interviews on how to increase your set point, plus a free recording of my discussion with Dr. Hyla Cass about how to use 5-HTP while weaning off antidepressants—but I'd recommend doing this under supervision of a knowledgeable clinician because of the risk of serotonin syndrome, which can be a life-threatening condition. You also have a risk of worsening depression, and we know that people with severe depression actually benefit from prescription antidepressants.

I was interviewed recently for an interesting article in O Magazine about the benefit of low-dose antidepressants in women; many women report that low doses really help them cope. If taking a low dose, you are in good company as many women find that a low dose—such as half or one quarter—is right for them. There is no shame in that. I am a fierce advocate of women finding what works best for them and being proud of it!

13. What are the top three most important blood tests we can do?

First of all, congratulations on taking your health into your own hands. Here are the top three tests I recommend to my patients:

1. Blood panel. Ask your doctor to order:

    • Comprehensive metabolic panel
    • VAP cholesterol (extended panel—includes subtypes of LDL and HDL plus lipo[a], VLDL)
    • Ferritin

- Thyroid panel: TSH, free T3, reverse T3
- Cortisol
- DHEA
- If overweight: add leptin, insulin, IGF-1 (growth hormone)
- If infertile: add free, bioavailable and total testosterone, progesterone day 21–23, fasting insulin, leptin, and glucose.

2. Omega-6/Omega-3 ratio. If you are having new symptoms of ADD in perimenopause, get the omega-6/omega-3 ratio test. Omega-3s are one of the most proven supplements we have, yet most people don't optimize their level. Learn where to order the home test at http://thehormonecurebook.com/labs/.

3. Complete Hormone Profile. If your doctor is the more open-minded type, check out my favorite hormone test, the Complete Hormone Profile (find it at http://thehormonecurebook.com/labs/). It will tell you about your adrenals, both short- and long-term adrenal health, and inform you of your estrogen metabolism—that is, do you have a modifiable tendency toward breast cancer or not?

If your doctor won't order these tests, you can still go to http://thehormonecurebook.com/labs/ to learn about the home tests that you can order yourself, and then consult with a practitioner who is more collaborative.

14. I can't seem to regulate my body temperature—I'm either freezing cold or sweating like a pig—what do you recommend?

Low body temperature is associated with low thyroid and, more specifically, free T3 (the active version of thyroid hormone). T3 is present in small but important amounts in your body. It plays a vital role in promoting weight loss, warm limbs, and a good mood. If your free T3 is low, it can be from a number of causes:

- Hashimoto's disease (thyroiditis)
- perimenopause
- environmental toxins
- stress
- genetics
- gluten sensitivity or celiac disease
- vitamin D deficiency
- cancer treatment
- goitrogens (compounds found in soy, millet, broccoli, and Brussels sprouts).

Luckily, testing your thyroid is simple and inexpensive. Just get your hands on a "basal body thermometer" that measures temperature at the lower scale, between 96 and 99 degrees F. Normal is between 97.8 and 98.2 degrees, but can vary quite a bit. Nevertheless, if your basal temperature in the morning is consistently below 97.8 degrees F, this is further evidence of low thyroid function.[9]

Low progesterone may also be a factor. Progesterone is "thermogenic"—it raises your body temperature and boosts your metabolism. If you're experiencing hot flashes, that could be a symptom of perimenopause or menopause, in which case you may want to look into vitamin E, magnesium oxide, maca, or rhubarb.

15. What is the best way to jump-start fertility if my partner and I are thinking about trying for a baby?

There are lots of ways you can upgrade your fertility if you and your partner are ready to have a baby.

The first step, as always, is balancing your hormones. Take the quiz at the beginning of the book and see what hormonal issues you should straighten out first. Stress, low thyroid, and especially sex hormone issues relating to estrogen and progesterone should be addressed to ensure your maximum fertility.

PCOS (polycystic ovary syndrome) is the number one reason women struggle to get pregnant. PCOS affects 20 percent of women and can interfere with fertility by blocking regular monthly ovulation. If you are trying to conceive, I recommend demanding that your doctor do a blood test to check your fasting insulin, glucose, progesterone on day 21, and leptin. This will clarify whether or not you have insulin resistance, a key marker for PCOS.[10] Before you go the übermedical route, you may be able to improve your fertility with a few small lifestyle and food changes specifically targeted to women who want to get pregnant.

The folks at the University of Arizona Center for Integrative Medicine have several excellent resources on fertility. I especially recommend their chapter on cortisol and fertility in the book *Integrative Women's Health*. I also recommend Dr. Victoria Maize's book on fertility, *Be Fruitful*. (She is a colleague of mine and coauthor of the above-mentioned book.)

16. My hair is falling out—what can I do?

Some 30 percent of women report serious hair loss by age 30. By age 50, that statistic climbs to 50 percent. This is a major problem, of both vanity and sanity.

Dramatic hair loss is often an early-warning sign of low thyroid, especially if your hair gets thinner, coarse, and brittle. Another cause of hair loss in women is high testosterone; this is usually the case when the symptom is male-pattern hair loss. The good news is that you can often stop and even reverse the symptoms of hair loss once you balance your hormones.

My advice is to try therapies aimed at the root cause of your hair loss first, and ask your doctor for my top blood tests, including:

- Complete blood count (a measure of whether you are anemic and your immune system is functioning)
- Ferritin (the most sensitive test for iron stores in your body)
- Thyroid-stimulating hormone (TSH), free T3, and possibly, reverse T3
- Cortisol
- Fasting insulin and glucose
- Testosterone (I prefer total and free testosterone in women with hair loss)
- Antinuclear antibody (tells you whether the hair loss is related to an autoimmune condition).

Treatment strategies include 1,000 mg per day of evening primrose oil, which inhibits the conversion of testosterone to dihydrotestosterone. It's also a good source of essential fatty acids—and the symptoms of hypothyroidism are quite similar to those for insufficient essential fatty acids.

You can also help hair loss with your fork: one study showed that 90 percent of women with thinning hair were deficient in iron and the amino acid lysine, which helps transport the iron that is essential for many metabolic processes.[11] You can add lysine to your diet with foods rich in protein, such as meat and poultry, soy, eggs, cheese (especially Parmesan), and some fish (cod, sardines). Grains contain small quantities of lysine, but legumes contain lots; therefore, meals that combine the two—Indian dal with rice, beans with rice and tortilla, falafel and hummus with pita bread—are a good way to get complete protein in your diet and keep hair on your head.

17. I have trouble staying asleep. What do you recommend?

Sleepless nights, a wonky circadian rhythm, and trouble falling asleep are classic signs of hormonal imbalance, and 80 percent of my patients suffer from a lack of quality sleep. I've got two recommendations: find a natural strategy that works for you (see more below) and don't resort to sleeping pills. Not only do they add an average of only 20 minutes of additional sleep per night, but they're also associated with so many additional health issues that I think they should be taken off pharmacy shelves for good.

High cortisol and low progesterone commonly affect sleep patterns, so following The Gottfried Protocol for those issues could be the solution to your bedtime woes. If you need a little additional help, here are my favorite recommendations for getting a restorative night's sleep, seven days a week:

- Set a technology curfew: the blue lights of television, phone, computer, and tablet screens confuse your brain and keep it in "daytime" mode.
- Cut alcohol and caffeine out of your diet. Alcohol may help you fall asleep faster, but it hijacks the quality of your sleep later in the night. Caffeine, taken even eight hours before bedtime, can still disrupt sleep.
- Keep your bedroom dark, cool, and comfortable. Turn it into your "sleep sanctuary."
- Consider valerian as a pill or tea. One trial in menopausal women showed that 530 mg of valerian[12] extract improved sleep in 30 percent of treated insomniacs.

ACKNOWLEDGMENTS

Hillary Clinton famously said that it takes a village to raise a child, and I'd add that in perimenopause, it takes a village to do most things. It took me years to learn her truth, which I now translate as *Get help and build your network before you need it.*

First, I need to acknowledge the true superstars of this book: my beloved patients and clients, whom I care for in my Berkeley integrative medicine office and also virtually in my online Mission Ignition e-courses and mentoring programs. You birthed this book—I was merely the midwife catching the baby. Thank you for sharing with me your narratives, many of which landed in this book (with changed names and no identifying data, of course). I am grateful for your partnership and trust, and for allowing me to be of service. You provide an incredible gift: you activate my inner healer, a wellspring of vitality and creativity. It's paradoxical that when I am of service, cortisol is better behaved, and I feel more energized, balanced, and ready to rock my mission.

Deep appreciation to my parents, Albert and Mary Lil Szal, for your unconditional love and support throughout my life, and especially over the past eighteen months of my writing this book, my labor of love. I'm grateful for your relentless love and support. Mom, your help with editing and caring for the girls (and me) were invaluable.

I am awestruck by my sisters: Anna Esterline and Justina Szal. Thank you both for your enduring love, calming words, honest advice when I need to take a chill pill, dance, share a cocktail—and especially for taking my daughters to the mall when I needed to write. When Mama is happy, everyone is happy!

Next, thanks to my growth friends, change agents, and revolutionaries: Ana Forrest of ForrestYoga.com; Susan Harrow of PRsecrets.com; Johanna Ilfeld, PhD, of SuccessReboot.com; Jennifer Landa, MD, of DrJenniferLanda.com; Danielle Laporte of DanielleLaporte.com; Todd Lepine, MD, of DrLepine.com; Alexis Neely of AlexisNeely.com; Mary Shomon of Thyroid-info.com; and the smartest nutritionist I know, JJ Virgin of JJVirgin.com. *You are pure synergy and my rad sauce.*

Thank you to the many bighearted people who wrote about *The Hormone Cure,* interviewed me, shared the love on social media, hosted me for a blog tour, joined the revolution, became a Hormone Cure Evangelista, and moved the conversation forward. Let's keep talking and offering up more solutions to women who need help and are too young to feel old. Big thanks also to our revolutionary group of Hormone Cure Practitioners—to learn more if you're a doctor, coach, nutritionist, or other allopathic or alternative health provider, go to http://www.saragottfriedmd.com/practitioners/.

Thank you to the countless people who were of service to me in my ongoing education, my spiritual inquiry, and my work on this book. I'm grateful to my early mentors, who taught me to relish evidence and to keep women safe, using the crucial yet underutilized tools of epidemiology and critical thinking. Thanks to Ellen Seely, MD, who was my erstwhile champion at Brigham and Women's Hospital during my research fellowship in endocrinology. Deep appreciation to Sarah Kilpatrick, MD/PhD—now chief of obstetrics and gynecology at Cedars-Sinai Medical Center in Los Angeles—for your endless rigor and for serving as my clinical guru, mentor, and research advisor during my obstetrics and gynecology residency. You taught me how to hold the bar high for women. Special thanks also to the inspiring Louann Brizendine, MD, author of the books *The Female Brain* and *The Male Brain* and founder of the University of California at San Francisco Women's Mood and Hormone Clinic. I'm full of gratitude also to Christiane Northrup, MD, who started the new meme about hormones decades ago. We are in magnificent agreement that connection to inner divinity is the most powerful epigenomic influence. Drs. Seely, Kilpatrick, Brizendine, and Northrup were my greatest influences when it comes to how I think of the matrix of the female body. You all taught me an exquisitely original form of synthesis and showed by your example how to craft an original conceptual model.

I'm indebted to a long list of careful and encouraging readers for *The Hormone Cure,* including my mom, Mary Lil Szal, and many dear friends and colleagues, including Kathleen Toup, MD; Marsha Nunley, MD; Rebecca Elia, MD; Johanna Ilfeld, PhD; Kathrin O'Sullivan; Susan Harrow; Emily Cronbach, MD; Nicole Daedone; Amy Fleischer; Linda Arnone; Marya Globig; Allison Hagey; Neha Sangwan, MD; Betty Suh-Burgmann, MD; Nori Hudson; Nathalie Bera-Miller, MD; and, of course, my husband, David Gottfried (who deserves an honorary "MD"). Thank you for spending your time and considerable intellect reading the text as it unfolded, and for your valuable contributions. As always, it was my darling husband who burned the midnight oil to clarify each chapter. For a guy, *he gets it.*

This book would not be possible without the enduring support of my agent, Katherine ("Kitty") Cowles. When we met, it was love at first sight. Through Kitty, I met Whitney Frick at Scribner, my brilliant editor with whom collaboration has been pure joy, every step of the way. Thanks also to my editorial team here in the Bay Area—Elaine Hooker, Nora Isaacs, Deborah Burstyn, and Pam Feinsilber: you propelled me forward and set me straight. Special thanks to Nancy Siller Wilson for excellent illustrations, designs, and reflections.

To my powerful support team: much love and gratitude. Thanks especially to Leslie Murphy for helping to keep the house running and picking up the girls from school, Jennifer Seligman for nourishing lunches and organizing principles, and my terrific assistants, including Cary Masin, Rachel Jurkowicz, and Liora Shachar.

To my awesome girlfriends who provide therapy, laughs, and endless oxytocin—thank you. To Jo Ilfeld, our weekly running date keeps me sane and inspired. You heard the blow-by-blow details for *The Hormone Cure* on a weekly basis yet doggedly hung in there with me, offering wise advice, laughter, and desperately needed coaching. Not only that, you *stepped up graciously* every time I asked, even when you had plenty on your own plate with three children and a thriving professional coaching practice. You are a magnificent friend.

Leslye Robbins, you keep me laughing and happily married, and always *floor me* with your insights. Julia Hill Hanrahan, MD, you are my first and best doctor friend. Meryl Rosofsky, MD, you are my inspiration to be bold and curious, even with the distraction of a conventional medical degree. Ariella Chezar, *I crazypants miss you* since you moved back to the Berkshires, but please know you were as potent an influence on my ideas of natural ways to heal the female body, and healthier alternatives for neurohormonal balancing, as any doctor or book. You were there, Sister, in those insane years, nudging me to walk with you and think differently about conventional paradigms of health. To my Saturday-morning walking group—especially Leslye Robbins, Rachel Engel, Sue Proctor, Jennifer Panish, and Hana Rotman—thank you for your unwavering support, fantastic parenting and husband-management advice, and for the warmest welcome to the school community. I'm honored to grow old with all of you (in a neurohormonally optimized way), walking and dishing our lives every Saturday!

Gratitude also to my uncle, Chuck Teubner, for your perpetual support and enthusiasm throughout my career. You've always been there when I needed you, from that first medical school interview through to current strategy. Thanks as well to Aunt Lynda for your ongoing and influential support combined with soulful marketing mojo. You both rock, and I love you.

One last serotonin-drenched shout-out to the earliest trio of mentors who instilled in me a love for learning, eternal optimism, and delight in thinking for myself: Mom, Grandpa, and Mud. I'm blessed by a mighty genetic tree.

My grandfather, General Harold C. Teubner, exercised, stretched, and popped supplements—similar to Mud (his mother), back in the 1960s—before it was trendy. He extolled the virtues of lifestyle management decades prior to Tim Ferriss, and recommended that I study science because his own calling, as an aeronautical/astronautical engineer, was so fulfilling to him. My aunt, Tricia Crisp, describes aptly his rare ability to make one feel like his favorite, even though he didn't play favorites among his four children and many grandchildren. He died peacefully in his sleep at age ninety-three, while I completed this book in 2012. Even though he lived a long life, his death is a severe loss for me and my family. I hope to carry on his important legacy, and I'm grateful to live on with his DNA in my every cell. Grandpa was one of those gritty men whom Winston Churchill described: "We sleep safely at night because rough men stand ready to visit violence on those who would harm us."

My deep appreciation to my great-grandmother, Lillian Teubner Dietz (also known as "Mud"), who left me with deep murmurings of a novel way to conceive health and longevity, and introduced me to yoga, the best system I've encountered for extraordinary living. Mud encouraged me to dream big and go against the grain.

To my magical daughters, thank you for your patience with my very long process of writing my first book, which I know felt like another sibling for the past eighteen months. I missed many field trips, forgot lunches, and had spotty attendance (at best) at volleyball, soccer, and softball games—yet you endured my borderline neglectful and distracted attention. Thank you for your love, for your honest protests (I encourage the protests especially), and for the important mirror you offer me as your mom. You enliven me to grow as a mother and caretaker, and help me stretch in my awareness, insight, and occasionally, radical presence. I am blessed by you both and sharing in your joy every day.

Most importantly, I want to acknowledge my true love, *beshert,* and life partner, David Gottfried. You are the most important influence in my life, on a daily basis and for more than a decade. You funded and subsidized, both literally and metaphorically, every part of making my dreams come true—you talked endlessly with me about hormones, pitched me to your editors and publisher, strategized my professional shift in focus, and paved the way for my creativity to unfold. Thank you for that priceless gift. I know the journal articles, more than one thousand of them, strewn all over the house, were not part of your idea of a sacred home, but you persisted in seeing beyond the clutter to who I am, at the deepest level. Your relentless pursuit of living your values inspires and guides me. You are a healer, genius, and shaman, and I'm blessed to be on the sacred path of marriage with you. Your mind, depth, and abiding love are deeply nurturing and grounding for me. Finally, I must add: *I still think you're the hottest man on the planet.*

NOTES

CHAPTER 4: HIGH AND/OR LOW CORTISOL

1 McEwan BS. "Stressed or stressed out: what is the difference?" *Journal of Psychiatry and Neuroscience* 30 (5) (2005): 315–18.

2 Tamres LK, Janicki D, Helgeson VS. "Sex Differences in Coping Behavior: A Meta-Analytic Review and an Examination of Relative Coping." *Personality and Social Psychology Review* 6 (2002): 2–30. doi: 10.1207/S15327957PSPR0601_1.

3 Ross CE, Mirowsky J, Goldsteen K. "The impact of the family on health: the decade in review." *Journal of Marriage and Family* 52 (1990): 1059–78; Cutrona CE, Russell DW, Gardner KA. "The relationship enhancement model of social support" in Kayser K, Bodenmann G, Revenson TA, eds. "Couples Coping with Stress: Emerging Perspectives on Dyadic Coping." *American Psychological Association* (2005): 73–95.

4 Undén AL, Orth-Gomér K, Elofsson S. "Cardiovascular effects of social support in the workplace: twenty-four-hour ECG monitoring of men and women." *Psychosomatic Medicine* 53 (1) (1991): 50–60.

5 Slatcher RB, Robles TF, Repetti RL, Fellows MD. "Momentary work worries, marital disclosure, and salivary cortisol among parents of young children." *Psychosomatic Medicine* 72 (9) (2010): 887–96.

6 Klumb P, Hoppmann C, Staats M. "Work hours affect spouse's cortisol secretion—for better and for worse." *Psychosomatic Medicine* 68 (2006): 742–46.

7 Saxbe DE, Repetti RL, Graesch AP. "Time spent in housework and leisure: links with parents' physiological recovery from work." *Journal of Family Psychology* 25 (2) (2011): 271–81.

8 Hyman M. *The UltraMind Solution.* New York: Scribner, 2009.

9 Woods NF, Mitchell ES, Smith-DiJulio K. "Cortisol Levels During the Menopausal Transition and Early Postmenopause: Observations from the Seattle Midlife Women's Health Study." *Menopause* 16 (4) (2009): 708–18. doi: 10.1097/gme.0b013e318198d6b2.

10 Laughlin GA, Barrett-Connor E. "Sexual Dimorphism in the Influence of Advanced Aging on Adrenal Hormone Levels: The Rancho Bernardo Study." *Journal of Clinical Endocrinology & Metabolism* 85 (10) (2000): 3561–68.

11 Pace-Schott EF, Spencer RM. "Age-related changes in the cognitive function of sleep." *Progress Brain Research* 191 (2011): 75–89.

12 Stone AA, Schwartz JE, Broderick JE, Deaton A. "A snapshot of the age distribution of psychological well-being in the United States." *Proceedings of the National Academy of Sciences of the United States of America* 107 (22) (2010): 9985–90. Epub 2010 May 17.

13 Nieman LK, Biller BM, Findling JW, et al. "The diagnosis of Cushing's syndrome: an Endocrine Society Clinical Practice Guideline." *Journal of Clinical Endocrinology and Metabolism* 93 (5) (2008): 1526–40.

14 Tsagarakis S, Vassiliadi D, Thalassinos N. "Endogenous subclinical hypercortisolism: diagnostic uncertainties and clinical implications." *Journal of Endocrinological Investigation* 29 (5) (2006): 471–82.

15 Gold SM, Dziobek I, Rogers K, et al. "Hypertension and hypothalamo-pituitary-adrenal axis hyperactivity affect frontal lobe integrity." *Journal of Clinical Endocrinology and Metabolism* 90 (6) (2005): 3262–67.

16 Wolfram M, Bellingrath S, Kudielka BM. "The cortisol awakening response (CAR) across the female menstrual cycle." *Psychoneuro-endocrinology* 36 (6) (2011): 905–12.

17 Portner M. "The Orgasmic Mind: The Neurological Roots of Sexual Pleasure." *Scientific American Mind* 19 (2008): 66–71.

18 Epel ES, Blackburn EH, Lin J, et al. "Accelerated telomere shortening in response to life stress." *Proceedings of the National Academy of Sciences of the United States of America* 101 (49) (2004): 17312–15.

19 Epel E, Daubenmier J, Moskowitz JT, et al. "Can meditation slow rate of cellular aging? Cognitive stress, mindfulness, and telomeres." *Annals of New York Academy of Sciences* 1172 (2009): 34–53; Jacobs TL, Epel ES, Lin J, et al. "Intensive meditation training, immune cell telomerase activity, and psychological mediators." *Psychoneuroendocrinology* 36 (5) (2011): 664–81. PMID: 21035949.

20 Banderet LE, Lieberman HR. "Treatment with tyrosine, a neurotransmitter precursor, reduces environmental stress in humans." *Brain Research Bulletin* 22 (4) (1989): 759–62.

21 Jacobs GD. *Say Good Night to Insomnia.* New York: Holt Paperbacks, 2009.

22 Norager CB, Jensen MB, Weimann A, Madsen MR. "Metabolic effects of caffeine ingestion and physical work in 75-year-old citizens. A randomized, double-blind, placebo-controlled, cross-over study." *Clinical Endocrinology (Oxford)* 65 (2) (2006): 223–28; MacKenzie T, Comi R, Sluss P, Keisari R, et al. "Metabolic and hormonal effects of caffeine: randomized, double-blind, placebo-controlled, crossover trial." *Metabolism* 56 (12) (2007): 1694–98.

23 Bjorntorp P, Rosmond R. "Obesity and cortisol." *Nutrition* 16 (2000):

924–36. doi: 10.1016/S0899-9007(00)00422-6; Daubenmier J, Kristeller J, Hecht FM, et al. "Mindfulness Intervention for Stress Eating to Reduce Cortisol and Abdominal Fat among Overweight and Obese Women: An Exploratory Randomized Controlled Study." *Journal of Obesity* (2011): 651936.

24 Janković D, Wolf P, Anderwald CH, et al. "Prevalence of Endocrine Disorders in Morbidly Obese Patients and the Effects of Bariatric Surgery on Endocrine and Metabolic Parameters." *Obesity Surgery* 22 (1) (2011): 62–69.

25 Langenecker SA, Weisenbach SL, Giordani B, et al. "Impact of chronic hypercortisolemia on affective processing." *Neuropharmacology* 62 (1) (2012): 217–25.

26 Gold PW, Goodwin FK, Chrousos GP. "Clinical and biochemical manifestations of depression. Relation to the neurobiology of stress." *New England Journal of Medicine* 319 (7) (1988): 413–20; Barden N, Reul JM, Holsboer F. "Do antidepressants stabilize mood through actions on the hypothalamic-pituitary-adrenocortical system?" *Trends in Neurosciences* 18 (1) (1995): 6–11; Holsboer F. "The corticosteroid receptor hypothesis of depression." *Neuropsychopharmacology* 23 (5) (2000): 477–501; Pariante CM, Miller AH. "Glucocorticoid receptors in major depression: relevance to pathophysiology and treatment." *Biological Psychiatry* 49 (5) (2001): 391–404; Irwin MR, Miller AH. "Depressive disorders and immunity: 20 years of progress and discovery." *Brain Behavior and Immunity* 21 (4) (2007): 374–83; McGirr A, Diaconu G, Berlim MT, et al. "Dysregulation of the sympathetic nervous system, hypothalamic-pituitary-adrenal axis and executive function in individuals at risk for suicide." *Journal of Psychiatry and Neuroscience* 35 (6) (2010): 399–408; Howland RH. "Use of endocrine hormones for treating depresssion." *Journal of Psychosocial Nursing and Mental Health Service* 48 (12) (2010): 13–16.

27 Doecke JD, Laws SM, Faux NG, et al. "Blood-Based Protein Biomarkers for Diagnosis of Alzheimer's Disease." *Archives of Neurology* (July 16, 2012):1–8. doi: 10.1001/archneurol.2012.1282.

28 Gold SM, Dziobek I, Rogers K, et al. "Hypertension and hypothalamo-pituitary-adrenal axis hyperactivity affect frontal lobe integrity." *Journal of Clinical Endocrinology and Metabolism* 90 (6) (2005): 3262–67; Heesen C, Mohr DC, Huitinga I, et al. "Stress regulation in multiple sclerosis: current issues and concepts." *Multiple Sclerosis* 13 (2) (2007): 143–48; Ysrraelit MC, Gaitán MI, Lopez AS, Correale J. "Impaired hypothalamic-pituitary-adrenal axis activity in patients with multiple sclerosis." *Neurology* 71 (24) (2008): 1948–54; Kern S, Schultheiss T, Schneider H, et al. "Circadian cortisol, depressive

symptoms and neurological impairment in early multiple sclerosis."
Psychoneuroendocrinology 36 (10) (2011): 1505–12.

29 Ebrecht M, Hextall J, Kirtley LG, et al. "Perceived stress and cortisol
levels predict speed of wound healing in healthy male adults."
Psychoneuroendocrinology 29 (6) (2004): 798–809.

30 Milutinovic DV, Macut D, Božić I, et al. "Hypothalamic-pituitary-
adrenocortical axis hypersensitivity and glucocorticoid receptor
expression and function in women with polycystic ovarian syndrome."
Experimental and Clinical Endocrinology and Diabetes 119 (10) (2011):
636–43.

31 Vgontzas AN, Bixler EO, Lin HM, et al. "Chronic insomnia is
associated with nyctohemeral activation of the hypothalamic-
pituitary-adrenal axis: clinical implications." *Journal of Clinical and
Endocrinological Metabolism* 86 (8) (2001): 3787–94; Rodenbeck A,
Huether G, Rüther E, Hajak G. "Interactions between evening and
nocturnal cortisol secretion and sleep parameters in patients with
severe chronic primary insomnia." *Neuroscience Letters* 324 (2) (2002):
159–63.

32 Greendale GA, Unger JB, Rowe JW, Seeman TE. "The relation between
cortisol excretion and fractures in healthy older people: results from
the MacArthur studies-Mac." *Journal of the American Geriatrics Society*
47 (7) (1999): 799–803; Morelli V, Eller-Vainicher C, Salcuni AS, et al.
"Risk of new vertebral fractures in patients with adrenal incidentaloma
with and without subclinical hypercortisolism: a multicenter
longitudinal study." *Journal of Bone and Mineral Research* 26 (8) (2011):
1816–21. doi: 10.1002/jbmr.398.

33 Björnsdottir S, Sääf M, Bensing S, et al. "Risk of hip fracture in
Addison's disease: a population-based cohort study." *Journal of
Internal Medicine* 270 (2) (2011): 187–95. doi: 10.1111/j.1365-
2796.2011.02352.x.

34 Juster RP, Sindi S, Marin MF, et al. "A clinical allostatic load index is
associated with burnout symptoms and hypocortisolemic profiles in
healthy workers." *Psychoneuroendocrinology* 36 (6) (2011): 797–805.

35 Izawa S, Saito K, Shirotsuki K, et al. "Effects of prolonged stress on
salivary cortisol and dehydroepiandrosterone: a study of a two-week
teaching practice." *Psychoneuroendocrinology* 37 (6) (2012): 852–58.

36 Fournier JC, DeRubeis RJ, Hollon SD, et al. "Antidepressant drug
effects and depression severity: a patient-level meta-analysis." *Journal
of the American Medical Association* 303 (1) (2010): 47–53.

37 Meloun M, Hill M, Vceláková-Havlíková H. "Minimizing the effects of
multicollinearity in the polynomial regression of age relationships and sex
differences in serum levels of pregnenolone sulfate in healthy subjects."
Clinical Chemistry and Laboratory Medicine 47 (4) (2009): 464–70.

38 Martin FP, Rezzi S, Peré-Trepat E, et al. "Metabolic effects of dark chocolate consumption on energy, gut microbiota, and stress-related metabolism in free-living subjects." *Journal of Proteome Research* 8 (12) (2009): 5568–79.

39 Välimäki MJ, Härkönen M, Eriksson CJ, Ylikahri RH. "Sex hormones and adrenocortical steroids in men acutely intoxicated with ethanol." *Alcohol* 1 (1) (1984): 89–93.

40 Kiefer F, Jahn H, Otte C, Naber D, Wiedemann K. "Hypothalamic-pituitary-adrenocortical axis activity: a target of pharmacological anticraving treatment?" *Biology Psychiatry* 60 (1) (2006): 74–76.

41 Freedman ND, Park Y, Abnet CC, et al. "Association of Coffee Drinking with Total and Cause-Specific Mortality." *New England Journal of Medicine* 366 (2012): 1891–1904.

42 Rapaport MH, Schettler P, Bresee C. "A Preliminary Study of the Effects of a Single Session of Swedish Massage on Hypothalamic-Pituitary-Adrenal and Immune Function in Normal Individuals." *Journal of Alternative and Complementary Medicine* 16 (10) (2010): 1079–88. doi: 10.1089/acm.2009.0634.

43 Khalsa DS, Amen D, Hanks C, et al. "Cerebral blood flow changes during chanting meditation." *Nuclear Medicine Communications* 30 (12) (2009): 956–61; Kalyani BG, Venkatasubramanian G, Arasappa R, et al. "Neurohemodynamic correlates of 'OM' chanting: a pilot functional magnetic resonance imaging study." *International Journal of Yoga* 4 (1) (2011): 3–6.

44 Painovich JM, Shufelt CL, Azziz R, et al. "A pilot randomized, single-blind, placebo-controlled trial of traditional acupuncture for vasomotor symptoms and mechanistic pathways of menopause." *Menopause* 19 (1) (2011): 54–61.

45 Gerra G, Avanzini P, Zaimovic A, et al. "Neurotransmitter and endocrine modulation of aggressive behavior and its components in normal humans." *Behavioral Brain Research* 81 (1–2) (1996): 19–24; Harris AH, Luskin F, Norman SB, et al. "Effects of a group forgiveness intervention on forgiveness, perceived stress, and trait-anger." *Journal of Clinical Psychology* 62 (6) (2006): 715–33.

46 Tibbits D, Ellis G, Piramelli C, et al. "Hypertension reduction through forgiveness training." *Journal of Pastoral Care and Counseling* 60 (1–2) (2006): 27–34.

47 Toussaint L. "Physiological correlates of forgiveness: findings from a radically and socio-economically diverse sample of community residents." Abstract presented at Scientific Findings of Forgiveness Conference, 2003 (http://www.forgiving.org/conference_archive/conference_2.htm accessed 12/28/11).

48 Blank J. "Toys: Sex Toys" in *Human Sexuality: An Encyclopedia,* eds. VL

Bullough and B Bullough. New York: Garland, 1994; Komisaruk BR, Beyer-Flores C, Whipple B. *The Science of Orgasm*. Baltimore: Johns Hopkins University Press, 2006.

49 Tull ES, Sheu YT, Butler C, Cornelious K. "Relationships between perceived stress, coping behavior and cortisol secretion in women with high and low levels of internalized racism." *Journal of the National Medical Association* 97 (2) (2005): 206–12.

50 Onuki M, Suzawa A. "Effect of pantethine on the function of the adrenal cortex. 2. Clinical experience using pantethine in cases under steroid hormone treatment." *Horumon To Rinsho Clinical Endocrinology* 18 (11) (1970): 937–40 [article in Japanese].

51 Gromova EG, Sviridova SP, Kushlinskiĭ NE, et al. "Regulation of the indices of neuroendocrine status in surgical patients with lung cancer using optimal doses of ascorbic acid." *Anesteziologiia Reanimatologiia* 5 (1990): 71–74 [article in Russian]; Liakakos D, Doulas NL, Ikkos D, et al. "Inhibitory effect of ascorbic acid (vitamin C) on cortisol secretion following adrenal stimulation in children." *Clinica Chimica Acta: International Journal of Clinical Chemistry* 65 (1975): 251–55.

52 Liakakos D, Doulas NL, Ikkos D, et al. "Inhibitory effect of ascorbic acid (vitamin C) on cortisol secretion following adrenal stimulation in children." *Clinica Chimica Acta: International Journal of Clinical Chemistry* 65 (1975): 251–55.

53 Peters EM, Anderson R, Nieman DC, et al. "Vitamin C supplementation attenuates the increases in circulating cortisol, adrenaline and anti-inflammatory polypeptides following ultramarathon running." *International Journal of Sports Medicine* 22 (7) (2001): 537–43.

54 Monteleone P, Beinat L, Tanzillo C, et al. "Effects of phosphatidylserine on the neuroendocrine response to physical stress in humans." *Neuroendocrinology* 52 (3) (1990): 243–48; Monteleone P, Maj M, Beinat L, et al. "Blunting by chronic phosphatidylserine administration of the stress-induced activation of the hypothalamo-pituitary-adrenal axis in healthy men." *European Journal of Clinical Pharmacology* 42 (1992): 385–88.

55 Benton D, Donohoe RT, Sillance B, Nabb S. "The influence of phosphatidylserine supplementation on mood and heart rate when faced with an acute stressor." *Nutritional Neuroscience* 4 (3) (2001): 169–78.

56 Noreen EE, Sass MJ, Crowe ML, et al. "Effects of supplemental fish oil on resting metabolic rate, body composition, and salivary cortisol in healthy adults." *Journal of the International Society of Sports Nutrition* 7 (31) (2010): 1–7.

57 Delarue J, Matzinger O, Binnert C, et al. "Fish oil prevents the adrenal

activation elicited by mental stress in healthy men." *Diabetes and Metabolism* 29 (3) (2003): 289–95.

58 Kimura K, Ozeki M, Juneja LR, Ohira H. "L-Theanine reduces psychological and physiological stress responses." *Biological Psychology* 74 (1) (2007): 39–45.

59 Miodownik C, Maayan R, Ratner Y, et al. "Serum levels of brain-derived neurotrophic factor and cortisol to sulfate of dehydroepiandrosterone molar ratio associated with clinical response to L-theanine as augmentation of antipsychotic therapy in schizophrenia and schizoaffective disorder patients." *Clinical Neuropharmacology* 34 (4) (2011): 155–60.

60 Smriga M, Ando T, Akutsu M, et al. "Oral treatment with L-lysine and L-arginine reduces anxiety and basal cortisol levels in healthy humans." *Biomedical Research* 28 (2) (2007): 85–90.

61 Banderet LE, Lieberman HR. "Treatment with tyrosine, a neurotransmitter precursor, reduces environmental stress in humans." *Brain Research Bulletin* 22 (4) (1989): 759–62.

62 Thomas JR, Lockwood PA, Singh A, Deuster PA. "Tyrosine improves working memory in a multitasking environment." *Pharmacology, Biochemistry and Behavior* 64 (3) (1999): 495–500.

63 Hanson R, Mendius R. *Buddha's Brain: The Practical Neuroscience of Happiness, Love, and Wisdom.* Oakland, CA: New Harbinger, 2009.

64 Martarelli D, Cocchioni M, Scuri S, Pompei P. "Diaphragmatic Breathing Reduces Exercise-induced Oxidative Stress." *Evidence-Based Complementary and Alternative Medicine* 49 (1) (2009): 122–27.

65 Benson H. *The Relaxation Response.* New York: Harper Collins, 1975.

66 Pawlow LA, Jones GE. "The impact of abbreviated progressive muscle relaxation on salivary cortisol and salivary immunoglobulin A (SIgA)." *Applied Psychophysiological and Biofeedback* 30 (4) (2005): 375–87.

67 Gopal A, Mondal S, Gandhi A, et al. "Effect of integrated yoga practices on immune responses in examination stress—a preliminary study." *International Journal of Yoga* 4 (1) (2011): 26–32.

68 Smith JA, Greer T, Sheets T, Watson S. "Is there more to yoga than exercise?" *Alternative Therapies in Health and Medicine* 17 (3) (2011): 22–29.

69 Banasik J, Williams H, Haberman M, et al. "Effect of Iyengar yoga practice on fatigue and diurnal salivary cortisol concentration in breast cancer survivors." *Journal of the American Academy of Nurse Practitioners* 23 (3) (2011): 135–42. doi: 10.1111/j.1745-7599.2010.00573.x; Bijlani RL, Vempati RP, Yadav RK, et al. "A brief but comprehensive lifestyle education program based on yoga reduces risk factors for cardiovascular disease and diabetes mellitus." *Journal of Alternative and Complementary Medicine* 11 (2) (2005): 267–74.

70 Nidich SI, Rainforth MV, Haaga DA, Hagelin J, et al. "A randomized controlled trial on effects of the Transcendental Meditation program on blood pressure, psychological distress, and coping in young adults." *American Journal of Hypertension* 22 (12) (2009):1326–31; Schneider R, Nidich S, Kotchen JM, et al. "Abstract 1177: Effects of Stress Reduction on Clinical Events in African Americans with Coronary Heart Disease: A Randomized Controlled Trial." *American Heart Association, Inc.* 120 (2009): S461; Campbell TS, Labelle LE, Bacon SL, et al. "Impact of mindfulness-based stress reduction (MBSR) on attention, rumination and resting blood pressure in women with cancer: a waitlist-controlled study." *Journal of Behavioral Medicine* 35 (3) (2011): 262–71.

71 Kabat-Zinn J. *Wherever You Go, There You Are: Mindfulness Meditation in Everyday Life.* New York: Hyperion, 1999.

72 Hölzel BK, Carmody J, Evans KC, et al. "Stress reduction correlates with structural changes in the amygdala." *Social, Cognitive and Affective Neuroscience* 5 (1) (2010): 11–17.

73 West J, Otte C, Geher K, et al. "Effects of Hatha yoga and African dance on perceived stress, affect, and salivary cortisol." *Annals of Behavioral Medicine* 28 (2) (2004): 114–18; Matousek RH, Dobkin PL, Pruessner J. "Cortisol as a marker for improvement in mindfulness-based stress reduction." *Complementary Therapies in Clinical Practice* 16 (2010): 13–19; Smith JA, Greer T, Sheets T, Watson S. "Is there more to yoga than exercise?" *Alternative Therapies in Health and Medicine* 17 (3) (2011): 22–29; Winbush NY, Gross CR, Kreitzer MJ. "The effects of mindfulness-based stress reduction on sleep disturbance: a systematic review." *Explore (NY)* 3 (6) (2007): 585–91; Bohlmeijer E, Prenger R, Taal E, Cuijpers P. "The effects of mindfulness-based stress reduction therapy on mental health of adults with a chronic medical disease: a meta-analysis." *Journal of Psychosomatic Research* 68 (2010): 539–44.

74 Daubenmier J, Kristeller J, Hecht FM, et al. "Mindfulness Intervention for Stress Eating to Reduce Cortisol and Abdominal Fat among Overweight and Obese Women: An Exploratory Randomized Controlled Study." *Journal of Obesity* (2011): 651936.

75 Upadhyay Dhungel K, Malhotra V, Sarkar D, Prajapati R. "Effect of alternate nostril breathing exercise on cardiorespiratory functions." *Nepal Medical College Journal* 10 (1) (2008): 25–27; Telles S, Raghuraj P, Maharana S, Nagendra HR. "Immediate effect of three yoga breathing techniques on performance on a letter-cancellation task." *Perceptual and Motor Skills* 104 (3 Pt 2) (2007): 1289–96.

76 Shannahoff-Khalsa DS. "Selective Unilateral Autonomic Activation: Implications for Psychiatry." *CNS Spectrums* 12 (8) (2007): 625–34.

77 Caso Marasco A, Vargas Ruiz R, Salas Villagomez A, Begoña Infante C. "Double-blind study of a multivitamin complex supplemented with ginseng extract." *Drugs under Experimental and Clinical Research* 2 (1996): 323–29.

78 Garay Lillo J, Caballero Garcia JC, Cabeza Mauricios G., et al. "Long-term multicenter study with Pharmaton Complex in adult patients." *Geriatrika* 8 (6) (1992): 69–74; Scaglione F, Weiser K, Alessandria M. "Effects of the standardized ginseng extract G115® in patients with chronic bronchitis: a nonblinded, randomised, comparative pilot study." *Clinical Drug Investigation [New Zealand]* 21 (2001): 41–45.

79 Reay JL, Scholey AB, Kennedy DO. "Panax ginseng (G115) improves aspects of working memory performance and subjective ratings of calmness in healthy young adults." *Human Psychopharmacology* 25 (6) (2010): 462–71.

80 Ernst E. "The risk-benefit profile of commonly used herbal therapies: Ginkgo, St. John's Wort, Ginseng, Echinacea, Saw Palmetto, and Kava." *Annals of Internal Medicine* 136 (1) (2002): 42–53.

81 Tode T, Kikuchi Y, Hirata J, et al. "Effect of Korean red ginseng on psychological functions in patients with severe climacteric syndromes." *International Journal of Gynaecology and Obstetrics* 67 (3) (1999): 169–74.

82 Cooley K, Szczurko O, Perri D, et al. "Naturopathic care for anxiety: a randomized controlled trial ISRCTN78958974." *PLoS One* 4 (8) (2009): e6628.

83 Olsson EM, von Schéele B, Panossian AG. "A randomised, double-blind, placebo-controlled, parallel-group study of the standardised extract SHR-5 of the roots of *Rhodiola rosea* in the treatment of subjects with stress-related fatigue." *Planta Medica* 75 (2) (2009): 105–12.

84 Zhang ZJ, Tong Y, Zou J, et al. "Dietary supplement with a combination of *Rhodiola crenulata* and *Ginkgo biloba* enhances the endurance performance in healthy volunteers." *Chinese Journal of Integral Medicine* 15 (3) (2009): 177–83.

85 Dwyer AV, Whitten DL, Hawrelak JA. "Herbal medicines, other than St. John's Wort, in the treatment of depression: a systematic review." *Alternative Medicine Review* 16 (16) (2011): 40–49.

86 Howland RH. "Use of endocrine hormones for treating depresssion." *Journal of Psychosocial Nursing and Mental Health Service* 48 (12) (2010): 13–16.

87 Stangle B, Hirshman E, Verbalis J. "Administration of dehydroepiandrosterone (DHEA) enhances visual-spatial performance in postmenopausal women." *Behavioral Neuroscience* 125 (5) (2011): 742–52.

88 Wolkowitz OM, Reus VI, Keebler A, et al. "Double-blind treatment of major depression with dehydroepiandrosterone." *American Journal of Psychiatry* 156 (4) (1999): 646–49; Schmidt PJ, Daly RC, Bloch M, et al. "Dehydroepiandrosterone monotherapy in midlife-onset major and minor depression." *Archives of General Psychiatry* 62 (2) (2005): 154–62.

89 West J, Otte C, Geher K, et al. "Effects of Hatha yoga and African dance on perceived stress, affect, and salivary cortisol." *Annals of Behavioral Medicine* 28 (2) (2004): 114–18.

90 Shelygina NM, Spivak RIa, Zaretskiï MM, et al. "Influence of vitamins C, B_1, and B_6 on the diurnal periodicity of the glucocorticoid function of the adrenal cortex in patients with atherosclerotic cardiosclerosis." *Voprosy Pitaniia* 2 (1975): 25–29 [article in Russian].

91 Epstein MT, Espiner EA, Donald RA, et al. "Licorice raises urinary cortisol in man." *Journal of Clinical Endocrinology and Metabolism* 47 (2) (1978): 397–400.

92 Räikkönen K, Seckl JR, Heinonen K, et al. "Maternal prenatal licorice consumption alters hypothalamic-pituitary-adrenocortical axis function in children." *Psychoneuroendocrinology* 35 (10) (2010): 1587–93.

93 Methlie P, Husebye EE, Hustad S, et al. "Grapefruit juice and licorice increase cortisol availability in patients with Addison's disease." *European Journal of Endocrinology* 165 (5) (2011): 761–69.

CHAPTER 5: LOW-PROGESTERONE BLUES

1 Brizendine L. *The Female Brain.* New York: Broadway Books, 2006.

2 Nillni YI, Toufexis DJ, Rohan KJ. "Anxiety sensitivity, the menstrual cycle, and panic disorder: a putative neuroendocrine and psychological interaction." *Clinical Psychology & Review* 31 (7) (2011): 1183–91.

3 Rapkin AJ, Akopians AL. "Pathophysiology of premenstrual syndrome and premenstrual dysphoric disorder." *Menopause International* 18 (2) (2012): 52–59.

4 Personal communication with PMS expert Dr. Andrea Rapkin on June 5, 2012. Department of Obstetrics and Gynecology, David Geffen School of Medicine at UCLA.

5 Branch DW, Gibson M, Silver RM. "Clinical practice. Recurrent miscarriage." *New England Journal of Medicine* 363 (18) (2010): 1740–47.

6 De Souza MJ. "Menstrual disturbances in athletes: a focus on luteal phase defects." *Medicine and Science in Sports and Exercise* 35 (9) (2003): 1553–63.

7   Santoro N, Crawford SL, Lasley WL. "Factors related to declining luteal function in women during the menopausal transition." *Journal of Clinical Endocrinology and Metabolism* 93 (5) (2008): 1711–21.

8   Cauley JA. "Elevated serum estradiol and testosterone concentrations are associated with a high risk for breast cancer. Study of Osteoporotic Fractures Research Group." *Annals of Internal Medicine* 130 (4 Pt 1) (1999): 270–77; Farhat GN, Cummings SR, Chlebowski RT, et al. "Sex hormone levels and risks of estrogen receptor-negative and estrogen receptor-positive breast cancers." *Journal of the National Cancer Institute* 103 (7) (2011): 562–70.

9   He C, Kraft P, Chen C. "Genome-wide association studies identify loci associated with age at menarche and age at natural menopause." *Nature Genetics* 41 (6) (2009): 724–28.

10 Giudice LC. "Clinical practice: Endometriosis." *New England Journal of Medicine* 362 (25) (2010): 2389–98.

11 Zhang YW, Ji H, Han ML, et al. "Luteal function in patients with endometriosis." *Proceedings of the Chinese Academy of Medical Sciences Peking Union Medical College* 4 (2) (1989): 96–101.

12 Bulun SE, Cheng YH, Pavone ME, et al. "Estrogen receptor-beta, estrogen receptor-alpha, and progesterone resistance in endometriosis." *Seminars in Reproductive Medicine* 28 (1) (2010): 36–43.

13 Bulun SE, Cheng YH, Yin P, et al. "Progesterone resistance in endometriosis: link to failure to metabolize estradiol." *Molecular and Cellular Endocrinology* 248 (1–2) (2006): 94–103.

14 Gorchev G, Maleeva A. "Serum E2 and progesterone levels in patients with atypical hyperplasia and endometrial carcinoma." *Akusherstvo i Ginekologiia* 32 (2) (1993): 23–24 [article in Bulgarian]; Modan B, Ron E, Lerner-Geva L, et al. "Cancer incidence in a cohort of infertile women." *American Journal of Epidemiology* 147 (1998): 1038–42.

15 Freeman EW, Purdy RH, Coutifaris C, et al. "Anxiolytic metabolites of progesterone: correlation with mood and performance measures following oral progesterone administration to healthy female volunteers." *Neuroendocrinology* 58 (4) (1993): 478–84.

16 Andréen L, Sundström-Poromaa I, Bixo M, et al. "Allopregnanolone concentration and mood—a bimodal association in postmenopausal women treated with oral progesterone." *Psychopharmacology* 187 (2) (2006): 209–21.

17 "IMS Health," accessed March 24, 2012, http://www.imshealth.com and sleep data originally cited by http://well.blogs.nytimes.com/2012/03/12/new-worries-about-sleeping-pills/. IMS data are proprietary and not reported in a peer-reviewed journal.

18 Kripke DF, Langer RD, Kline LE. "Hypnotics' association with mortality or cancer: a matched cohort study." *British Medical Journal Open* 2 (1) (2012): e000850.

19 Caufriez A, Leproult R, L'Hermite-Balériaux M, et al. "Progesterone prevents sleep disturbances and modulates GH, TSH, and melatonin secretion in postmenopausal women." *Journal of Clinical Endocrinology and Metabolism* 96 (4) (2011): E614–23.

20 Henmi H, Endo T, Kitajima Y, et al. "Effects of ascorbic acid supplementation on serum progesterone levels in patients with a luteal phase defect." *Fertility and Sterility* 80 (2) (2003): 459–61.

21 Brown SL, Fredrickson BL, Wirth MM, et al. "Social Closeness Increases Salivary Progesterone in Humans." *Hormones and Behavior* 56 (1) (2009): 108–11.

22 Rossignol AM. "Caffeine-containing beverages and premenstrual syndrome in young women." *American Journal of Public Health* 75 (1985): 1335–37; Rossignol AM, Zhang J, Chen Y, Xiang Z. "Tea and premenstrual syndrome in the People's Republic of China." *American Journal of Public Health* 79 (1989): 66–67.

23 Gold EB, Bair Y, Block G, et al. "Diet and lifestyle factors associated with premenstrual symptoms in a racially diverse community sample: Study of Women's Health Across the Nation (SWAN)." *Journal of Women's Health* 16 (5) (2007): 641–56.

24 Li CI, Chlebowski RT, Freiberg M, et al. "Alcohol consumption and risk of postmenopausal breast cancer by subtype: the women's health initiative observational study." *Journal of the National Cancer Institute* 102 (18) (2010): 1422–31; Chen WY, Rosner B, Hankinson SE, et al. "Moderate alcohol consumption during adult life, drinking patterns, and breast cancer risk." *Journal of the American Medical Association* 306 (17) (2011): 1884–90.

25 Bergmann MM, Schütze M, Steffen A, et al. "The association of lifetime alcohol use with measures of abdominal and general adiposity in a large-scale European cohort." *European Journal of Clinical Nutrition* 65 (10) (2011): 1079–87. doi: 10.1038/ejcn.2011.70.

26 Brown DJ. "*Vitex-agnus-castus* clinical monograph." *Quarterly Review of Natural Medicine* (1994): 111–21.

27 Wuttke W, Jarry H, Christoffel V, et al. "Chasteberry tree (*Vitex agnus-castus*)—pharmacology and clinical indications." *Phytomedicine* 10 (4) (2003): 348–57; Natural Medicines Comprehensive Database. Accessed 7/1/12. http://naturaldatabase.therapeuticresearch.com.

28 Blumenthal M, Gruenwald J, Hall T, Risters RS. "The Complete German E Commission monographs: therapeutic guide to herbal medicine." Boston: Integrative Medicine Communications (1998), 108; Halaska M, Beles P, Gorkow C, Sieder C. "Treatment of cyclical

mastalgia with a solution containing a *Vitex agnus castus* extract: results of a placebo-controlled double-blind study." *Breast* 8 (4) (1999): 175–81.

29 Westphal LM, Polan ML, Trant, AS. "Double-blind, placebo-controlled study of Fertilityblend: a nutritional supplement for improving fertility in women." *Clinical and Experimental Obstetrics and Gynecology* 33 (4) (2006): 205–8.

30 Turner S, Mills S. "A double-blind clinical trial on a herbal remedy for premenstrual syndrome: a case study." *Complementary Therapies in Medicine* 1 (1993): 73–77; Lauritzen CH, Reuter HD, Repges RM, et al. "Treatment of premenstrual tension syndrome with *Vitex agnus-castus.* Controlled, double-blind study versus pyridoxine." *Phytomedicine* 4 (1997): 183–89; Schellenberg R. "Treatment for the premenstrual syndrome with agnus castus fruit extract: prospective, randomized, placebo-controlled study." *British Medical Journal* 322 (2001): 134–37; Westphal LM, Polan ML, Trant, AS. "Double-blind, placebo-controlled study of Fertilityblend: a nutritional supplement for improving fertility in women." *Clinical and Experimental Obstetrics and Gynecology* 33 (4) (2006): 205–8; Zamani M, Neghab N, Torabian S. "Therapeutic effect of *Vitex agnus castus* in patients with premenstrual syndrome." *Acta Medica Iranica* 50 (2) (2012): 101–6.

31 Westphal LM, Polan ML, Trant, AS. "Double-blind, placebo-controlled study of Fertilityblend: a nutritional supplement for improving fertility in women." *Clinical and Experimental Obstetrics and Gynecology* 33 (4) (2006): 205–8; Loch EG, Selle H, Boblitz N. "Treatment of premenstrual syndrome with a phytopharmaceutical formulation containing *Vitex agnus-castus.*" *Journal of Women's Health & Gender-Based Medicine* 9 (3) (2000): 315–20.

32 Skibola CF. "The effect of *Fucus vesiculosus,* an edible brown seaweed, upon menstrual cycle length and hormonal status in three pre-menopausal women: a case report." *BMC Complementary and Alternative Medicine* 4 (2004): 10.

33 Nahid K, Fariborz M, Ataolah G, Solokian S. "The effect of an Iranian herbal drug on primary dysmenorrhea: a clinical controlled trial." *Journal of Midwifery & Women's Health* 54 (2009): 401–4; Agha-Hosseini M, Kashani L, Aleyaseen A, et al. "*Crocus sativus L.* (saffron) in the treatment of premenstrual syndrome: a double-blind, randomised and placebo-controlled trial." *BJOG: An International Journal of Obstetrics and Gynecology* 115 (2008): 515–19.

34 Dwyer AV, Whitten DL, Hawrelak JA. "Herbal medicines, other than St. John's Wort, in the treatment of depression: a systematic review." *Alternative Medicine Review* 16 (1) (2011): 40–49.

35 Komesaroff PA, Black CV, Cable V, Sudhir K. "Effects of wild yam

extract on menopausal symptoms, lipids and sex hormones in healthy menopausal women." *Climacteric* 4 (2001): 144–50.

36 Leonetti HB, Longo S, Anasti JN. "Transdermal progesterone cream for vasomotor symptoms and postmenopausal bone loss." *Obstetrics and Gynecology* 94 (1999): 225–28.

37 Wren BG, Champion SM, Willetts K, et al. "Transdermal progesterone and its effect on vasomotor symptoms, blood lipid levels, bone metabolic markers, moods, and quality of life for postmenopausal women." *Menopause* 10 (1) (2003): 13–18.

38 Benster B, Carey A, Wadsworth F, et al. "A double-blind placebo-controlled study to evaluate the effect of Progestelle progesterone cream on postmenopausal women." *Menopause International* 15 (2) (2009): 63–69.

39 PEPI Writing Group. "Effects of estrogen or estrogen/progestin regimens on heart disease risk factors in postmenopausal women. The Postmenopausal Estrogen/Progestin Interventions (PEPI) Trial. The Writing Group for the PEPI Trial." *Journal of the American Medical Association* 273 (3) (1995): 199–208.

40 Fournier A, Berrino F, Clavel-Chapelon F. "Unequal risks for breast cancer associated with different hormone replacement therapies: results from the E3N cohort study." *Breast Cancer Research and Treatment* 107 (1) (2008): 103–11. Erratum in *Breast Cancer Research and Treatment* 107 (2) (2008): 307–8.

41 Pullon SR, Reinken JA, Sparrow MJ. "Treatment of premenstrual symptoms in Wellington women." *New Zealand Medical Journal* 102 (862) (1989): 72–74.

42 Thys-Jacobs S. "Micronutrients and the premenstrual syndrome: the case for calcium." *Journal of the American College of Nutrition* 19 (2000): 220–27.

43 Walker AF, De Souza MC, Vickers MF, et al. "Magnesium supplementation alleviates premenstrual symptoms of fluid retention." *Journal of Women's Health* 7 (9) (1998): 1157–65; Wyatt KM, Dimmock PW, Jones PW, Shaughn O'Brien PM. "Efficacy of vitamin B_6 in the treatment of premenstrual syndrome: systematic review." *British Medical Journal* 318 (7195) (1999): 1375–81.

44 De Souza MC, Walker AF, Robinson PA, Bolland K. "A synergistic effect of a daily supplement for 1 month of 200 mg magnesium plus 50 mg vitamin B_6 for the relief of anxiety-related premenstrual symptoms: a randomized, double-blind, crossover study." *Journal of Women's Health and Gender-Based Medicine* 9 (2) (2000): 131–39.

45 Chocano-Bedoya PO, Manson JE, Hankinson SE, et al. "Dietary B vitamin intake and incident premenstrual syndrome." *American Journal of Clinical Nutrition* 93 (5) (2011): 1080–86; Bertone-Johnson

ER, Chocano-Bedoya PO, Zagarins SE, et al. "Dietary vitamin D intake, 25-hydroxyvitamin D3 levels and premenstrual syndrome in a college-aged population." *Journal of Steroid Biochemistry and Molecular Biology* 121 (1–2) (2010): 434–37.

46 Abraham GE. "Nutritional factors in the etiology of premenstrual tension syndromes." *Journal of Reproductive Medicine* 28 (1983): 446–64.

47 Kim SY, Park HJ, Lee H, Lee H. "Acupuncture for premenstrual syndrome: a systematic review and meta-analysis of randomised controlled trials." *BJOG: An International Journal of Obstetrics and Gynaecology* 118 (8) (2011): 899–915. doi: 10.1111/j.1471-0528.2011.02994.x.

48 Stoddard JL, Dent CW, Shames I, Bernstein L. "Exercise training effects on premenstrual distress and ovarian steroid hormones." *European Journal of Applied Physiology* 99 (1) (2007): 27–37.

49 Van Zak DB. "Biofeedback treatments for premenstrual and premenstrual affective syndromes." *International Journal of Psychosomatics* 41 (1–4) (1994): 53–60.

50 Yakir M, Kreitler S, Brzezinski A, et al. "Effects of homeopathic treatment in women with premenstrual syndrome: a pilot study." *British Homeopathic Journal* 90 (3) (2001): 148–53.

51 Lam RW, Carter D, Misri S, et al. "A controlled study of light therapy in women with late luteal phase dysphoric disorder." *Psychiatry Research* (1999) 86 (3): 185–92.

52 Canning S, Waterman M, Orsi N, et al. "The efficacy of *Hypericum perforatum* (St John's wort) for the treatment of premenstrual syndrome: a randomized, double-blind, placebo-controlled trial." *CNS Drugs* 24 (3) (2010): 207–25. doi: 10.2165/11530120-000000000-00000.

53 Van Die MD, Bone KM, Burger HG, et al. "Effects of a combination of *Hypericum perforatum* and *Vitex agnus-castus* on PMS-like symptoms in late-perimenopausal women: findings from a subpopulation analysis." *Journal of Alternative and Complementary Medicine* 15 (9) (2009): 1045–48.

54 Linde K, Ramirez G, Mulrow CD, et al. "St John's wort for depression—an overview and meta-analysis of randomised clinical trials." *British Medical Journal* (7052) (1996): 253–58.

55 Ford O, Lethaby A, Roberts H, Mol BW. "Progesterone for premenstrual syndrome." *Cochrane Database of Systematic Reviews* 14 (3) (2012): CD003415.

CHAPTER 6: EXCESS ESTROGEN

1 Quinlan MG, Duncan A, Loiselle C, et al. "Latent inhibition is affected by phase of estrous cycle in female rats." *Brain and Cognition*, 2010. doi: 10.1016/j.bandc.2010.08.003.

2 Schneider J, Kinne D, Fracchia A, et al. "Abnormal oxidative metabolism of estradiol in women with breast cancer." *Proceedings of the National Academy of Sciences* 79 (1982): 3047–51; Fishman J, Schneider J, Hershcope RJ, Bradlow HL. "Increased estrogen 16 alpha-hydroxylase activity in women with breast and endometrial cancer." *Journal of Steroid Biochemistry* 20 (4B) (1984): 1077–81; Zumoff B. "Hormonal profiles in women with breast cancer." *Obstetrics and Gynecology Clinics of North America* 21 (4) (1994): 751–72; Cauley JA, Zmuda JM, Danielson ME, et al. "Estrogen metabolites and the risk of breast cancer in older women." *Epidemiology* 14 (6) (2003): 740–44; Kabat GC, O'Leary ES, Gammon MD, et al. "Estrogen metabolism and breast cancer." *Epidemiology* 17 (1) (2006): 80–88; Im A, Vogel VG, Ahrendt G, et al. "Urinary estrogen metabolites in women at high risk for breast cancer." *Carcinogenesis* 30 (9) (2009): 1532–35; Fishman J, Schneider J, Hershcope RJ, Bradlow HL. "Increased estrogen 16 alpha-hydroxylase activity in women with breast and endometrial cancer." *Journal of Steroid Biochemistry* 20 (4B) (1984): 1077–81; Eliassen AH, Spiegelman D, Xu X, et al. "Urinary estrogens and estrogen metabolites and subsequent risk of breast cancer among premenopausal women." *Cancer Research* 72 (3) (2012): 696–706.

3 Sepkovic DW, Bradlow HL. "Estrogen hydroxylation—the good and the bad." *Annals of the New York Academy of Sciences* 1155 (2009): 57–67.

4 Seifert-Klauss V, Laakmann J, Rattenhuber J, et al. "Bone metabolism, bone density and estrogen levels in perimenopause: a prospective 2-year study." *Zentralbl Gynakol* 127 (3) (2005): 132–39 [article in German].

5 Kalleinen N, Polo-Kantola P, Irjala K, et al. "24-hour serum levels of growth hormone, prolactin, and cortisol in pre- and postmenopausal women: the effect of combined estrogen and progestin treatment." *Journal of Clinical Endocrinology and Metabolism* 93 (5) (2008): 1655–61.

6 Jamieson DJ, Terrell ML, Aguocha NN, et al. "Dietary exposure to brominated flame retardants and abnormal Pap test results." *Journal of Women's Health* (9) (2011):1269–78.

7 Komori S, Ito Y, Nakamura Y, et al. "A long-term user of cosmetic cream containing estrogen developed breast cancer and endometrial hyperplasia." *Menopause* 15 (6) (2008): 1191–92.

8 Massart F, Parrino R, Seppia P, et al. "How do environmental estrogen disruptors induce precocious puberty?" *Minerva Pediatrica* 58 (3) (2006): 247–54; Schoeters G, Den Hond E, Dhooge W, et al. "Endocrine disruptors and abnormalities of pubertal development." *Basic and Clinical Pharmacology and Toxicology* 102 (2) (2008): 168–75;

Roy JR, Chakraborty S, Chakraborty TR. "Estrogen-like endocrine disrupting chemicals affecting puberty in humans—a review." *Medical Science Monitor* 15 (6) (2009): RA137–45; Ozen S, Darcan S. "Effects of environmental endocrine disruptors on pubertal development." *Journal of Clinical Research in Pediatric Endocrinology* 3 (1) (2011): 1–6.

9 McLachlan JA, Simpson E, Martin M. "Endocrine disrupters and female reproductive health." *Best Practice and Research: Clinical Endocrinology and Metabolism* 20 (1) (2006): 63–75.

10 Environmental Working Group. "Bisphenol A: Toxic Plastics Chemical in Canned Food" (2007). http://www.ewg.org/reports/bisphenola.

11 Calafat AM, Ye X, Wong LY, et al. "Exposure of the U.S. population to bisphenol A and 4-tertiary-octylphenol: 2003–2004." *Environmental Health Perspectives* 116 (1) (2008): 39.

12 Lang IA, Galloway TS, Scarlett A, et al. "Association of urinary bisphenol A concentration with medical disorders and laboratory abnormalities in adults." *Journal of the American Medical Association* 300 (11) (2008): 1303–10.

13 Clayton EM, Todd M, Dowd JB, et al. "The impact of bisphenol A and triclosan on immune parameters in the U.S. population, NHANES 2003–2006." *Environmental Health Perspectives* 119 (3) (2011): 390–96.

14 Peretz J, Gupta RK, Singh J, et al. "Bisphenol A impairs follicle growth, inhibits steroidogenesis, and downregulates rate-limiting enzymes in the estradiol biosynthesis pathway." *Toxicological Sciences* 119 (1) (2011): 209–17.

15 Bolli A, Bulzomi P, Galluzzo P, et al. "Bisphenol A impairs estradiol-induced protective effects against DLD-1 colon cancer cell growth." *International Union of Biochemistry and Molecular Biology Life* 62 (9) (2010): 684–87.

16 Neel BA, Sargis RM. "The paradox of progress: environmental disruption of metabolism and the diabetes epidemic." *Diabetes* 60 (7) (2011): 1838–48.

17 Zoeller RT. "Environmental chemicals impacting the thyroid: targets and consequences." *Thyroid* 17 (9) (2007): 9811–17.

18 Jurewicz J, Hanke W. "Exposure to phthalates: Reproductive outcome and children health. A review of epidemiological studies." *International Journal of Occupational Medicine and Environmental Health* 24 (2) (2011): 115–41.

19 Lovekamp-Swan T, Davis BJ. "Mechanisms of phthalate ester toxicity in the female reproductive system." *Environmental Health Perspectives* 111 (2) (2003): 139–45.

20 Junger A. *Clean: The Revolutionary Program to Restore the Body's Natural Ability to Heal Itself.* New York: HarperOne, 2009.

21 Freeman EW, Sammel MD, Lin H, Gracia CR. "Obesity and reproductive hormone levels in the transition to menopause." *Menopause* 17 (4) (2010): 718–26.

22 Ibid.

23 Grodin JM, Siiteri PK, MacDonald PC. "Source of estrogen production in postmenopausal women." *Journal of Clinical Endocrinology and Metabolism* 36 (2) (1973): 207–14.

24 Key TJ, Pike MC. "The dose-effect relationship between 'unopposed' oestrogens and endometrial mitotic rate: its central role in explaining and predicting endometrial cancer risk." *British Journal of Cancer* 57 (1988): 205–12.

25 Chang SC, Lacey JV Jr, Brinton LA, et al. "Lifetime weight history and endometrial cancer risk by type of menopausal hormone use in the NIH-AARP diet and health study." *Cancer Epidemiology: Biomarkers and Prevention* 16 (4) (2007): 723–30.

26 Miller PE, Lesko SM, Muscat JE, et al. "Dietary patterns and colorectal adenoma and cancer risk: a review of the epidemiological evidence." *Nutrition and Cancer* 62 (4) (2010): 413–24.

27 Aldercreutz H, Pulkkinen MO, Hamalainin EK, Korpela JT. "Studies on the role of intestinal bacteria in metabolism of synthetic and natural steroid hormones." *Journal of Steroid Biochemistry* 20 (1) (1984) 20: 217–29; Winter J, Bokkenheuser VD. "Bacterial metabolism of natural and synthetic sex hormones undergoing enterohepatic circulation." *Journal of Steroid Biochemistry* 27 (4–6) (1987): 1145–49; Orme ML, Back DJ. "Factors affecting the enterohepatic circulation of oral contraceptive steroids." *American Journal of Obstetrics and Gynecology* 163 (6 Pt 2) (1990): 2146–52.

28 Dorgan J, Baer D, Albert P, et al. "Serum hormones and the alcohol-breast cancer association in postmenopausal women." *Journal of the National Cancer Institute* 93 (2001): 710–15; Mahabir S, Baer DJ, Johnson LL, et al. "The effects of moderate alcohol supplementation on estrone sulfate and DHEAS in postmenopausal women in a controlled feeding study." *Nutrition Journal* 3 (11) (2004).

29 Muneyyirci-Delale O, Nacharaju VL, Altura BM, Altura BT. "Sex steroid hormones modulate serum ionized magnesium and calcium levels throughout the menstrual cycles in women." *Fertility and Sterility* 69 (5) (1998): 958–62; Muneyyirci-Delale O, Nacharaju VL, Dalloul M, et al. "Serum ionized magnesium and calcium in women after menopause: inverse relation of estrogen with ionized magnesium." *Fertility and Sterility* 71 (5) (1999): 869–72.

30 Hightower JM, Moore D. "Mercury levels in high-end consumers of fish." *Environmental Health Perspectives* 111 (4) (2003): 604–8.

31 Ibid.

32 Zhang X, Wang Y, Zhao Y, Chen X. "Experimental study on the estrogen-like effect of mercuric chloride." *Biometals* 21 (2) (2007): 143–50.

33 Key TJ. "Endogenous oestrogens and breast cancer risk in premenopausal and postmenopausal women." *Steroids* 76 (8) (2011): 812–15.

34 Key TJ. "Serum oestradiol and breast cancer risk." *Endocrine-Related Cancer* 6 (2) (1999): 175–80.

35 Eliassen AH, Missmer SA, Tworoger SS, et al. "Endogenous steroid hormone concentrations and risk of breast cancer among premenopausal women." *Journal of the National Cancer Institute* 98 (19) (2006): 1406–15.

36 Key TJ. "Endogenous oestrogens and breast cancer risk in premenopausal and postmenopausal women." *Steroids* 76 (8) (2011): 812–15.

37 Cummings SR, Tice JA, Bauer S, et al. "Prevention of breast cancer in postmenopausal women: approaches to estimating and reducing risk." *Journal of the National Cancer Institute* 101 (6) (2009): 384–98.

38 Farhat GN, Cummings SR, Chlebowski RT, et al. "Sex hormone levels and risks of estrogen receptor-negative and estrogen receptor-positive breast cancers." *Journal of the National Cancer Institute* 103 (7) (2011): 562–70.

39 Cummings SR, Tice JA, Bauer S, et al. "Prevention of breast cancer in postmenopausal women: approaches to estimating and reducing risk." *Journal of the National Cancer Institute* 101 (6) (2009): 384–98.

40 Use the following link to find the latest guidelines: http://www.guideline.gov/content.aspx?id=15429.

41 This link with give you more information on the U.S. Preventive Services Task Force Agency: http://www.ahrq.gov/clinic/uspstfix.htm.

42 Schousboe JT, Kerlikowske K, Loh A, Cummings SR. "Personalizing mammography by breast density and other risk factors for breast cancer: analysis of health benefits and cost-effectiveness." *Annals of Internal Medicine* 155 (1) (2011): 10–20.

43 Shepherd JA, Kerlikowske K, Ma L, et al. "Volume of mammographic density and risk of breast cancer." *Cancer Epidemiology, Biomarkers and Prevention* 20 (7) (2011): 1473–82.

44 Nagata C, Kabuto M, Shimizu H. "Association of coffee, green tea, and caffeine intakes with serum concentrations of estradiol and sex hormone-binding globulin in premenopausal Japanese women." *Nutrition and Cancer* 30 (1) (1998): 21–24; Schliep KC, Schisterman EF, Mumford SL, et al. "Caffeinated beverage intake and reproductive hormones among premenopausal women in the BioCycle Study." *American Journal of Clinical Nutrition* 95 (2) (2012): 488–97.

45 Alexander DD, Morimoto LM, Mink PJ, Cushing CA. "A review and meta-analysis of red and processed meat consumption and breast cancer." *Nutrition Research Reviews* 23 (2) (2010): 349–65.

46 Brinkman MT, Baglietto L, Krishnan K, et al. "Consumption of animal products, their nutrient components and postmenopausal circulating steroid hormone concentrations." *European Journal of Clinical Nutrition* 64 (2) (2010): 176–83.

47 Ibid.

48 Aubertin-Leheudre M, Hämäläinen E, Adlercreutz H. "Diets and hormonal levels in postmenopausal women with or without breast cancer." *Nutrition and Cancer* 63 (4) (2011): 514–24; Aubertin-Leheudre M, Gorbach S, Woods M, et al. "Fat/fiber intakes and sex hormones in healthy premenopausal women in USA." *Journal of Steroid Biochemistry and Molecular Biology* 112 (1–3) (2008): 32–39; Bagga D, Ashley JM, Geffrey SP, et al. "Effects of a very low fat, high fiber diet on serum hormones and menstrual function. Implications for breast cancer prevention." *Cancer* 76 (12) (1995): 2491–96; Gaskins AJ, Mumford SL, Zhang C, et al., BioCycle Study Group. "Effect of daily fiber intake on reproductive function: the BioCycle Study." *American Journal of Clinical Nutrition* 90 (4) (2009): 1061–69; Gann PH, Chatterton RT, Gapstur SM, et al. "The effects of a low-fat/high-fiber diet on sex hormone levels and menstrual cycling in premenopausal women: a 12-month randomized trial (the Diet and Hormone Study)." *Cancer* 98 (9) (2003): 1870–79; Goldin BR, Woods MN, Spiegelman DL, et al. "The effect of dietary fat and fiber on serum estrogen concentrations in premenopausal women under controlled dietary conditions." *Cancer* 74 (suppl. 3) (1994): 1125–31; Kaneda N, Nagata C, Kabuto M, Shimizu H. "Fat and fiber intakes in relation to serum estrogen concentration in premenopausal Japanese women." *Nutrition and Cancer* 27 (3) (1997): 279–83; Rose DP, Goldman M, Connolly JM, Strong LE. "High-fiber diet reduces serum estrogen concentrations in premenopausal women." *American Journal of Clinical Nutrition* 54 (3) (1991): 520–25; Woods MN, Barnett JB, Spiegelman D, et al. "Hormone levels during dietary changes in premenopausal African-American women." *Journal of the National Cancer Institute* 88 (19) (1996): 1369–74; Wu AH, Pike MC, Stram DO. "Meta-analysis: dietary fat intake, serum estrogen levels, and the risk of breast cancer." *Journal of the National Cancer Institute* 91 (6) (1999): 529–34.

49 Ganji V, Kuo J. "Serum lipid responses to psyllium fiber: differences between pre- and post-menopausal, hypercholesterolemic women." *Nutrition Journal* 7 (22) (2012). doi: 10.1186/1475-2891-7-22; Vega-López S, Vidal-Quintanar RL, Fernandez ML. "Sex and hormonal

status influence plasma lipid responses to psyllium." *American Journal of Clinical Nutrition* 74 (4) (2001): 435–41.

50 Cummings SR, Tice JA, Bauer S, et al. "Prevention of breast cancer in postmenopausal women: approaches to estimating and reducing risk." *Journal of the National Cancer Institute* 101 (6) (2009): 384–98.

51 Ibid.

52 Del Priore G, Gudipudi DK, Montemarano N, et al. "Oral diindolylmethane (DIM): pilot evaluation of a nonsurgical treatment for cervical dysplasia." *Gynecologic Oncology* 116 (3) (2010): 464–67.

53 Kall MA, Vang O, Clausen J. "Effects of dietary broccoli on human in vivo drug metabolizing enzymes: evaluation of caffeine, oestrone and chlorzoxazone metabolism." *Carcinogenesis* 17 (4) (1996): 793–99.

54 Fowke JH, Longcope C, Hebert JR. "Brassica vegetable consumption shifts estrogen metabolism in healthy postmenopausal women." *Cancer Epidemiology: Biomarkers and Prevention* 9 (8) (2000): 773–79.

55 Reed GA, Sunega JM, Sullivan DK, et al. "Single-dose pharmacokinetics and tolerability of absorption-enhanced 3,3'-diindolylmethane in healthy subjects." *Cancer Epidemiology: Biomarkers and Prevention* 17 (10) (2008): 2619–24.

56 Bradlow HL. Review. "Indole-3-carbinol as a chemoprotective agent in breast and prostate cancer." *In Vivo* 22 (4) (2008): 441–45.

57 Teas J, Hurley TG, Hebert JR, et al. "Dietary seaweed modifies estrogen and phytoestrogen metabolism in healthy postmenopausal women." *Journal of Nutrition* 139 (5) (2009): 939–44.

58 Zahid M, Saeed M, Beseler C, et al. "Resveratrol and N-acetylcysteine block the cancer-initiating step in MCF-10F cells." *Free Radical Biology and Medicine* 50 (1) (2011): 78–85.

59 Dubey RK, Jackson EK, Gillespie DG, et al. "Resveratrol, a red wine constituent, blocks the antimitogenic effects of estradiol on human female coronary artery smooth muscle cells." *Journal of Clinical Endocrinology and Metabolism* 95 (9) (2010): E9–17.

60 Singh M, Singh N. "Curcumin counteracts the proliferative effect of estradiol and induces apoptosis in cervical cancer cells." *Molecular and Cellular Biochemistry* 347 (1–2) (2011): 1–11.

61 Monteiro R, Faria A, Azevedo I, Calhau C. "Modulation of breast cancer cell survival by aromatase inhibiting hop (*Humulus lupulus L.*) flavonoids." *Journal of Steroid Biochemistry and Molecular Biology* 105 (1–5) (2007): 124–30.

62 Pawlikowski M, Kolomecka M, Wojtczak A, Karasek M. "Effects of six months melatonin treatment on sleep quality and serum concentrations of estradiol, cortisol, dehydroepiandrosterone sulfate, and somatomedin C in elderly women." *Neuro Endocrinology Letters* 23 (Supplement 1) (2002): 17–19; Grant SG, Melan MA, Latimer JJ,

Witt-Enderby PA. "Melatonin and breast cancer: cellular mechanisms, clinical studies and future perspectives." *Expert Reviews in Molecular Medicine* 11 (2009): e5.

63 Tinelli A, Vergara D, Martignago R, et al. "Hormonal carcinogenesis and socio-biological development factors in endometrial cancer: a clinical review." *Acta Obstetricia et Gynecologica Scandinavica* 87 (11) (2008): 1101–13.

CHAPTER 7: LOW ESTROGEN

1 Gao Q, Mezei G, Nie Y, et al. "Anorectic estrogen mimics leptin's effect on the rewiring of melanocortin cells and Stat3 signaling in obese animals." *Nature Medicine* (1) (2007): 89–94; Hirschberg AL. "Sex hormones, appetite and eating behaviour in women." *Maturita* 71 (3) (2012): 248–56.

2 Harsh V, Meltzer-Brody S, Rubinow DR, Schmidt PJ. "Reproductive aging, sex steroids, and mood disorders." *Harvard Review of Psychiatry* 17 (2) (2009): 87–102.

3 Freedman RR, Woodward S. "Behavioral treatment of menopausal hot flushes: evaluation by ambulatory monitoring." *American Journal of Obstetric Gynecology* 167 (1992): 436–39.

4 Winther K, Rein E, Hedman C. "Femal, an herbal remedy made from pollen extracts, reduces hot flushes and improves quality of life in menopausal women: a randomized, placebo-controlled, parallel study." *Climacteric* 8 (2) (2005): 162–70.

5 Burger H. "The menopausal transition—endocrinology." *Journal of Sexual Medicine* 5 (10) (2008): 2266–73.

6 Broer SL, Eijkemans MJ, Scheffer GJ, et al. "Anti-Mullerian Hormone Predicts Menopause: A Long-Term Follow-Up Study in Normoovulatory Women." *Journal of Clinical Endocrinology and Metabolism* 96 (8) (2011): 2532–39.

7 Eliassen AH, Ziegler RG, Rosner B. "Reproducibility of fifteen urinary estrogens and estrogen metabolites over a 2- to 3-year period in premenopausal women." *Cancer Epidemiology, Biomarkers & Prevention* 18 (11) (2009): 2860–68.

8 Karelis AD, Fex A, Filion ME. "Comparison of sex hormonal and metabolic profiles between omnivores and vegetarians in pre- and post-menopausal women." *British Journal of Nutrition* 104 (2) (2010): 222–26; Dos Santos Silva I, Mangtani P, McCormack V, et al. "Lifelong vegetarianism and risk of breast cancer: a population-based case-control study among South Asian migrant women living in England." *International Journal of Cancer* 99 (2) (2002): 238–44.

9 Hirayama T. "Epidemiology of breast cancer with special reference to the role of diet." *Preventative Medicine* (2) (1978): 173–95; Iwasaki M,

Tsugane S. "Risk factors for breast cancer: epidemiological evidence from Japanese studies." *Cancer Science* 102 (9) (2011): 1607–14. doi: 10.1111/j.1349-7006.2011.01996.x.

10 Iwasaki M, Tsugane S. "Risk factors for breast cancer: epidemiological evidence from Japanese studies." *Cancer Science* 102 (9) (2011): 1607–14. doi: 10.1111/j.1349-7006.2011.01996.x.

11 O'Donnell E, Goodman JM, Harvey PJ. "Clinical review: cardiovascular consequences of ovarian disruption: a focus on functional hypothalamic amenorrhea in physically active women." *Journal of Clinical Endocrinology and Metabolism* (12) (2011): 3638–48.

12 Pellicano R, Astegiano M, Bruno M. "Women and celiac disease: association with unexplained infertility." *Minerva Medica* 98 (3) (2007): 217–19; Martinelli D, Fortunato F, Tafuri S. "Reproductive life disorders in Italian celiac women. A case-control study." *BMC Gastroenterology* 10 (2010): 89; Soni S, Badawy SZ. "Celiac disease and its effect on human reproduction: a review." *Journal of Reproductive Medicine* 55 (1–2) (2010): 3–8.

13 Martinelli D, Fortunato F, Tafuri S. "Reproductive life disorders in Italian celiac women. A case-control study." *BMC Gastroenterology* 10 (2010): 89; Soni S, Badawy SZ. "Celiac disease and its effect on human reproduction: a review." *Journal of Reproductive Medicine* 55 (1–2) (2010): 3–8.

14 Bykova S, Sabel'nikova E, Parfenov A, et al. "Reproductive disorders in women with celiac disease. Effect of the etiotropic therapy." *Experimental and Clinical Gastroenterology* 3 (2011): 12–18 [article in Russian]; Pradhan M, Manisha, Singh R, Dhingra S. "Celiac disease as a rare cause of primary amenorrhea: a case report." *Journal of Reproductive Medicine* 52 (5) (2007): 453–55; Feuerstein J. "Reversal of premature ovarian failure in a patient with Sjögren syndrome using an elimination diet protocol." *Journal of Alternative and Complementary Medicine* 16 (7) (2010): 807–9.

15 Armstrong D, Don-Wauchope AC, Verdu EF. "Testing for gluten-related disorders in clinical practice: the role of serology in managing the spectrum of gluten sensitivity." *Canadian Journal of Gastroenterology* 25 (4) (2011): 193–97.

16 Kotsopoulos J, Eliassen AH, Missmer SA, et al. "Relationship between caffeine intake and plasma sex hormone concentrations in premenopausal and postmenopausal women." *Cancer* 115 (12) (2009): 2765–74.

17 Nagata C, Shimizu H, Takami R, et al. "Hot flushes and other menopausal symptoms in relation to soy product intake in Japanese women." *Climacteric* 2 (1) (1999): 6–12; Wu AH, Stanczyk FZ, Seow A, et al. "Soy intake and other lifestyle determinants of serum estrogen

levels among postmenopausal Chinese women in Singapore." *Cancer Epidemiology: Biomarkers and Prevention* 11 (9) (2002): 844–51; Zhang X, Shu XO, Li H, et al. "Prospective cohort study of soy food consumption and risk of bone fracture among postmenopausal women." *Archives of Internal Medicine* 165 (16) (2005): 1890–95.

18 Hooper L, Ryder JJ, Kurzer MS. "Effects of soy protein and isoflavones on circulating hormone concentrations in pre- and post-menopausal women: a systematic review and meta-analysis." *Human Reproduction Update* 15 (4) (2009): 423–40.

19 Lethaby AE, Brown J, Marjoribanks J, et al. "Phytoestrogens for vasomotor menopausal symptoms." *Cochrane Database of Systematic Reviews* 17 (4) (2007): CD001395; Nelson HD, Vesco KK, Haney E, et al. "Nonhormonal therapies for menopausal hot flashes: systematic review and meta-analysis." *Journal of the American Medical Association* 295 (17) (2006): 2057–71; Pitkin J. "Alternative and complementary therapies for the menopause." *Menopause International* (1) (2012): 20–27; Taku K, Melby MK, Kronenberg F, et al. "Extracted or synthesized soybean isoflavones reduce menopausal hot flash frequency and severity: systematic review and meta-analysis of randomized controlled trials." *Climacteric.* 15 (2) (2012): 115–24; Trock BJ, Hilakivi-Clarke L, Clarke R. "Meta-analysis of soy intake and breast cancer risk." *Journal of the National Cancer Institute* 98 (7) (2006): 459–71; Villaseca P. "Non-estrogen conventional and phytochemical treatments for vasomotor symptoms: what needs to be known for practice." *Climacteric* 15 (2) (2012): 115–24.

20 Hooper L, Ryder JJ, Kurzer MS. "Effects of soy protein and isoflavones on circulating hormone concentrations in pre- and post-menopausal women: a systematic review and meta-analysis." *Human Reproduction Update* 15 (4) (2009): 423–40.

21 Pruthi SL, Thompson PJ, Novotny DL, et al. "Pilot evaluation of flaxseed for the management of hot flashes." *Journal for the Society of Integrative Oncology* 5 (3) (2007): 106–12.

22 van Anders SM, Brotto L, Farrell J, Yule M. "Associations among physiological and subjective sexual response, sexual desire, and salivary steroid hormones in healthy premenopausal women." *Journal of Sexual Medicine* 6 (3) (2009): 739–51.

23 Nicole Daedone, personal communication, founder of OneTaste.us, on May 18, 2012.

24 Azizi H, Feng Liu Y, Du L, Hua Wang C, et al. "Menopause-related Symptoms: Traditional Chinese Medicine vs Hormone Therapy." *Alternative Therapies in Health and Medicine* 17 (4) (2011): 48–53.

25 Sunay D, Ozdiken M, Arslan H, et al. "The effect of acupuncture on postmenopausal symptoms and reproductive hormones: a sham controlled clinical trial." *Acupuncture in Medicine* 29 (1) (2011): 27–31.

26 Auerbach L, Rakus J, Bauer C, et al. "Pomegranate seed oil in women with menopausal symptoms: a prospective randomized, placebo-controlled, double-blinded trial." *Menopause* 19 (4) (2012): 426–32.

27 Park H, Parker GL, Boardman CH, et al. "A pilot phase II trial of magnesium supplements to reduce menopausal hot flashes in breast cancer patients." *Supportive Care in Cancer* 19 (6) (2011): 859–63.

28 Meissner H, Kapczynski W, Mscisz A, et al. "Use of a gelatinized maca (*Lepidium peruvianum*) in early-postmenopausal women—a pilot study." *International Journal of Biomedical Science* I (1) (2005): 33–45; Meissner H, et al. "Hormone-balancing effect of pre-gelatinized organic maca (*Lepidium peruvianum Chacon*): (III) Clinical responses of early-postmenopausal women to maca in double-blind, randomized, crossover configuration, outpatient study." *International Journal of Biomedical Science* 2 (4) (2006): 375–94.

29 Brooks NA, Wilcox G, Walker KZ, et al. "Beneficial effects of *Lepidium meyenii* (maca) on psychological symptoms and measures of sexual dysfunction in postmenopausal women are not related to estrogen or androgen content." *Menopause* 15 (6) (2008): 1157–62.

30 Dording CM, Fisher L, Papakostas G, et al. "A double-blind, randomized, pilot dose-finding study of maca root (*L. meyenii*) for the management of SSRI-induced sexual dysfunction." *CNS Neuroscience and Therapeutics* 14 (3) (2008): 182–91.

31 Weaver CM, Martin BR, Jackson GS, et al. "Antiresorptive effects of phytoestrogen supplements compared with estradiol or risedronate in postmenopausal women using (41)Ca methodology." *Journal of Clinical Endocrinology and Metabolism* 94 (10) (2009): 3798–805; Okamura S, Sawada Y, Satoh T, et al. "*Pueraria mirifica* phytoestrogens improve dyslipidemia in postmenopausal women probably by activating estrogen receptor subtypes." *Tohoku Journal of Experimental Medicine* 216 (4) (2008): 341–51.

32 Heger M, Ventskovskiy BM, Borzenko I, et al. "Efficacy and safety of a special extract of *Rheum rhaponticum* (ERr 731) in perimenopausal women with climacteric complaints: a 12-week randomized, double-blind, placebo-controlled trial." *Menopause* 13 (5): 744–59; Kaszkin-Bettag M, Ventskovskiy BM, Solskyy S, et al. "Confirmation of the efficacy of ERr 731 in perimenopausal women with menopausal symptoms." *Alternative Therapies in Health and Medicine* 15 (1) (2009): 24–34.

33 Abdali K, Khajehei M, Tabatabaee HR. "Effect of St John's wort on severity, frequency, and duration of hot flashes in premenopausal, perimenopausal and postmenopausal women: a randomized, double-blind, placebo-controlled study." *Menopause* 17 (2) (2010): 326–31.

34 Grube B, Walper A, Wheatley D. "St. John's Wort extract: efficacy for menopausal symptoms of psychological origin." *Advances in Therapy* 16 (4) (1999): 177–86.

35 Uebelhack R, Blohmer JU, Graubaum HJ, et al. "Black cohosh and St. John's wort for climacteric complaints: a randomized trial." *Obstetrics and Gynecology* 107 (2 Pt 1) (2006): 247–55.

36 Rostock M, Fischer J, Mumm A, et al. "Black cohosh (*Cimicifuga racemosa*) in tamoxifen-treated breast cancer patients with climacteric complaints—a prospective observational study." *Gynecological Endocrinology* 27 (10) (2011): 844–48.

37 Kim SY, Seo SK, Choi YM, et al. "Effects of red ginseng supplementation on menopausal symptoms and cardiovascular risk factors in postmenopausal women: a double-blind randomized controlled trial." *Menopause* 19 (4) (2012): 461–66.

38 Tode T, Kikuchi Y, Hirata J, et al. "Effect of Korean red ginseng on psychological functions in patients with severe climacteric syndromes." *International Journal of Gynaecology and Obstetrics* 67 (3) (1999): 169–74.

39 Wiklund L, Mattsson L, Lindgren R, Limoni C. "Effects of a standardized ginseng on the quality of life and physiological parameters in symptomatic postmenopausal women: a double-blind, placebo-controlled trial." *International Journal of Clinical Pharmacology Research* 19 (3) (1999): 89–99.

40 Rister R, Klein S, Riggins C. *The Complete German Commission E Monographs: Therapeutic Guide to Herbal Medicines* (Austin, TX: American Botanical Council, 1998).

41 Taavoni S, Ekbatani N, Kashaniyan M, Haghani H. "Effect of valerian on sleep quality in postmenopausal women: a randomized placebo-controlled clinical trial." *Menopause* 18 (9) (2011): 951–55.

42 Kuhlmann J, Berger W, Podzuweit H, Schmidt U. "The influence of valerian treatment on 'reaction time, alertness and concentration' in volunteers." *Pharmacopsychiatry* 32 (1999): 235–41.

43 Taavoni S, Ekbatani N, Kashaniyan M, Haghani H. "Effect of valerian on sleep quality in postmenopausal women: a randomized placebo-controlled clinical trial." *Menopause* 18 (9) (2011): 951–55.

44 Hirata JD, Swiersz LM, Zell B. "Does dong quai have estrogenic effects in postmenopausal women? A double-blind, placebo-controlled trial." *Fertility and Sterility* 68 (1997): 981–86.

45 Zhu DP. "Dong quai." *American Journal of Chinese Medicine* 15 (3–4) (1987): 117–25; Zava DT, Dollbaum CM, Blen M. "Estrogen and progestin bioactivity of foods, herbs, and spices." *Proceedings of the Society for Experimental Biology and Medicine* 217 (3) (1998): 369–78; Amato P, Christophe S, Mellon PL. "Estrogenic activity of herbs commonly used as remedies for menopausal symptoms." *Menopause* 9 (2002): 145–50.

46 Baber RJ, Templeman C, Morton T, et al. "Randomized placebo-controlled trial of isoflavone supplement on menopausal symptoms in women." *Climacteric* 2 (2) (1999): 85–92; Tice JA, Ettinger B, Ensrud K. "Phytoestrogen supplements for the treatment of hot flashes: the Isoflavone Clover Extract (ICE) Study: a randomized controlled trial." *Journal of the American Medical Association* 290 (2) (2003): 207–14; Knight DC, Howes JB, Eden JA. "The effect of Promensil, an isoflavone extract, on menopausal symptoms." *Climacteric* (2) (1999): 79–84.

47 Cosgrove L, Shi L, Creasey DE, et al. "Antidepressants and breast and ovarian cancer risk: a review of the literature and researchers' financial associations with industry." *PLoS One* 6 (4) (2011): e18210.

48 Lindheim SR, Legro RS, Bernstein L, et al. "Behavioral stress responses in premenopausal and postmenopausal women and the effects of estrogen." *American Journal of Obstetrics and Gynecology* 167 (6) (1992): 1831–36.

49 Lokuge S, Frey BN, Foster JA, et al. "Depression in women: windows of vulnerability and new insights into the link between estrogen and serotonin." *Journal of Clinical Psychiatry* 72 (11) (2011): e1563–69.

50 Soares CN, Almeida OP, Joffe H, Cohen LS. "Efficacy of estradiol for the treatment of depressive disorders in perimenopausal women: a double-blind, randomized, placebo-controlled trial." *Archives of General Psychiatry* 58 (6) (2001): 529–34.

51 Rossouw JE, Anderson GL, Prentice RL, et al.; Writing Group for the Women's Health Initiative Investigators. "Risks and benefits of estrogen plus progestin in healthy postmenopausal women: principal results from the Women's Health Initiative randomized controlled trial." *Journal of the American Medical Association* 288 (3) (2002): 321–33.

52 Gorney C. "The Estrogen Dilemma." *New York Times Magazine,* April 14, 2010. http://www.nytimes.com/2010/04/18/magazine/18estrogen-t.html?pagewanted=all.

53 Somers S. *Ageless: The Naked Truth About Bioidentical Hormones.* New York: Crown Publishers, 2006.

54 Yong M, Atkinson C, Newton KM. "Associations between endogenous sex hormone levels and mammographic and bone densities in premenopausal women." *Cancer Causes Control* 20 (7) (2009): 1039–53.

55 Huang Y, Malone KE, Cushing-Haugen KL, et al. "Relationship between menopausal symptoms and risk of postmenopausal breast cancer." *Cancer Epidemiology Biomarkers & Prevention* 20 (2) (2011): 379–88.

56 Szmuilowicz ED, Manson JE, Rossouw JE, et al. "Vasomotor symptoms and cardiovascular events in postmenopausal women." *Menopause* 18 (6) (2011): 603–10.

57 Files JA, Ko MG, Pruthi S. "Bioidentical Hormone Therapy." *Mayo Clinic Proceedings* 86 (7) (2011): 673–80.

CHAPTER 8: EXCESS ANDROGENS

1 March WA, Moore VM, Willson KJ, et al. "The prevalence of polycystic ovary syndrome in a community sample assessed under contrasting diagnostic criteria." *Human Reproduction* 25 (2010): 544–51. doi: 10.1093/humrep/dep399.

2 Dabbs JM Jr, Hargrove MF. "Age, testosterone, and behavior among female prison inmates." *Psychosomatic Medicine* 59 (5) (1997): 477–80.

3 Bromberger JT, Schott LL, Kravitz HM, et al. "Longitudinal change in reproductive hormones and depressive symptoms across the menopausal transition: results from the Study of Women's Health Across the Nation (SWAN)." *Archives of General Psychiatry* 67 (6) (2010): 598–607.

4 Sapienza P, Zingales L, Maestripieri D. "Gender differences in financial risk aversion and career choices are affected by testosterone." *Proceedings of the National Academy of Sciences of the United States of America* 106 (36) (2009): 15268–73.

5 Morrison MF, Freeman EW, Lin H, Sammel MD. "Higher DHEA-S (dehydroepiandrosterone sulfate) levels are associated with depressive symptoms during the menopausal transition: results from the PENN Ovarian Aging Study." *Archives of Women's Mental Health* 14 (5) (2011): 375–82. doi: 10.1007/s00737-011-0231-5; Chen MJ, Chen CD, Yang JH, et al. "High serum dehydroepiandrosterone sulfate is associated with phenotypic acne and a reduced risk of abdominal obesity in women with polycystic ovary syndrome." *Human Reproduction* 26 (1) (2011): 227–34; Villareal DT, Holloszy JO. "Effect of DHEA on abdominal fat and insulin action in elderly women and men: a randomized controlled trial." *Journal of the American Medical Association* 292 (18) (2004): 2243–48.

6 Panjari M, Davis SR. "Vaginal DHEA to treat menopause-related atrophy: a review of the evidence." *Maturitas* 70 (1) (2011): 22–25.

7 Camacho-Martínez FM. "Hair loss in women." *Seminars in Cutaneous Medicine and Surgery* 28 (1) (2009): 19–32.

8 Legro RS. "Insulin resistance in polycystic ovary syndrome:

treating a phenotype without a genotype." *Molecular and Cellular Endocrinology* 145 (1–2) (1998): 103–10.

9 Wild RA, Carmina E, Diamanti-Kandarakis E, et al. "Assessment of cardiovascular risk and prevention of cardiovascular disease in women with the polycystic ovary syndrome: a consensus statement by the Androgen Excess and Polycystic Ovary Syndrome (AE-PCOS) Society." *Journal of Clinical Endocrinology and Metabolism* 95 (5) (2010): 2038–49.

10 Boudarene M, Legros JJ, Timsit-Berthier M. "Study of the stress response: role of anxiety, cortisol and DHEAs." *Encephale* 28 (2) (2002): 139–46 [article in French].

11 Rosenfield RL, Bordini B. "Evidence that obesity and androgens have independent and opposing effects on gonadotropin production from puberty to maturity." *Brain Research* 1364 (2010): 186–97.

12 Huang A, Brennan K, Azziz R. "Prevalence of hyperandrogenemia in the polycystic ovary syndrome diagnosed by the National Institutes of Health 1990 criteria." *Fertility and Sterility* 93 (6) (2010): 1938–41; Azziz R, Sanchez LA, Knochenhauer ES, et al. "Androgen excess in women: experience with over 1,000 consecutive patients." *Journal of Clinical Endocrinology and Metabolism* 89 (2) (2004): 453–62.

13 Yildiz BO. "Diagnosis of hyperandrogenism: clinical criteria." *Best Practice and Research: Clinical Endocrinology & Metabolism* 20 (2) (2006): 167–76.

14 Sathyapalan T, Atkin SL. "Mediators of inflammation in polycystic ovary syndrome in relation to adiposity." *Mediators of Inflammation* 758656 (2010); Escobar-Morreale HF, Luque-Ramírez M, González F. "Circulating inflammatory markers in polycystic ovary syndrome: a systematic review and metaanalysis." *Fertility and Sterility* 95 (3) (2011): 1048–58. e1–2; Repaci A, Gambineri A, Pasquali R. "The role of low-grade inflammation in the polycystic ovary syndrome." *Molecular and Cellular Endocrinology* 335 (1) (2011): 30–41.

15 Lambrinoudaki I. "Cardiovascular risk in postmenopausal women with the polycystic ovary syndrome." *Maturitas* 68 (1) (2011): 13–16.

16 Puurunen J, Piltonen T, Morin-Papunen L, et al. "Unfavorable hormonal, metabolic, and inflammatory alterations persist after menopause in women with PCOS." *Journal of Clinical Endocrinology and Metabolism* 96 (6) (2011): 1827–34.

17 de França Neto AH, Rogatto S, Do Amorim MM, et al. "Oncological repercussions of polycystic ovary syndrome." *Gynecological Endocrinology* 26 (10) (2010): 708–11; Hardiman P, Pillay OS, Atiomo A. "Polycystic ovary syndrome and endometrial carcinoma." *Lancet* 361 (2003): 1810–12. Erratum in *Lancet* 362 (9389) (2003): 1082.

18 Barry JA, Hardiman PJ, Saxby BK, Kuczmierczyk A. "Testosterone

and mood dysfunction in women with polycystic ovarian syndrome compared to subfertile controls." *Journal of Psychosomatic Obstetrics and Gynaecology* 32 (2) (2011): 104–11; Himelein MJ, Thatcher SS. "Polycystic ovary syndrome and mental health: a review." *Obstetrical and Gynecological Survey* 61 (11) (2006): 723–32; Pastore LM, Patrie JT, Morris WL, et al. "Depression symptoms and body dissatisfaction association among polycystic ovary syndrome women." *Journal of Psychosomatic Research* 71 (4) (2011): 270–76.

19 Livadas S, Chaskou S, Kandaraki AA, et al. "Anxiety is associated with hormonal and metabolic profile in women with polycystic ovarian syndrome." *Clinical Endocrinology (Oxford)* 75 (5) (2011): 698–703. doi: 10.1111/j.1365–2265.2011.04122.x.

20 Schwimmer JB, Khorram O, Chiu V, Schwimmer WB. "Abnormal aminotransferase activity in women with polycystic ovary syndrome." *Fertility and Sterility* 83 (2005): 494–97; Economou F, Xyrafis X, Livadas S, et al. "In overweight/obese but not in normal-weight women, polycystic ovary syndrome is associated with elevated liver enzymes compared to controls." *Hormones (Athens)* 8 (3) (2009): 199–206.

21 Sheehan MT. "Polycystic ovarian syndrome: diagnosis and management." *Clinical Medicine and Research* 2 (1) (2004): 13–27.

22 Lass N, Kleber M, Winkel K, et al. "Effect of Lifestyle Intervention on Features of Polycystic Ovarian Syndrome, Metabolic Syndrome, and Intima-Media Thickness in Obese Adolescent Girls." *Journal of Clinical Endocrinology and Metabolism* 96 (11) (2011): 3533–40.

23 Smith RN, Mann NJ, Braue A, et al. "The effect of a high-protein, low glycemic-load diet versus a conventional, high glycemic-load diet on biochemical parameters associated with acne vulgaris: a randomized, investigator-masked, controlled trial." *Journal of the American Academy of Dermatology* 57 (2) (2007): 247–56; Smith R, Mann N, Mäkeläinen H, et al. "A pilot study to determine the short-term effects of a low glycemic load diet on hormonal markers of acne: a nonrandomized, parallel, controlled feeding trial." *Molecular Nutrition and Food Research* 52 (6) (2008): 718–26.

24 Marsh K, Brand-Miller J. "The optimal diet for women with polycystic ovary syndrome?" *British Journal of Nutrition* 94 (2) (2005): 154–65.

25 Simopoulos AP. "The importance of the ratio of omega-6/omega-3 essential fatty acids." *Biomedicine and Pharmacotherapy* 56 (8) (2002): 365–79.

26 Phelan N, O'Connor A, Kyaw Tun T, et al. "Hormonal and metabolic effects of polyunsaturated fatty acids in young women with polycystic ovary syndrome: results from a cross-sectional analysis and a randomized, placebo-controlled, crossover trial." *American Journal of Clinical Nutrition* 93 (3) (2011): 652–62.

27 Nidhi R, Padmalatha V, Nagarathna R, Ram A. "Effect of a yoga program on glucose metabolism and blood lipid levels in adolescent girls with polycystic ovary syndrome." *International Journal of Gynaecology and Obstetrics* 24 (4) (2012): 223–27.

28 Anderson RA. "Chromium and polyphenols from cinnamon improve insulin sensitivity." *Proceedings of the Nutrition Society* 67 (1) (2008): 48–53.

29 No author listed. "A scientific review: the role of chromium in insulin resistance." *The Diabetes Educator* (2004): Supplement 2–14.

30 Nordio M, Proietti E. "The combined therapy with myo-inositol and D-chiro-inositol reduces the risk of metabolic disease in PCOS overweight patients compared to myo-inositol supplementation alone." *European Review for Medical and Pharmacological Sciences* 16 (5) (2012): 575–81.

31 Nestler JE, Jakubowicz DJ, Reamer P, et al. "Ovulatory and metabolic effects of D-chiro-inositol in the polycystic ovary syndrome." *New England Journal of Medicine* 340 (17) (1999): 1314–20.

32 Iuorno MJ, Jakubowicz DJ, Baillargeon JP, et al. "Effects of d-chiro-inositol in lean women with the polycystic ovary syndrome." *Endocrine Practice* 8 (6) (2002): 417–23.

33 Li HW, Brereton RE, Anderson RA, et al. "Vitamin D deficiency is common and associated with metabolic risk factors in patients with polycystic ovary syndrome." *Metabolism* 60 (10) (2011): 1475–81.

34 Stener-Victorin E, Waldenström U, Tägnfors U, et al. "Effects of electro-acupuncture on anovulation in women with polycystic ovary syndrome." *Acta Obstetricia et Gynecologica Scandinavica* 79 (3) (2000): 180–88.

35 Diamanti-Kandarakis E, Piperi C, Spina J, et al. "Polycystic ovary syndrome: the influence of environmental and genetic factors." *Hormones (Athens)* 5 (1) (2006): 17–34; Kandaraki E, Chatzigeorgiou A, Livadas S, et al. "Endocrine disruptors and polycystic ovary syndrome (PCOS): elevated serum levels of bisphenol A in women with PCOS." *Journal of Clinical Endocrinology and Metabolism* 96 (3) (2011): E480–84.

36 Zhang J, Li T, Zhou L, et al. "Chinese herbal medicine for subfertile women with polycystic ovarian syndrome." *Cochrane Database of Systematic Reviews* 9 (2010): CD007535.

37 Anderson RA. "Chromium and polyphenols from cinnamon improve insulin sensitivity." *Proceedings of the Nutrition Society* 67 (1) (2008): 48–53.

38 Ziegenfuss TN, Hofheins JE, Mendel RW, et al. "Effects of a water-soluble cinnamon extract on body composition and features of the

metabolic syndrome in pre-diabetic men and women." *Journal of the International Society of Sports Nutrition* 3 (2006): 45–53.

39 Kuek S, Wang WJ, Gui SQ. "Efficacy of Chinese patent medicine Tian Gui Capsule in patients with polycystic ovary syndrome: a randomized controlled trial." *Zhong Xi Yi Jie He Xue Bao (Journal of Chinese Integrative Medicine)* 9 (9) (2011): 965–72.

CHAPTER 9: LOW THYROID

1 Kritz-Silverstein D, Schultz ST, Palinska LA, et al. "The association of thyroid stimulating hormone levels with cognitive function and depressed mood: the Rancho Bernardo study." *Journal of Nutrition Health and Aging* 13 (4) (2009): 317–21.

2 Gold MS, Pottash AL, Extein I. "Hypothyroidism and depression. Evidence from complete thyroid function evaluation." *Journal of the American Medical Association* 245 (19) (1981): 1919–22; Hickie I, Bennett B, Mitchell P, et al. "Clinical and subclinical hypothyroidism in patients with chronic and treatment-resistant depression." *Australian and New Zealand Journal of Psychiatry* 30 (2) (1996): 246–52.

3 Canaris GJ, Manowitz NR, Mayor G, Ridgway EC. "The Colorado Thyroid Disease Prevalence Study." *Archives of Internal Medicine* 160 (2000): 526–34; Empson M, Flood V, Ma G, et al. "Prevalence of thyroid disease in an older Australian population." *International Medical Journal* 37 (7) (2007): 448–55.

4 "Oxford Companion to the Body: thyroid gland," accessed 2012 http://www.answers.com/topic/thyroid-1, http://www.netplaces.com/thyroid-disease/hypothyroidism/blood-tests.htm.

5 Shifren JL, Desindes S, McIlwain M, et al. "A randomized, open-label, crossover study comparing the effects of oral versus transdermal estrogen therapy on serum androgens, thyroid hormones, and adrenal hormones in naturally menopausal women." *Menopause* 14 (6) (2007): 985–94.

6 Van den Beld AW, Visser TJ, Feelders RA, et al. "Thyroid hormone concentrations, disease, physical function, and mortality in elderly men." *Journal of Clinical Endocrinology and Metabolism* 90 (12) (2005): 6403–9.

7 Parle J, Roberts L, Wilson S, et al. "A randomized controlled trial of the effect of thyroxine replacement on cognitive function in community-living elderly subjects with subclinical hypothyroidism: the Birmingham Elderly Thyroid study." *Journal of Clinical Endocrinology and Metabolism* 95 (8) (2010): 3623–32; Pollock MA, Sturrock A, Marshall K, et al. "Thyroxine treatment in patients with symptoms of hypothyroidism but thyroid function tests within the reference range: randomised double blind placebo controlled

crossover trial." *British Medical Journal* 323 (7318) (2001): 891–95; Surks MI, Ortiz E, Daniels GH, et al. "Subclinical thyroid disease: scientific review and guidelines for diagnosis and management." *Journal of the American Medical Association* 291 (2) (2004): 228–38; Villar HC, Saconato H, Valente O, Atallah AN. "Thyroid hormone replacement for subclinical hypothyroidism." *Cochrane Database of Systematic Reviews* 3 (2007): CD003419.

8 Cai Y, Ren Y, Shi J. "Blood pressure levels in patients with subclinical thyroid dysfunction: a meta-analysis of cross-sectional data." *Hypertension Research* 34 (10) (2011): 1098–105. doi: 10.1038/hr.2011.91; Magri F, Buonocore M, Camera A, et al. "Improvement of intra-epidermal nerve fiber density in hypothyroidism after L-thyroxine therapy." *Clinical Endocrinology (Oxford)* (2012), doi: 10.1111/j.1365–2265.2012.04447.x; Razvi S, Weaver JU, Butler TJ, Pearce SH. "Levothyroxine Treatment of Subclinical Hypothyroidism, Fatal and Nonfatal Cardiovascular Events, and Mortality." *Archives of Internal Medicine* 172 (10) (2012): 811–17; Reid SM, Middleton P, Cossich MC, Crowther CA. "Interventions for clinical and subclinical hypothyroidism in pregnancy." *Cochrane Database of Systematic Reviews* 7 (2010): CD007752; Van den Boogaard E, Vissenberg R, Land JA, et al. "Significance of (sub)clinical thyroid dysfunction and thyroid autoimmunity before conception and in early pregnancy: a systematic review." *Human Reproduction Update* 17 (5) (2011): 605–19; Villar HC, Saconato H, Valente O, Atallah AN. "Thyroid hormone replacement for subclinical hypothyroidism." *Cochrane Database of Systematic Reviews* 3 (2007): CD 003419.

9 Wartofsky L, Dickey RA. "The evidence for a narrower thyrotropin reference range is compelling." *Journal of Clinical Endocrinology and Metabolism* 90 (9) (2005): 5483–88.

10 Brent GA. "Clinical practice. Graves' disease." *New England Journal of Medicine* 358 (24) (2008): 2594–605.

11 Pearce EN, Farwell AP, Braverman LE. "Thyroiditis." *New England Journal of Medicine* 348 (2003): 2646–55.

12 Tan ZS, Beiser A, Vasan RS, et al. "Thyroid Function and the Risk of Alzheimer Disease: The Framingham Study." *Archives of Internal Medicine* 168 (14) (2008): 1514–20.

13 Hak AE, Pols HA, Visser TJ, et al. "Subclinical hypothyroidism is an independent risk factor for atherosclerosis and myocardial infarction in elderly women: the Rotterdam Study." *Annals of Internal Medicine* 132 (4) (2000): 270–78.

14 Martins RM, Fonseca RH, Duarte MM, et al. "Impact of subclinical hypothyroidism treatment in systolic and diastolic cardiac function." *Arquivos Brasileiros de Endocrinologia e Metabologia* 55 (7) (2011): 460–67.

15 Diamanti-Kandarakis E, Bourguignon JP, Giudice LC, et al. "Endocrine-Disrupting Chemicals: An Endocrine Society Scientific Statement." *Endocrine Reviews* 30 (4) (2009): 293–342.

16 Sund-Levander M, Forsberg C, Wahren LK. "Normal oral, rectal, tympanic and axillary body temperature in adult men and women: a systematic literature review." *Scandinavian Journal of Caring Science* 16 (2) (2002): 122–28.

17 Marwaha RK, Tandon N, Garg MK, et al. "Thyroid status two decades after salt iodisation: Country-wide data in school children from India." *Clinical Endocrinology (Oxford)* (2011). doi: 10.1111/j.1365-2265.2011.04307.x.

18 Mazzoccoli G, Carughi S, Sperandeo M, et al. "Neuro-endocrine correlations of hypothalamic-pituitary-thyroid axis in healthy humans." *Journal of Biological Regulators and Homeostatic Agents* 25 (2) (2011): 249–57.

19 Roelfsema F, Pereira AM, Biermasz NR, et al. "Diminished and irregular TSH secretion with delayed acrophase in patients with Cushing's syndrome." *European Journal of Endocrinology* 161 (5) (2009): 695–703.

20 Kivity S, Agmon-Levin N, Zisappl M, et al. "Vitamin D and autoimmune thyroid diseases." *Cellular and Molecular Immunology* 8 (3) (2011): 243–47; Tamer G, Arik S, Tamer I, Coksert D. "Relative vitamin D insufficiency in Hashimoto's thyroiditis." *Thyroid* 21 (8) (2011): 891–96.

21 Assimakopoulos SF, Papageorgiou I, Charonis A. "Enterocytes' tight junctions: From molecules to diseases." *World Journal of Gastrointestinal Pathophysiology* 2 (6) (2011): 123–37.

22 Metso S, Hyytiä-Ilmonen H, Kaukinen K, et al. "Gluten-free diet and autoimmune thyroiditis in patients with celiac disease. A prospective controlled study." *Scandinavian Journal of Gastroenterology* 47 (1) (2012): 43–48.

23 Ibid.; Sategna-Guidetti C, Volta U, Ciacci C, et al. "Prevalence of thyroid disorders in untreated adult celiac disease patients and effect of gluten withdrawal: an Italian multicenter study." *American Journal of Gastroenterology* 96 (3) (2001): 751–57.

24 Reid JR, Wheeler SF. "Hyperthyroidism: Diagnosis and Treatment." *American Family Physician* 72 (4) (2005): 623–30.

25 Rushton DH, Dover R, Sainsbury AW, et al. "Iron deficiency is neglected in women's health." *British Medical Journal* 325 (7373) (2002): 1176.

26 Nishiyama S, Futagoishi-Suginohara Y, Matsukura M, et al. "Zinc supplementation alters thyroid hormone metabolism in disabled patients with zinc deficiency." *Journal of the American College of Nutrition* 13 (1) (1994): 62–67.

27 Toulis KA, Anastasilakis AD, Tzellos TG, et al. "Selenium supplementation in the treatment of Hashimoto's thyroiditis: a systematic review and a meta-analysis." *Thyroid* 20 (10) (2010): 1163–73.

28 Schomburg L. "Selenium, selenoproteins and the thyroid gland: interactions in health and disease." *Nature Reviews Endocrinology* 8 (3) (2011):160–71. doi: 10.1038/nrendo.2011.174.

29 Olivieri O, Girelli D, Azzini M, et al. "Low selenium status in the elderly influences thyroid hormones."*Clinical Science (London)* 89 (6) (1995): 637–42; Olivieri O, Girelli D, Stanzial AM, et al. "Selenium, zinc, and thyroid hormones in healthy subjects: low T3/T4 ratio in the elderly is related to impaired selenium status." *Biological Trace Element Research* 51 (1) (1996): 31–41.

30 Hess SY. "The impact of common micronutrient deficiencies on iodine and thyroid metabolism: the evidence from human studies." *Best Practice and Research: Clinical Endocrinology and Metabolism* 24 (1) (2010): 117–32.

31 Rushton DH, Dover R, Sainsbury AW, et al. "Iron deficiency is neglected in women's health." *British Medical Journal* 325 (7373) (2002): 1176.

32 "University of Maryland: Hypothyroidism," http://www.umm.edu/altmed/articles/hypothyroidism-000093.htm.

33 Bowthorpe J. *Stop the Thyroid Madness: A Patient Revolution Against Decades of Inferior Treatment* (Fredericksburg, TX: Laughing Grape Publishing, 2011); Shomon MJ. *Living Well with Hypothyroidism: What Your Doctor Doesn't Tell You . . . That You Need to Know (Revised Edition)* (New York: William Morrow Paperbacks, 2005); Shomon MJ. *The Thyroid Diet Revolution: Manage Your Master Gland of Metabolism for Lasting Weight Loss* (New York: William Morrow Paperbacks, 2012).

CHAPTER 10: COMMON COMBINATIONS OF HORMONAL IMBALANCES

1 Abdullatif HD, Ashraf AP. "Reversible subclinical hypothyroidism in the presences of adrenal insufficiency." *Endocrine Practice* 12 (5) (2006): 572; Doshi SR. "Relative adrenal insufficiency masquerading hypothyroidism." *Journal of Clinical and Diagnostic Research* 4 (4) (2010): 2907–9; Fitzgerald KN. *Case Studies in Integrative and Functional Medicine.* Duluth, GA: Metametrix Institute: 2011; Mathioudakis N, Thapa S, Wand GS, Salvatori R. "ACTH-secreting pituitary microadenomas are associated with a higher prevalence of central hypothyroidism compared to other microadenoma types." *Clinical Endocrinology (Oxford)* (2012). doi: 10.1111/j.1365-2265.2012.04442.x; Mazzoccoli G, Carughi S, Sperandeo M, et al. "Neuro-endocrine correlations of hypothalamic-pituitary-thyroid axis in healthy humans." *Journal of Biological Regulators and Homeostatic*

Agents 25 (2) (2011): 249–57; Roelfsema F, Pereira AM, Biermasz NR, et al. "Diminished and irregular TSH secretion with delayed acrophase in patients with Cushing's syndrome." *European Journal of Endocrinology* 161 (5) (2009): 695–703.

2 Mazzoccoli G, Carughi S, Sperandeo M, et al. "Neuro-endocrine correlations of hypothalamic-pituitary-thyroid axis in healthy humans." *Journal of Biological Regulators and Homeostatic Agents* 25 (2) (2011): 249–57.

3 Boas M, Feldt-Rasmussen U, Main KM. "Thyroid effects of endocrine disrupting chemicals." *Molecular Cellular Endocrinology* 355 (2) (2012): 240–48; Boas M, Main KM, Feldt-Rasmussen U. "Environmental chemicals and thyroid function: an update." *Current Opinion in Endocrinology, Diabetes and Obesity* 16 (5) (2009): 385–91; Patrick L. "Thyroid disruption: mechanism and clinical implications in human health." *Alternative Medicine Review* 14 (4) (2009): 326–46; Jugan ML, Levi Y, Blondeau JP. "Endocrine disruptors and thyroid hormone physiology." *Biochemical Pharmacology* 79 (7) (2010): 939–47.

4 Cohen S, Janicki-Deverts D, Doyle WJ, et al. "Chronic stress, glucocorticoid receptor resistance, inflammation, and disease risk." *Proceedings of the National Academy of Sciences of the United States of America* 109 (16) (2012): 5995–99.

5 Cole SW. "Social regulation of leukocyte homeostasis: the role of glucocorticoid sensitivity." *Brain Behavior and Immunity* 22 (7) (2008): 1049–55; Meagher MW, Johnson RR, Good E, Welsh TH. "Social stress alters the severity of a virally initiated model of multiple sclerosis." *Psychoneuroimmunology* 4th ed. Ader R, Felton D, Cohen N, eds. *Academic*, vol II (2006): 1107–24.

6 Cohen S, Janicki-Deverts D, Doyle WJ, et al. "Chronic stress, glucocorticoid receptor resistance, inflammation, and disease risk." *Proceedings of the National Academy of Sciences of the United States of America* 109 (16) (2012): 5995–99.

7 Goosens KA, Sapolsky RM. "Stress and Glucocorticoid Contributions to Normal and Pathological Aging." In Riddle DR, ed. *Brain Aging: Models, Methods, and Mechanisms* in *Frontiers in Neuroscience*. Boca Raton, Fl: CRC Press, 2007: Chapter 13.

8 Stone AA, Schwartz JE, Broderick JE, Deaton A. "A snapshot of the age distribution of psychological well-being in the United States." *Proceedings of the National Academy of Sciences of the United States of America* 107 (22) (2010): 9985–90.

9 Terzidis K, Panoutsopoulos A, Mantzou A, Tourli P, et al. "Lower early morning plasma cortisol levels are associated with thyroid autoimmunity in the elderly." *European Journal of Endocrinology* 162 (2) (2010): 307–13.

10   Conley C. *Emotional Equations: Simple Truths for Creating Happiness and Success.* New York: Free Press, 2012; Mathioudakis N, Thapa S, Wand GS, Salvatori R. "ACTH-secreting pituitary microadenomas are associated with a higher prevalence of central hypothyroidism compared to other microadenoma types." *Clinical Endocrinology (Oxford)* (2012). doi: 10.1111/j.1365–2265.2012.04442.x.

11   Abdullatif HD, Ashraf AP. "Reversible subclinical hypothyroidism in the presence of adrenal insufficiency." *Endocrine Practice* 12 (5) (2006): 572.

12   Baumgartner A, Hiedra L, Pinna G, et al. "Rat brain type II 5'-iodothyronine deiodinase activity is extremely sensitive to stress." *Journal of Neurochemistry* 71 (1998): 817–26; Bradley DJ, Towle HC, Young WS. "3rd Spatial and temporal expression of alpha- and beta-thyroid hormone receptor mRNAs, including the beta 2-subtype, in the developing mammalian nervous system." *Journal of Neuroscience* 12 (1992): 2288–302; Puymirat J, Miehe M, Marchand R, et al. "Immunocytochemical localization of thyroid hormone receptors in the adult rat brain." *Thyroid* (1991): 173–84.

13   Dluhy RG. "The adrenal cortex in thyrotoxicosis" in Braverman L, Utiger R, eds. *Werner and Ingbar's The Thyroid: A Fundamental and Clinical Text,* 9th ed. Philadelphia: Lippincott, Williams & Wilkins, 2005: 602–5.

14   Doshi SR. "Relative adrenal insufficiency masquerading hypothyroidism." *Journal of Clinical and Diagnostic Research* 4 (4) (2010): 2907–9; Fitzgerald KN. *Case Studies in Integrative and Functional Medicine.* Duluth, GA: Metametrix Institute, 2011; Mathioudakis N, Thapa S, Wand GS, Salvatori R. "ACTH-secreting pituitary microadenomas are associated with a higher prevalence of central hypothyroidism compared to other microadenoma types." *Clinical Endocrinology (Oxford)* (2012). doi: 10.1111/j.1365-2265.2012.04442.x.

15   Danhof-Pont MB, van Veen T, Zitman FG. "Biomarkers in burnout: a systematic review." *Journal of Psychosomatic Research* 70 (6) (2011): 505–24; Endocrine Society (2010), http://www.hormone.org/public/myths_facts.cfm; Nippoldt T. "Mayo Clinic office visit. Adrenal fatigue. An interview with Todd Nippoldt, M.D." *Mayo Clinic Women's Healthsource* 14 (3) (2010): 6.

16   Lewis G, Wessely S. "The epidemiology of fatigue: more questions than answers." *Journal of Epidemiology and Community Health* 46 (2) (1992): 92–97.

17   American College Health Association (2011), http://www.achancha.org/docs/ACHA-NCHA-II_ReferenceGroup_ExecutiveSummary_Spring2011.pdf.

18 Rabin RC. "Sleeping Pills Rising in Popularity Among Young Adults." *New York Times,* January 14, 2009. http://www.nytimes.com/2009/01/15/health/15sleep.html.

19 Leproult R, Van Cauter E. "Role of sleep and sleep loss in hormonal release and metabolism." *Endocrine Development* 17 (2010): 11–21; Lovallo WR, Farag NH, Vincent AS, et al. "Cortisol responses to mental stress, exercise, and meals following caffeine intake in men and women." *Pharmacology, Biochemistry and Behavior* 83 (3) (2006): 441–47.

20 Dean BB, Borenstein JE. "A prospective assessment investigating the relationship between work productivity and impairment with premenstrual syndrome." *Journal of Occupational and Environmental Medicine* 46 (2004): 649–56; Hourani LL, Yuan H, Bray RM. "Psychosocial and lifestyle correlates of premenstrual symptoms among military women." *Journal of Women's Health* 13 (2004): 812–21; Tabassum S, Afridi B, Aman Z, et al. "Premenstrual syndrome: frequency and severity in young college girls." *Journal of the Pakistan Medical Association* 55 (2005): 546–49.

21 Maruo T, Katayama K, Barnea ER, Mochizuki M. "A role for thyroid hormone in the induction of ovulation and corpus luteum function." *Hormone Research* 37 Suppl. 1 (1992): 12–18.

22 Leonard JL, Koehrle J. "Intracellular, Pathways of Iodothyronine Metabolism" in Braverman LE, Utiger RD, eds. *Werner and Ingbar's The Thyroid: A Fundamental and Clinical Text,* 9th ed. Philadelphia: Lippincott, Williams & Wilkins, 2005: 119; Stavreus Evers A. "Paracrine Interactions of Thyroid Hormones and Thyroid Stimulation Hormone in the Female Reproductive Tract Have an Impact on Female Fertility." *Frontiers in Endocrinology (Lausanne)* 3 (2012): 50.

23 Hatsuta M, Abe K, Tamura K, et al. "Effects of hypothyroidism on the estrous cycle and reproductive hormones in mature female rat." *European Journal of Pharmacology* 486 (3) (2004): 343–48; Jahagirdar V, Zoeller TR, Tighe DP, et al. "Maternal hypothyroidism decreases progesterone receptor expression in the cortical subplate of fetal rat brain." *Journal of Neuroendocrinology* (2012). doi: 10.1111/j.1365-2826.2012.02318.x.

24 Zagrodzki P, Przybylik-Mazurek E. "Selenium and hormone interactions in female patients with Hashimoto disease and healthy subjects." *Endocrine Research* 35 (1) (2010): 24–34; Zagrodzki P, Ratajczak R. "Selenium status, sex hormones, and thyroid function in young women." *Journal of Trace Elements in Medicine and Biology* 22 (4) (2008): 296–304; Zagrodzki P, Ratajczak R, Wietecha-Posłuszny R. "The interaction between selenium status, sex hormones, and thyroid metabolism in adolescent girls in the luteal phase of their menstrual cycle." *Biological Trace Element Research* 120 (1–3) (2007): 51–60.

APPENDIX H

1. Olsson EM, von Schéele B, Panossian AG. "A randomised, double-blind, placebo-controlled, parallel-group study of the standardised extract shr-5 of the roots of *Rhodiola rosea* in the treatment of subjects with stress-related fatigue." *Planta Medica* 75 (2) (2009): 105–12.

2. Amen D. *Unleash the Power of the Female Brain: Supercharging Yours for Better Health, Energy, Mood, Focus, and Sex* (New York: Harmony Books, 2013).

3. Noreen EE, Buckley JG, Lewis SL, et al. "The effects of an acute dose of Rhodiola rosea on endurance exercise performance." *Journal of Strength and Conditioning Research* 3 (March 27, 2013): 839–47.

4. Chavarro JE, Rich-Edwards JW, Rosner BA, et al. "Caffeinated and alcoholic beverage intake in relation to ovulatory disorder infertility." *Epidemiology* (2009): 374–81.

5. Chutkan, R. *Gutbliss: A 10-Day Plan to Ban Bloat, Flush Toxins, and Dump Your Digestive Baggage* (New York: Avery, 2013).

6. Chavarro JE, Rich-Edwards JW, Rosner BA, et al. "Use of multivitamins, intake of B vitamins, and risk of ovulatory infertility." *Journal of Fertility and Sterility* (2008): 668–76; Wilson RD, Johnson JA, Wyatt P, et al. Genetics Committee of the Society of Obstetricians and Gynaecologists of Canada and The Motherrisk Program, "Pre-conceptional vitamin/folic acid supplementation 2007: the use of folic acid in combination with a multivitamin supplement for the prevention of neural tube defects and other congenital anomalies." *Journal of Obstetrics and Gynaecology Canada* (2007): 1003–26.

7. Anagnostis P, Karras S, Goulis DG. "Vitamin D in human reproduction: a narrative review." *Integrative Journal of Clinical Practice* (2013).

8. Westphal LM, Polan ML, Trant AS. "Double-blind, placebo-controlled study of Fertilityblend: a nutritional supplement for improving fertility in women." *Clinical and Experimental Obstetrics and Gynecology* 33 (4) (2006): 205–8.

9. http://www.ahpa.org; Dugoua JJ, Seely D, Perri D, et al. "Safety and efficacy of chastetree (Vitex agnus-castus) during pregnancy and lactation." *Canadian Journal of Clinical Pharmacology* 15 (1) (Winter 2008): e74–e79; Daniele C, Thompson Coon J, Pittler MH, et al. "Vitex agnus castus: a systematic review of adverse events." *Drug Safety* 28 (4) (2005): 319–32.

10. Buie T, Winter H, Kushak R. "Preliminary findings in gastrointestinal investigation of autistic patients." Summary: Harvard University and Mass General Hospital (2002); Valicenti-McDermott M, McVicar K, Rapin I, et al. "Frequency of gastrointestinal symptoms in children with autism spectrum disorders and association with family history of autoimmune disease." *Journal of Developmental Behavior &*

Pediatrics (2006): 128–36; Green M, et al. "Public health implications of the microbial pesticide Bacillus thuringiensis: an epidemiological study, Oregon, 1985–86." *American Journal of Public Health* 80 (7) (1990): 848–52; http://www.againstthegrainnutrition.com/newsandnotes/2009/04/14/genetically-engineered-corn-may-cause-allergies-infertility-and-disease/#sthash.SHd4fgys.dpuf; Velimirov A, et al. "Biological effects of transgenic maize NK603xMON810 fed in long-term reproduction studies in mice." *Forschungsberichte der Sektion* (2008): http://www.againstthegrainnutrition.com/newsand notes/2009/04/14/genetically-engineered-corn-may-cause-allergies-infertility-and-disease/#sthash.SHd4fgys.dpuf; Kay VR, Chambers C, Foster WG. "Reproductive and developmental effects of phthalate diesters in females." *Critical Review of Toxicology* (2013): 200–19.

11. Samsel A, Seneff S. "Glyphosate's suppression of cytochrome P450 enzymes and amino acid biosynthesis by the gut microbiome: pathways to modern diseases." *Entropy* 15 (4) (April 2013): 1416–63.

12. Joensen UN, Frederiksen H, Jensen MB, et al. "Phthalate excretion pattern and testicular function: a study of 881 healthy Danish men." *Environmental Health Perspectives* (2012): 1397–403.

13. Cobellis L, Latini G, De Felice C, et al. "High plasma concentrations of di-(2-ethylhexyl)-phthalate in women with endometriosis." *Journal of Human Reproduction* 18 (7) (2003): 1512–15; Mendola P, Messer LC, Rappazzo K. "Science linking environmental contaminant exposures with fertility and reproductive health impacts in the adult female." *Journal of Fertility and Sterility* (2008): e81–e94; Hoppin JA, Jaramillo R, London SJ, et al. "Phthalate exposure and allergy in the U.S. population: results from NHANES 2005–2006." *Environmental Health Perspectives* (2013).

14. Bauquis C. "Adverse effects of phthalates on ovarian response to IVF." *European Society of Human Reproduction and Embryology* (2013).

15. United States Consumer Product Safety Commission, http://cs.cpsc.gov/ConceptDemo/SearchCPSC.aspx?query=http://www.cpsc.gov/info/toysafety/phthalates.html&OldURL=true&autodisplay=true.

16. O'Connor PJ, Poudevigne MS, Cress ME, et al. "Safety and efficacy of supervised strength training adopted in pregnancy." *Journal of Physical and Active Health* (2011): 309–20; Dye TD, Knox KL, Artal R, et al. "Physical activity, obesity, and diabetes in pregnancy." *American Journal of Epidemiology* (1997): 961–65.

17. Rakhshani A, Nagarathna R, Mhaskar R, et al. "The effects of yoga in prevention of pregnancy complications in high-risk pregnancies: a randomized controlled trial." *Preventive Medicine* 55 (4) (October 2012): 333–40, doi: 10.1016/j.ypmed.2012.07.020, epub August 2, 2012; Deshpande C, Rakshani A, Nagarathna R, et al. "Yoga for high-

risk pregnancy: a randomized controlled trial." *Annals of Medical and Health Sciences Research* 3 (3) (July 2013): 341–44.

PAPERBACK Q AND A

1. Caso Marasco A, Vargas Ruiz R, Salas Villagomez A, et al. "Double blind study of a multivitamin complex supplemented with ginseng extract." *Drugs under Experimental and Clinical Research* 2 (1996): 323–29; Olsson EM, von Schéele B, Panossian AG. "A randomised, double-blind, placebo-controlled, parallel-group study of the standardised extract shr-5 of the roots of Rhodiola rosea in the treatment of subjects with stress-related fatigue." *Planta Medica* 75 (2) (2009): 105–12.
2. Parker WH, Broder MS, Liu Z, et al. "Ovarian conservation at the time of hysterectomy for benign disease." *Obstetrics & Gynecology* (2005): 219–26.
3. Tode T, Kikuchi Y, Hirata J, et al. "Effect of Korean red ginseng on psychological functions in patients with severe climacteric syndromes." *International Journal of Gynaecology and Obstetrics* 67 (3) (1999): 169–74.
4. Dorgan J, Baer D, Albert P, et al. "Serum hormones and the alcohol-breast cancer association in postmenopausal women." *Journal of the National Cancer Institute* 93 (2001): 710–15; Mahabir S, Baer DJ, Johnson LL, et al. "The effects of moderate alcohol supplementation on estrone sulfate and DHEAS in postmenopausal women in a controlled feeding study." *Nutrition Journal* 3 (11) (2004).
5. Grodin JM, Siiteri PK, MacDonald PC. "Source of estrogen production in postmenopausal women." *Journal of Clinical Endocrinology and Metabolism* 36 (2) (1973): 207–14.
6. Shah D, Bansal S. "Polycystic ovaries—beyond menopause." *Climacteric* (October 2013).
7. Del Priore G, Gudipudi DK, Montemarano N, et al. "Oral diindolylmethane (DIM): pilot evaluation of a nonsurgical treatment for cervical dysplasia." *Gynecologic Oncology* 116 (3) (2010): 464–67; Brooks NA, Wilcox G, Walker KZ, et al. "Beneficial effects of Lepidium meyenii (Maca) on psychological symptoms and measures of sexual dysfunction in postmenopausal women are not related to estrogen or androgen content." Menopause 15 (6) (2008): 1157–62.
8. Schneider J, Kinne D, Fracchia A, et al. "Abnormal oxidative metabolism of estradiol in women with breast cancer." *Proceedings of the National Academy of Sciences* 79 (1982): 3047–51; Fishman J, Schneider J, Hershcope RJ, Bradlow HL. "Increased estrogen 16 alpha-hydroxylase activity in women with breast and endometrial cancer." *Journal of Steroid Biochemistry* 20 (4B) (1984): 1077–81; Zumoff B. "Hormonal profiles in women with breast cancer." *Obstetrics and*

Gynecology Clinics of North America 21 (4) (1994): 751–72; Cauley JA, Zmuda JM, Danielson ME, et al. "Estrogen metabolites and the risk of breast cancer in older women." *Epidemiology* 14 (6) (2003): 740–44; Kabat GC, O'Leary ES, Gammon MD, et al. "Estrogen metabolism and breast cancer." *Epidemiology* 17 (1) (2006): 80–88; Im A, Vogel VG, Ahrendt G, et al. "Urinary estrogen metabolites in women at high risk for breast cancer." *Carcinogenesis* 30 (9) (2009): 1532–35; Fishman J, Schneider J, Hershcope RJ, et al. "Increased estrogen 16 alpha-hydroxylase activity in women with breast and endometrial cancer." *Journal of Steroid Biochemistry* 20 (4B) (1984): 1077–81; Eliassen AH, Spiegelman D, Xu X, et al. "Urinary estrogens and estrogen metabolites and subsequent risk of breast cancer among premenopausal women." *Cancer Research* 72 (3) (2012): 696–706.

9. Sund-Levander M, Forsberg C, Wahren LK. "Normal oral, rectal, tympanic and axillary body temperature in adult men and women: a systematic literature review." *Scandinavian Journal of Caring Science* 16 (2) (2002): 122–28.

10. Huang A, Brennan K, Azziz R. "Prevalence of hyperandrogenemia in the polycystic ovary syndrome diagnosed by the National Institutes of Health 1990 criteria." *Fertility and Sterility* 93 (6) (2010): 1938–41; Azziz R, Sanchez LA, Knochenhauer ES, et al. "Androgen excess in women: experience with over 1,000 consecutive patients." *Journal of Clinical Endocrinology and Metabolism* 89 (2) (2004): 453–62.

11. Rushton DH. Dover R, Sainsbury AW, et al. "Iron deficiency is neglected in women's health." *British Medical Journal* 325 (7373) (2002): 1176.

12. Taavoni S, Ekbatani N, Kashaniyan M, et al. "Effect of valerian on sleep quality in postmenopausal women: a randomized placebo-controlled clinical trial." *Menopause* 18 (9) (2011): 951–55

INDEX

Page numbers in *italics* refer to tables and charts.